T0327565

# Integrative Play Therapy

Edited by

Athena A. Drewes
Sue C. Bratton
Charles E. Schaefer

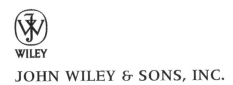

WILEY

JOHN WILEY & SONS, INC.

Copyright © 2011 by John Wiley & Sons, Inc. All rights reserved.

Published by John Wiley & Sons, Inc., Hoboken, New Jersey.
Published simultaneously in Canada.

*Library of Congress Cataloging-in-Publication Data:*
  Integrative play therapy / edited by Athena A. Drewes, Sue C. Bratton, and Charles E. Schaefer.
     p. ; cm.
  Includes bibliographical references and index.
  ISBN 978-0-470-61792-2 (cloth : alk. paper)
  ISBN 978-1-118-06425-2 (ebk)
  ISBN 978-1-118-06426-9 (ebk)
  ISBN 978-1-118-06424-5 (ebk)
  ISBN 978-1-118-09479-2 (obk)
  1.  Play therapy. I. Drewes, Athena A., 1948- editor. II. Bratton, Sue C., editor. III. Schaefer, Charles E., 1933- editor.
  [DNLM: 1. Play Therapy—methods. 2. Child. 3. Mental Disorders—therapy. WS 350.4]
  RJ505.P6I568 2011
  618.92'891653—dc22                                                    2010051400

Printed in the United States of America

10 9 8 7 6 5 4 3 2 1

# TABLE OF CONTENTS

# PREFACE

The necessity for *Integrative Play Therapy* has evolved out of each of our personal experiences and approaches in the field of play therapy. We have each found that the complex and difficult treatment cases we encountered often required a more comprehensive treatment approach involving the blending of theories and techniques. Many of our play therapy colleagues have also moved away from a one-size-fits-all treatment approach that uses a single theoretical approach for all or most treatment cases. Until recently, play therapists tended to remain wedded to the original theoretical framework they learned in their graduate training. Alternative conceptualizations and potentially superior evidence-informed interventions have now become available. In addition, there has been a growing movement within both the child and adult psychotherapy fields toward an integrative treatment approach. Indeed, the use of a multitheoretical framework as a foundation for practice has become the prevailing zeitgeist.

We believe that this book will help play therapists learn from the descriptions of how other therapists have integrated various theoretical approaches in resolving the common psychological disorders of childhood. The ultimate goal of this book is to heighten awareness of the necessity, efficacy, and wide applicability of a multitheoretical treatment approach. We hope that as play therapists become committed to integration, they will move away from identifying themselves with a particular school and toward an identification as an integrative play therapist.

Athena A. Drewes
Sue C. Bratton
Charles E. Schaefer

# About the Editors

**Athena A. Drewes**, PsyD, RPT-S is Director of Clinical Training, APA-Accredited Doctoral Internship and a clinician at the Astor Services for Children & Families, a large nonprofit multiservice mental health agency in New York. She is a Registered Play Therapist and Supervisor, past Director of the Association for Play Therapy and founder/past president of the New York Association for Play Therapy. She is Editor and chapter author of *School-based Play Therapy*; *School-based Play Therapy, Second Edition*; *Blending Play Therapy with Cognitive Behavioral Therapy* (Wiley); *Cultural Issues in Play Therapy*; and *Supervision Can Be Playful*. Dr. Drewes is a nationally and internationally renowned guest lecturer on a variety of play therapy topics.

**Sue C. Bratton**, Ph.D., LPC, RPT-S is Director of the Center for Play Therapy and Professor at The University of North Texas. Dr. Bratton is nationally and internationally known for her work in the area of play therapy and Child Parent Relationship Therapy (CPRT). She is a frequent speaker around the world, and has published over 60 articles, books, chapters, videos and other publications in the field of play therapy, the majority of which are research–based. Her most recent books are *Child Parent Relationship Therapy (CPRT): A 10-Session Filial Therapy Model, Child Parent Relationship Therapy (CPRT) Treatment Manual, Child-Centered Play Therapy Research: The Evidence Base for Practitioners,* and *Integrative Play Therapy.* Her research agenda focuses on CPRT and play therapy effectiveness. Dr. Bratton is a Past President of the Association for Play Therapy, recipient of the 2007 Outstanding Research Award for Association for Play Therapy, and the 2005 Nancy Guillory Award for Outstanding Service and Contribution to the Field of Play Therapy from the Texas Association for Play Therapy.

**Charles E. Schaefer**, Ph.D., RPT-S is Professor Emeritus of Psychology at Fairleigh Dickinson University in Teaneck, New Jersey. He is co-founder and Director-Emeritus of the Association for Play Therapy. He is also founder and co-director of the Play Therapy Training Institute in New Jersey. Dr. Schaefer coordinates an International Play Therapy Study Group held annually in Wroxton, England. Among his books on Play Therapy are: *Play Therapy for Preschool Children*; *Empirically-Based Play Interventions for Children*; *Contemporary Play Therapy*; *Short-term Play Therapy for Children*; *The Playing Cure: Individualized Play Therapy for Specific Childhood Problems*; *Game Play*; *101 Favorite Play Therapy Techniques*; *Play Therapy With Adults*; *Play Therapy With Adolescents*; *Play Therapy for Very Young Children, and Play Diagnosis and Assessment.* In 2006, he received the Lifetime Achievement Award from the Association for Play Therapy. Dr. Schaefer is a frequent presenter at national and international Play Therapy conferences. He has been a guest on the Good Morning America, Today, and Oprah Winfrey TV shows. His private practice in clinical child psychology is located in Hackensack, New Jersey.

# CONTRIBUTORS

**Jeffrey S. Ashby Ph.D., ABPP**
Professor
Counseling Psychology
Counseling & Psychological Services
Georgia State University
Atlanta, Georgia

**Sue C. Bratton, Ph.D., LPC, RPT-S**
Professor & Director
Center for Play Therapy
University of North Texas
Denton, Texas

**Karina G. Campos, M.A.**
Psychology Intern
Doctoral Candidate at Pepperdine
    University
Los Angeles, California

**Kara Carnes-Holt, Ph.D., LPC,
NCC, RPT-S**
Assistant Professor
University of Wyoming
Laramie, Wyoming

**Peggy L. Ceballos, Ph.D.**
Assistant Professor
University of North Carolina
    at Charlotte
Charlotte, North Carolina

**Karishma Chengappa, M.S.**
Graduate Student
Clinical Child Doctoral Program
Department of Psychology
West Virginia University
Morgantown, West Virginia

**Amanda H. Costello, B.S.**
Graduate Student
Clinical Child Doctoral Program
Department of Psychology
West Virginia University
Morgantown, West Virginia

**Marie-José Dhaese, Ph.D., RPT-S,
ATR, CPT-S**
Centre for Expressive Therapy,
    Counseling and Consulting
Parksville, British Columbia, Canada

**Athena A. Drewes, Psy.D.,
RPT-S**
Director of Clinical Training and APA-
    Accredited Doctoral Psychology
    Internship
Astor Services for Children and
    Families
Poughkeepsie, New York

**Paris Goodyear-Brown, LCSW,
RPT-S**
Private Practice
Paris and Me Counseling for Kids
Brentwood, Tennessee

**Sarah Hamil, LCSW, RPT-S,
ATR-BC**
Private Practice
Jackson, Tennessee

**Jessica Jäger, Ph.D.**
Child and Adolescent Mental Health
    Service (CAMHS)
Lewes, East Sussex, England

**Victoria A. McGuinness, LMHC, RPT**
Private Practice
Bellingham, Washington

**Cheryl B. McNeil, Ph.D.**
Professor, Clinical Child Psychology
West Virginia University
Morgantown, West Virginia

**Evangeline Munns, Ph.D., RPT-S**
Private Practice
King City, Ontario, Canada

**Julie Blundon Nash, Ph.D.**
Foster Care Clinic Coordinator
Community Mental Health Center
Chester, Connecticut

**Christina Noble, M.A., M.S., LAPC, NCC**
Doctoral Candidate
Georgia State University
Atlanta, Georgia

**Kevin O'Connor, Ph.D., RPT-S**
Distinguished Professor
Clinical Ph.D. and Clinical Psy.D.
    Programs
California School of Professional
    Psychology at Alliant International
    University
Fresno, California

**Dale-Elizabeth Pehrsson, Ph.D., RPT-S**
Associate Professor and Associate
    Dean
College of Education
University of Nevada – Las Vegas
Henderson, Nevada

**Virginia Ryan, Ph.D.**
Play Therapist and Play Therapy
    Supervisor
Ryan Children's Services
Hull, East Yorkshire, England

**Charles E. Schaefer, Ph.D., RPT-S**
Professor Emeritus
Fairleigh Dickinson University
Teaneck, New Jersey
Director Emeritus of the Association
    for Play Therapy

**John W. Seymour, Ph.D., LMFT, CCMHC, ACS, RPT-S**
Associate Professor
Department of Counseling and
    Student Personnel
Minnesota State University, Mankato
Mankato, Minnesota

**Janine Shelby, Ph.D., RPT-S**
Assistant Professor
Director of Child Psychology Training
    and Child Trauma Clinic
Department of Psychiatry, Geffen
    School of Medicine
University of California at Los Angeles
Torrance, California

**Jocelyn O. Stokes, B.A.**
Graduate Student
Clinical Child Doctoral Program
Department of Psychology
West Virginia University
Morgantown, West Virginia

**Daniel S. Sweeney, Ph.D., LMFT, LPC, RPT-S**
Professor of Counseling
Director, Northwest Center for Play
    Therapy Studies
Graduate Department of Counseling
George Fox University
Portland, Oregon

**Ashley B. Tempel, M.S.**
Graduate Student
Clinical Child Doctoral Program
Department of Psychology
West Virginia University
Morgantown, West Virginia

**Glade Topham, Ph.D., LMFT**
Assistant Professor
Department of Human Development
    and Family Science
Oklahoma State University
Stillwater, Oklahoma

**Risë VanFleet, Ph.D., RPT-S**
President, Private Practice
Family Enhancement and Play
    Therapy Center, Inc.
Boiling Springs, Pennsylvania

**Kyle N. Weir, Ph.D., LMFT**
Associate Professor
Program Coordinator
Department of Counseling, Special
    Education and Rehabilitation
California State University
Interim Director – Fresno Family
    Counseling Center
Fresno, California

# Introduction: Importance of an Integrative Approach to Child Therapy

*1*

*Section*

# History of Psychotherapy Integration and Related Research

## John W. Seymour

## Introduction

Psychotherapy has been a formal discipline in Western cultures for more than 100 years, with roots stretching back to the beginning of human civilization (Ellenberger, 1970; Frank & Frank, 1993). Since the early models of Freud, Adler, and Jung, the field has expanded to more than 400 models (Norcross & Newman, 1992), with models ascending and descending in usage and importance, and with some disappearing altogether while others have continued in forms that would be both familiar and unfamiliar to the model founder(s). This proliferation of models has often confounded practitioners, researchers, and recipients of psychotherapy with the variety of assumptions, terminologies, and applications. In *The Structure of Scientific Revolutions*, Kuhn (1973), building on concepts developed by Polanyi (1964a/1946, 1964b) and others, outlined how scientific inquiry evolves in a kind of ebb-and-flow pattern in a professional scientific community. Kuhn's model can be applied to the history of psychotherapy integration to better understand the issues that have repeatedly arisen through years of dialogue, to better inform current efforts in psychotherapy integration during the first part of the 21st century.

Kuhn (1973) suggested that professional scientific communities are based on accumulated facts and assumptions about the field of inquiry, and over time they create an explanatory model, or *paradigm*, founded on this set of *received beliefs*. For psychotherapy, this model has typically included philosophical assumptions about methods of knowing (epistemology), the psychological components of human nature (philosophy of the mind), identifying the dynamic processes that move humans toward and away from mental health (etiology of health and unhealth), and identifying and encouraging professional practice methods of enhancing mental health (applied ethics). Through reflection and research, new data and experiences (*anomalies*) challenge the older model in a kind of ebb-and-flow pattern, with periods characterized by creative discovery and advancing those claims as well as conserving existing traditions by defending those claims, punctuated by periods of quiescence.

Applied and theoretical responses to these differences have spawned many years of efforts to resolve the debate, through both research and rhetoric, to either prove a current method right or create a new blend of theory and practice to create a newer right way. Kuhn (1973) has emphasized that in this process, "The problems of paradigm articulation are simultaneously theoretical and experimental" (p. 33). Psychotherapists and psychotherapy researchers have used several major ways to develop these newer right ways: some have opted for an approach built more on challenging the differences and maintaining an existing paradigm, whereas others have opted for an approach built more on identifying and advancing the similarities, which has been the typical approach of psychotherapy integration.

Stricker and Gold (2008) point out that *psychotherapy integration* in some form is a part of every clinical and research process, as part of the learning process of psychotherapists working from a particular model and considering new ideas or techniques for possible incorporation into their existing model. Prochaska and Norcross (2010) describe the motivation of psychotherapy integration to be that of "a spirit of open inquiry and a zest for transtheoretical dialogue" (p. 455). The term *integrative psychotherapy* is more often reserved to refer "to a new and particular form of psychotherapy with a set of theories and clinical practices that synthesizes concepts and methods from two or more schools of psychotherapy" (Stricker & Gold, 2008, p. 390). Since the mid-1970s, integrative psychotherapy has grown into an important branch in the study of psychotherapy, with multiple articles and textbooks written on the topic, as well as a professional society. More recently, integrative psychotherapy has been applied to special populations, including multicultural psychotherapy (Fischer, Jome, & Atkinson, 1998a, 1998b), couples, family, and relational therapy (Feldman & Pinsof, 1982; Pinsof, 1983, 1994, 1995; Sparks & Duncan, 2009), and psychotherapy with children (Gold, 1992; Kelley, Bickman, & Norwood, 2009). A review of the history of psychotherapy integration identifies the issues of epistemology, philosophy of the mind, etiology of health, and professional applied ethics to inform the efforts of psychotherapy integration within the field of play therapy.

## The Early Roots of Integrative Psychotherapy

Medical anthropologists (Dow, 1986; Kleinman, 1980, 1988) and historians of psychotherapy (Ellenberger, 1970; Frank and Frank, 1993; Torrey, 1986), begin the history of psychotherapy with the efforts of the earliest humans to understand and heal various maladies of the human condition (Ellenberger, 1970). As Frank and Frank (1993) stated, "psychotherapeutic methods have existed since time immemorial" (p. 1). Studies of both ancient and contemporary folk medicine reveal some striking similarities in the healing traditions of psychotherapy and folk medicine. Kleinman (1988) pointed out that both traditions include an evolving conceptual system centered on the social and experiential dimensions of sickness and healing, with emphases on the efficacy of the treatments and the meanings given to each dimension. Both traditions are what Kleinman termed Explanatory Models, which provided the etiology, onset, pathophysiology, treatment, and prognosis for classifications of conditions. Both traditions involve symbolic healing, which bridges the personal experience of the suffering person with social support and cultural meanings.

Prochaska and Norcross (2010) point out that psychotherapy integration is likely as old as the earliest dialogues in what would become philosophy and psychology, motivated by the desire to look beyond the obvious and explore the unexplained. To the ancient and contemporary folk practitioners (as well as many contemporary psychotherapists in Eastern traditions), the concept of psychotherapy integration is incorporated into the Explanatory Models of those traditions. The mental and physical are intertwined in a nonlinear system of cause and effect mediated by the social cultural context. There is no either/or, psychological/physical divide, no question of "Is it psychological or physical?" as found in many discussions of Western psychotherapy (Kleinman 1980, 1988). Most Western traditions, under the historical influence of a dualistic view of mental and physical processes, have struggled more with this tension, which has been addressed through intentional pursuits of psychotherapy integration.

It could be said that the three earliest models of Freud, Adler, and Jung were integrative in spirit. All were, to various degrees, building on, reacting to, or extending the theories and techniques from diverse resources in philosophy, psychology, and medicine, into a coherent approach that to the developers made the best explanatory sense of the causes and treatments of mental illness.

Freud built on earlier contributions such as those of Messmer, Puysèger, Charcot, and Janet, incorporating this with his own study and clinical experience in medicine and his interests in culture and evolution (Ellenberger, 1970). Through hosting regular meetings of professionals with similar interests (such as the Vienna Study Group of the early 1900s), he was not only shaped by the views of his contemporaries, such as Adler and Jung, but he also influenced the development of their theories. Along with stimulating a creative process that created an enormous shift in the study of human behavior, these differences and challenges also fueled intense debates that over time solidified psychotherapy models into warring camps of ideology and practice. Kuhn (1973) described the beginnings of scientific revolution and paradigm shift as "the tradition-shattering complements to the tradition-bound activity of normal science" (p. 6).

The emerging assumptions of Freud and his contemporaries challenged the understandings of human behavior in their day, leading to a backlash of paradigm-preserving responses from the established science. Over time, the differences even among the Vienna Group became so great that a series of rifts occurred, with Adler and then Jung parting ways with Freud, with all three advancing their models both through promoting their approaches and challenging the others (Ellenberger, 1970). This pattern of a developing science, outlined by Kuhn (1973), has repeated itself many times in the 100-plus-year history of psychotherapy, in what Saltzman and Norcross described as *therapy wars*, where efforts are made to prove once and for all the correctness of a particular model (and the incorrectness of others).

The history of psychotherapy integration has had several shifting points so far, beginning with periods of ascendancy of a particular model and the conserving and creative responses to it. Psychoanalysis, founded from the 19th-century foundations of philosophy, science, and medicine, was challenged by Adler, Jung, and others and began a period of ascendancy that would later be challenged by behaviorism, which began to peak in the 1950s. The ascendancy of behaviorism challenged not only the epistemology, psychology of mind, and etiology of health implied in psychoanalysis but also the dominant paradigm by questioning the effectiveness in the lives of people, a significant issue of applied ethics. Efforts of psychotherapy integration, practically stated, answer the basic question of "What therapy to use, when to use it, and to whom should you use it with?" (Ivey, 1980).

## First Efforts at Psychotherapy Integration

As a documented professional effort, psychotherapy integration began in 1930, with the publishing of a paper by Ischolonsky of Germany that drew parallels between Pavlovian conditioning and psychoanalysis (Arkowitz, 1984). French (1933) extended those parallels with his own comparison, which was presented at a meeting of the American Psychiatric Association and then published with mixed reviews from all sides (Arkowitz, 1984). Three years later, Rosenzweig (1936) published a paper, "Some Implicit Common Factors in Diverse Methods of Psychotherapy," and in 1940 presented the paper at a professional conference hosted by the American Orthopsychiatric Association on commonalities of different psychotherapies. His initial description of common factors was predictive of what would later be identified in common factors research many years later (Duncan, 2009). Rosenzweig (1936) also suggested that "the yet undefined effect of the personality of the good therapist" (p. 425) was also a key factor in successful psychotherapy. His contributions were significant in the development of the field, but they were not well documented until more recently (Duncan, 2009). It should be noted that one of the other presenters was Rogers, who two years later referenced the conference and Rosenzweig in his first book, *Counseling and Psychotherapy* (Rogers, 1942), and later collaborated with Rosenzweig in other endeavors. Most of these early efforts at integration aimed at synthesizing ideas from psychoanalysis, and over time these efforts converged into what would become trends toward eclectic and integrated models.

Since the 1930s, efforts have been made to identify similarities among the two psychotherapy models of the time, behaviorism/learning theory and psychoanalysis, such as Sears' (1944) examination of the role of reinforcement of the therapeutic relationship. Better known today is Dollard and Miller's (1950) *Personality and Psychotherapy*, a synthesis of psychoanalytic concepts with laboratory-based learning theories of Hull, Tolman, and others. Alexander and French (1946) reevaluated psychoanalytic theory to accommodate the use of more behavior-based active interventions by the therapist, giving a more directive role to the therapist and a more prescriptive function in guiding the therapy process. Although the purpose of these interventions was to increase insight in the psychoanalytic sense, the updated model was the first to suggest multiple interactive and therapeutic factors that were summarized in the construct "corrective emotional experience," which has found wide application in several psychotherapy approaches. Alexander continued this line of inquiry with additional study on the role of the therapist's approval and affection as reinforcers of the therapeutic relationship and better therapy outcome (Gold & Stricker, 2006; Stricker & Gold, 2008; Wampold, 2001).

## Psychotherapy Integration and the Call for Accountability

With the ascendancy of behaviorism and learning theory in the late 1940s, the publishing of Eysenck's (1952) critique of the effectiveness of psychotherapy (more specifically psychoanalysis) was a crisis of accountability for psycho-analysis, which proved to be a significant catalyst to research and rhetoric on all sides of the issue, including those defending the still-young field of psycho-therapy and those asking fundamental questions of integrity in the research and delivery of psychotherapy of all types, which continue to be raised today by psychotherapy researchers (Arkowitz, 1984; Eysenck, 1978; Glass & Kliegl, 1983; Glass & Smith, 1978; Saltzman & Norcross, 1990; Smith & Glass, 1977; Smith, Glass, & Milton, 1980; Wampold, 1997, 2001, 2009).

From the mid-1950s to the early 1970s, discussion of psychotherapy integration was characterized by competing forces as the ascendancy of behav-iorism influenced the discussion and was influenced by those in the discussion. Eysenck (1952, 1960, 1978, 1983) contributed to the debate over an extended period, raising both the issues as well as the competitive tone of the discussions (Arkowitz, 1984; Greenberg, 1986; Greenberg & Pinsof, 1986; Wampold, 1997, 2001, 2009). Many new psychotherapy models were proposed, and existing models were revised. Consistent with Kuhn's (1973) understanding of scientific revolution, these changes were greeted both with enthusiasm of new inquiry as well as protection of existing models by adherents. Many psychotherapists, who were weary or confused by the ongoing philosophical debates, adopted more practically based, less theoretically based eclecticism and embraced a wide range of eclectic approaches. Others held firmly to earlier models, often making a rhetorical appeal to the great leader myth of the founder of the approach (Brammer & Shostrom, 1977).

Rogers (1963), in addressing the Sixth Annual Conference of the American Academy of Psychotherapists, related a recent experience of his participation in a clinical presentation of diverse psychotherapy models applied to a particular case. While expecting the diverse group to come together at some point in the experience of what was helpful psychotherapy, he was surprised by the differ-ences reported, as examples of moments in the therapy that he would have labeled therapeutic were considered by others to be nontherapeutic or even countertherapeutic. In commenting on this experience, he concluded that:

> Psychotherapy at the present time is in a state of chaos. It is not however a meaningless chaos, but an ocean of confusion, teeming with life, spawning vital new ideas, approaches, procedures, and theories at an incredibly rapid rate. Hence the present is a period in which the most diverse methods are used, and which the most divergent explanations are given for a single event. This situation makes inevitable the development of a new fact-finding attitude—a more objective appraisal of different types of change in personality and behavior, and a more empirical understanding of the subtle subjective conditions which lead to these changes. (p. 15)

Psychotherapists who were bewildered with the proliferation of models and the conflicting claims of models developed pick-and-choose methods of selecting techniques of various models, with less emphasis on the theoretical consistency of the techniques and more emphasis on clinical utility in a given clinical situation.

A national survey of psychotherapists completed in the 1970s by Larson (1980) found strong support for an informal model of practical eclecticism, with 65% of therapists indicating that they practiced from multiple models, while 62% reported the belief that using a single model was a less effective practice. While supporting the concept of eclecticism, many of these therapists strongly followed the tenets of their primary school allegiance. Larson expressed concern with a professional culture of "dogma eat dogma" (p. 19) that valued loyalty to a model (termed *schoolism* by Larson) over openness to new ones. Ivey (1980) expressed the concern that psychotherapists were being limited into a choice of either being therapeutically exclusive or practicing an undisciplined "lazy eclecticism" (p. 14). Smith (1982) described "a hodgepodge of inconsistent concepts and techniques" (p. 802) that passed as an eclectic model. Patterson (1989b) cautioned that

> there are as many eclectic approaches as there are eclectic therapists. Each operates out of his or her unique bag of techniques, on the basis of his or her particular training, experiences, and biases, on a case-by-case basis, with no general theory or set of principles as guides. (p. 428)

This critique of eclecticism led later to more theory-based and research-based prescriptive psychotherapy adaptations, such as Lazarus's (1971, 1976, 2006) Multimodal Therapy model and Beutler's Systematic Prescriptive Psychotherapy (Beutler, Consoli, & Lane, 2005). More in the spirit of Roger's (1963) address, both sides showed increasing interest in a more disciplined way to find more common ground, with London (1972) and Lazarus (1971, 1976, 1977) suggesting an end to ideological loyalty in behaviorism to increase focus on effective treatments, whatever the source. Behaviorists such as Birk (1970) and Brinkley-Birk (Birk & Brinkley-Birk, 1974) proposed an integrated approach with behavioral, cognitive, and analytic contributions. Psychoanalysts such as Marmor (1971, 1976) noted that psychotherapy could be considered a learning procedure, building a connection between the two models, and suggesting operational factors that are present in all psychotherapeutic models, such as a good therapeutic relationship, the release of tension, cognitive learning, and identification with the therapist. Strupp (1979), in a review of the therapeutic relationship in psychoanalytic and behavior models, observed that they had more in common than different, suggesting that the therapeutic relationship might be a good starting point for integration.

## Psychotherapy Integration Moves Beyond Eclecticism

In the late 1970s and through the late 1980s, psychotherapy models proliferated, with Smith (1982) identifying just over 100 in 1982. Early models were promoted with an appeal to the great leader myth to promote the uniqueness and efficacy of those models (Brammer & Shostrom, 1977). Norcross (2005) has studied typical characteristics of eclectic practitioners, with eclectics more often voicing dissatisfaction with the current fragmentation in the field. However, the lack of theoretical basis and lack of treatment decision-making protocols for most eclectic approaches have contributed to eclecticism as having an ambivalent, if not negative, meaning in current thinking. Norcross clarified, though, that eclecticism per se is not the problem, but rather an uncritical and unsystematic approach that he suggests would be more accurately described as *syncretism*.

The publication of Wachtel's (1977) *Psychoanalysis and Behavior Therapy: Toward an Integration* was a pivotal point in the development of psychotherapy integration models, and he is credited with laying the foundation for an approach to integration that unified theory with practice, in response to the concerns for careless forms of nontheoretical eclecticism (Norcross, 2005; Stricker & Gold, 1996). Wachtel proposed a comprehensive model on both the theoretical and clinical levels in a variety of topic areas. By bringing together more recent interpersonal psychoanalytic views with recent behavioral therapies having more cognitive components, a synthesis was possible (Arkowitz, 1984).

Also during the 1970s, several important psychotherapy outcome studies questioned Eysenck's (1952) challenge to the effectiveness of psychotherapy. Bergin (1971), in a review of 23 controlled studies, and Luborsky, Singer, and Luborsky (1975), in a review of 40 controlled studies, concluded that psychotherapy was effective. Smith and Glass (1977) and Smith, Glass, and Milton (1980), using meta-analysis, did an extensive review of 475 controlled studies of psychotherapy, concluding that "psychotherapy is beneficial, consistently so and in many different ways" (p. 183). They went on to state that they "did not expect that the demonstrable benefits of quite different types of psychotherapy would be so little different," calling that finding "the most startling and intriguing finding we came across" (p. 185). They also suggested that further research should not focus as much on differences in types of therapy but on identifying underlying shared mechanisms of change. Their findings drew an immediate rhetorical response from Eysenck (1978), referring to their work as "an exercise in mega-silliness" (p. 517).

## Psychotherapy Integration Evolves Distinct Approaches

The publication of a comprehensive model by Wachtel provided the impetus for the next period of challenge and growth in psychotherapy integration. Formed from a loosely organized professional network of psychotherapy integrationists, the Society for the Exploration of Psychotherapy Integration (SEPI) was begun in 1983 and held its first conference in 1985 (Wolfe, 2001). The *Journal of Psychotherapy Integration* was founded to further develop research into the creation of truly integrative models (Arkowitz, 1991). At the Family Institute of Chicago, Feldman, Pinsof, and others began to formulate an integrative model that included relational therapies (Feldman & Pinsof, 1982; Pinsof, 1983).

New efforts were made to better define the research agenda for studying psychotherapy. In *The Psychotherapeutic Process: A Research Handbook* (Greenberg & Pinsof, 1986), Greenberg (1986) challenged the timing of earlier outcome research that focused on comparing model to model, when the same research was showing that it was not the models affecting outcomes, but some underlying and yet poorly understood factors. Greenberg (1986) stated "it is not that prediction is an unimportant goal but rather that we need rigorous description and explanation to illuminate prediction—to define what it is that leads to positive outcomes in psychotherapy" (p. 711), stating further that a new process research was needed "which actively focuses on providing an understanding of some of the specific mechanisms of change in different psychotherapeutic episodes could begin to help in the search for explanations of the active ingredients in therapeutic change" (p. 713).

Prochaska and DiClemente (1982, 1984) formulated a transtheoretical approach that attempted to describe the process and mechanisms of change shared by various models of psychotherapy, attempting to avoid the divisiveness of earlier model wars and respond to the concerns of what could be a haphazard eclecticism.

Norcross and Newman (1992) identified several reasons that psychotherapy integration has become more popular among a range of psychotherapy researchers and clinicians. With so many therapies (400-plus), it had simply become overwhelming to know which therapies to utilize. The diversity of clients and the consistently mixed results applying models to all people with all problems pointed to the limitations of models that are too narrowly defined in theory and application. Studies in therapeutic outcome had increasingly identified that the commonalities of psychotherapies have a greater effect on clinical outcome than do the unique elements of particular models. Proponents of very different models found themselves working together to address the greater role that third-party payers and policy makers have taken in evaluating the results of psychotherapy. Clinical training and supervision guided by treatment manuals, along with learning technologies, have allowed for varied methods to reach wider audiences of trainees. In addition to these factors, Gold (1993) suggested that with some models now several generations old, there was less emphasis on the purity of model and loyalty to the founder as had been described by Brammer and Shostrom (1977). As with virtually every aspect of social science research of this time period, the cultural forces of multiculturalism, feminism, and globalism were encouraging more open dialogue about differences and reevaluation of community-held assumptions of race, gender, and class, and possible interactions in psychotherapy.

As integrative models proliferated, several patterns of integration were identified as the most common approaches to psychotherapy integration: technical eclecticism, common factors integration, assimilative integration, and theoretical integration (Gold, 1996, 2006; Gold & Stricker, 2006; Grencavage & Norcross, 1990; Norcross & Goldfried, 2005; Prochaska & Norcross, 2010; Stricker & Gold, 1993, 1996). There is overlap among these approaches, but each has a slightly different emphasis in the linkage between theory and clinical practice and between clinical practice and approaches to outcome research. Norcross (2005) sees the distinctions as "largely semantic and conceptual, not particularly functional in practice" (p. 10).

Technical Eclecticism has been described by Norcross as more "actuarial than theoretical," with the research emphasis placed on predicting for whom particular interventions work well, rather than *why* they work well. Examples of technical eclecticism have included Lazarus's (1971, 1976, 2006) Multimodal Therapy model and Beutler's Systematic Prescriptive Psychotherapy (Beutler, Consoli, & Lane, 2005). Technical eclecticism has made an important contribution to psychotherapy integration by cataloguing the many techniques, both shared and unique, used in the various approaches to psychotherapy. It has been less successful in providing the theory needed to guide research and practice in the processes of psychotherapy.

Common Factors Integration looks at the intermediate level of psychotherapy, identifying clinical strategies and change processes shared by several psychotherapy models, the mechanisms of change. Frank and Frank's (1993) *Persuasion and Healing*, first published in the 1960s, was an early effort at an historical review of these commonalities. Hubble, Duncan, and Miller's (1999) common factors approach, updated by Duncan, Miller, Wampold, and Hubble (2009), greatly extended the research in identifying clinically significant approaches individualized to the experience of each individual and defined by client-defined outcomes. This focus on defining outcome through the lens of the recipient of psychotherapy has been mentioned by both supporters and detractors.

Assimilative Integration has functionally been a very common informal approach to integration, as psychotherapists working from a specific model have selectively introduced and then incorporated elements of other models into their primary working model. Messer (1992), as well as Stricker and Gold (2002), point out that the assimilative approach is derived from both theoretical integration and technical eclecticism. Therapists maintain a home theory and incorporate techniques from other theoretical orientations, often reinterpreting the meaning of the technique through the lens of the home theory.

Theoretical Integration has been perhaps the most daunting approach to integration, characterized by a comprehensive approach to integrating the theories of pathology and therapy techniques into a unified system. Wachtel's (1977) integration was an important example of this approach, but it was limited in the theories integrated (psychoanalysis and behaviorism/learning theory). Prochaska and DiClemente (1982, 1984) took a more comprehensive approach, developing a theory built on everyday processes of change and problem solving and expanding it to an application to psychotherapy. Stages of change (precontemplation, contemplation, decision, action, and maintenance) with 10 potential change processes in psychotherapy (consciousness raising, self-reevaluation, social reevaluation, self-liberation, social liberation, counter-conditioning, stimulus control, contingency management, dramatic relief, and helping relationship) contributing to a hierarchy of interventions (symptom/situational, maladaptive cognitions, current interpersonal conflicts, family systems conflicts, and intrapersonal conflicts). The Transtheoretical Model of Prochaska and DiClemente has been applied to many clinical issues, and research is ongoing.

## Psychotherapy Integration and Evidence-Based Practices

Ivey (1980), when asked to make 20-year predictions in psychotherapy, hoped that by 2000, "The final gasp of 'my theory is better and more perfect than your theory' will be heard" (p. 14). However, sociocultural and economic forces have impacted the movement toward psychotherapy integration and outcome research based on the underlying mechanisms shared by all psychotherapies (Henry, 1998; Mahoney, 2008). Although the emphasis on accountability of evidence-based therapy has been greatly needed, the use of medically based research approaches to outcome has diverted a great deal of attention to a new "therapy war," the battle of therapeutic outcome measurement (Norcross, 2005; Norcross, Beutler, & Levant, 2005; Orlinsky, 2006).

In the late 1990s, Norcross (1997, 2001, 2002, 2005) saw the psychotherapy integration movement as stalled, with "an abundance of awareness but a dearth of action" (Norcross, 1997, p. 86) in updating methods of research and application. He called for more consensus of understanding the concepts of psychotherapy integration, the development of more outcome research, and the updating of training programs to emphasize learning integrative methods.

## Psychotherapy Integration Into the Future

Norcross (2005) identified several obstacles that in the future will continue to influence the development of psychotherapy integration models. Despite efforts at rapprochement by many psychotherapists, partisan zealotry continues to some degree, partly maintained by the challenge that professional reputations and the resulting funding of research are rarely built on commonalities and consensus, but rather on competition. Millon and Grossman (2008) describe the current state of psychotherapy research as "stuck in a babble of conflict and confusion" (p. 362), which seems to hearken back to Rogers' (1963) "state of chaos" (p. 15) comments of a generation ago.

Although much has been done in psychotherapy training to promote theoretical orientation and basic professional skills, training approaches need to be better developed to reflect the process and mechanisms of psychotherapy, with careful attention to incorporating better measures of outcome (Andrews, Norcross, & Halgin, 1992; Norcross & Halgin, 2005; Norcross, 2005). Considering the importance of therapist factors identified in common factor research, one possible method would be to include the incorporation of self of therapist work with studies on integrative psychotherapy. Beitman and Soth (2006) have described the importance of self-observation as a core psychotherapy process, which includes an active scan of one's inner landscape, the ability for introspection, and a clear awareness of one's social and cultural environment. Training methods would need to include methods for incorporating self-observation in all of the dimensions of providing psychotherapy. Goldfried (2001), Norcross (2006), and Wolfe (2001) have all provided first-person accounts of the inter-relationship of personal and professional development as clinicians and researchers in psychotherapy integration, providing a resource for how self-observation has worked in their practice.

Further development of psychotherapy integration will need to continue to address the issues of epistemology and philosophy of mind. The contradictory assumptions of human nature, personality development, and the origins of psychopathology remain a roadblock to true integration (Norcross, 2005), much as Patterson (1989a, 1989b) had pointed out more than 15 years earlier. As Orlinsky (2009) stated

> *the epistemological situation in the human sciences is simply more complex than in the physical sciences because participant-observers (and external observers, in a different way) are inherently more extensively involved in constructing the reality they observe. (p. xxiii)*

The resolution may come from a more postmodern perspective on psychotherapy research (Safran & Messer, 1997), reflecting the suggestions of Polanyi (1964a/1946, 1964b) and Kuhn (1973) that even scientists never escape our perspectives, because the acts of observation and synthesis in scientific inquiry are always bound in the perceptual lens of the researcher. In every scientific endeavor, but particularly those studying human behavior, the researcher is forever a participant-observer, and the meanings are always shared meanings. This is consistent with Kelly's (1955, 1963, 2003/1970) Personal Construct Theory, which for many years has challenged the traditional methods of scientific inquiry applied to human behavior. It seems that the field of psychotherapy has not been able to escape the bind inherent in human investigation, that the desire to know and the incompleteness of knowledge are inescapably entwined.

Norcross (2005) has suggested that one approach to promoting psychotherapy integration would be to work toward common definitions of all of the units of study in the construct of psychotherapy. Perhaps the one consistency in psychotherapy theory and research has been the inconsistency of terminology in both developing theory and in operationalizing those theories into commonly understood units of experience that can be implemented in practice and measured by research. Messer (1987, 1992, 2001, 2008) has expressed support for the intention of the suggestion but believes that it would not be possible to completely define a common language, much less consolidate all of psychotherapy into a unified whole. He asserts that this desire to unify has much more to do with the comfort of the provider of psychotherapy in satisfying an internal desire to make sense of the work through traditional models. Unification has much less to do with the comfort of the recipients of psychotherapy, who typically are looking to make sense of their life rather than a model. Messer, along with Fishman, suggested that this is an opportunity to restore the case study to prominence in psychotherapy research and training, and he termed this a Pragmatic Case Study Method (Fishman, 2001; Fishman & Messer, 2005).

Continued psychotherapy integration researchers will need to remain active participants in the conversations on evidence-based practice (Norcross, Beutler, & Levant, 2005). Some have suggested that a needed corrective would be to consider the issues from a more nonlinear perspective than evidence-based practice, suggesting a meta-theory that is more circular, which would also include the standpoint of practice-based evidence. Theory would be not only the source of research but also a product of research, with research being a source of theory as well as a product. Anchin (2008) suggests that a biopsychosocial systems meta-theory might create the bridge for unifying the various approaches. Pinsof and Lebow (2005a, 2005b) proposed a Biopsychosocial Systems Theory (BST), which is built on an interactive constructivism and focuses on the therapeutic unit of the case study in developing theory and research.

Historical debates on the value of psychotherapy included primarily the practitioners and researchers in the field. The modern debate, represented by evidence-based practice research, involves the additional stakeholders of third-party payers, health policy leaders, and consumers of psychotherapy services (Norcross, Beutler, & Levant, 2005). Future discussions of outcome will need to include the concerns of all stakeholders, and respectful conversations will have to be held in language that translates to all participants. Much of the thinking—and much of the funding—on evidence-based practice has come from the medical field, and in doing so has not asked the epistemological question of whether medical model methods of research are best suited for study in human behavior. Wampold (2001) points to more than 30 years of psychotherapy outcome research that from the medical model perspective is deemed inconclusive but likely suggests that a more accurate conclusion is that medical model research is ineffective in measuring psychotherapy outcome.

Duncan, Miller, Wampold, and Hubble (2009) outline ways that psychotherapy outcome research can be developed that better reflects the epistemological assumptions in studying human behavior as opposed to physical processes.

Current writers in psychotherapy integration suggest that psychotherapy integration is moving into a new phase of development that will focus more on unification, as a part of a larger movement aimed at the unification of the clinical sciences (Magnavita, 2008), while others caution that substantial differences exist in epistemology and philosophy of mind to slow the process considerably (Anchin, 2008; Knoblauch, 2008). Whatever the next conceptualization of integration will be, it will inevitably include application to a variety of special populations served by psychotherapy, including the psychotherapy of children.

# References

Alexander, F., & French, T. (1946). *Psychoanalytic therapy*. New York, NY: Ronald Press.

Anchin, J. C. (2008). Pursuing a unifying paradigm for psychotherapy: Tasks, dialectical considerations, and biopsychosocial systems metatheory. *Journal of Psychotherapy Integration, 18,* 310–349.

Andrews, J. D. W., Norcross, J. C., & Halgin, R. P. (1992). Training in psychotherapy integration. In J. C. Norcross and M. R. Goldfried (Eds.), *Handbook of psychotherapy integration* (pp. 563–592). New York, NY: Basic Books.

Arkowitz, H. (1984). Historical perspective on the integration of psychoanalytic therapy and behavior therapy. In H. Arkowitz & S. Messer (Eds.), *Psychoanalytic therapy and behavioral therapy: Is integration possible?* (pp. 1–30). New York, NY: Plenum.

Arkowitz, H. (1991). Introductory statement: Psychotherapy integration comes of age. *Journal of Psychotherapy Integration, 1,* 1–4.

Beitman, B. D., & Soth, A. M. (2006). Activation of self-observation: A core process among the psychotherapies. *Journal of Psychotherapy Integration, 16,* 383–397.

Bergin, A. E. (1971). The evaluation of therapeutic outcomes. In A. E. Bergin & S. I Garfield (Eds.), *Handbook of psychotherapy and behavior change*. New York, NY: John Wiley.

Beutler, L. E., Consoli, A. J., & Lane, G. (2005). Systematic treatment selection and prescriptive psychotherapy. In J. C. Norcross & M. R. Goldfried (Eds.), *Handbook of psychotherapy integration* (2nd ed., pp. 121–143). New York, NY: Oxford University Press.

Birk, L. (1970). Behavior therapy: Integration with dynamic psychiatry. *Behavior Therapy, 1,* 522–526.

Birk, L., & Brinkley-Birk, A. (1974). Psychoanalysis and behavior therapy. *American Journal of Psychiatry, 131,* 499–510.

Brammer, L., & Shostrom, E. (1977). *Therapeutic psychology: Fundamentals of counseling and psychotherapy* (3rd ed.). Englewood Cliffs, NJ: Prentice Hall.

Dollard, J., & Miller, N. E. (1950). *Personality and psychotherapy: An analysis in terms of learning, thinking, and culture*. New York, NY: McGraw-Hill.

Dow, J. (1986). Universal aspects of symbolic healing: A theoretical synthesis. *American Anthropologist, 88,* 56–69.

Duncan, B. L. (2009). Prologue: Saul Rosenzweig: The founder of the common factors. In B. L. Duncan, S. D. Miller, B. E. Wampold, & Hubble, M. A. (Eds.), *The heart and soul of change: Delivering what works in therapy* (2nd ed.). Washington, DC: American Psychological Association Press.

Duncan, B. L., Miller, S. D., Wampold, B. E., & Hubble, M. A. (Eds.). (2009). *The heart and soul of change: Delivering what works in therapy* (2nd ed.). Washington, DC: American Psychological Association Press.

Ellenberger, H. F. (1970). *The discovery of the unconscious: The history and evolution of dynamic psychiatry*. New York, NY: Basic Books.

Eysenck, H. J. (1952). The effects of psycho-therapy: An evaluation. *Journal of Counseling Psychology, 16,* 319–324.

Eysenck, H. J. (1960). Learning theory and behavior therapy. In H. J. Eysenck (Ed.), *Behaviour therapy and the neuroses.* London, England: Pergamon.

Eysenck, H. J. (1978). An exercise in mega-silliness. *American Psychologist, 33,* 517.

Eysenck, H. J. (1983). The effectiveness of psychotherapy: The specter at the feast. *Behavioral and Brain Sciences, 6,* 290.

Feldman, L. B., & Pinsof, W. M. (1982). Problem maintenance in family systems: An integrative model. *Journal of Marital and Family Therapy, 8,* 295–308.

Fischer, A. R., Jome, L. M., & Atkinson, D. R. (1998a). Back to the future of multicultural psychotherapy with a common factors approach. *Counseling Psychologist, 26,* 602–606.

Fischer, A. R., Jome, L. M., & Atkinson, D. R. (1998b). Reconceptualizing multicultural counseling: Universal healing conditions in a culturally specific context. *Counseling Psychologist, 26,* 525–588.

Fishman, D. R. (2001). From single case to database: A new method for enhancing psychotherapy, forensic, and other psychological practice. *Applied & Preventive Psychology, 10,* 275–304.

Fishman, D. R., & Messer, S. B. (2005). Case-based studies as a source of unity in applied psychology. In R. J. Sternberg (Ed.), *The unification of psychology: Prospect or pipedream?* (pp. 37–59). Washington, DC: American Psychological Association Press.

Frank, J. D., & Frank, J. B. (1993). *Persuasion and healing* (3rd ed.). Baltimore, MD: Johns Hopkins University Press.

French, T. M. (1933). Interrelations between psychoanalysis and the experimental work of Pavlov. *American Journal of Psychiatry, 89,* 1165–1203.

Glass, G. V., & Kliegl, R. M. (1983). An apology for research integration in the study of psychotherapy. *Journal of Consulting and Clinical Psychology, 51,* 28–41.

Glass, G. V., & Smith, M. L. (1978). Reply to Eysenck. *American Psychologist, 33,* 517–519.

Gold, J. R. (1992). An integrative-systemic approach to severe psychopathology in children and adolescents. *Journal of Integrative and Eclectic Psychotherapy, 11,* 67–78.

Gold, J. R. (1993). The sociohistorical context of psychotherapy integration. In G. Stricker & J. R. Gold (Eds.), *Comprehensive handbook of psychotherapy integration* (pp. 3–8). New York, NY: Plenum Press.

Gold, J. R. (1996). *Key concepts in psychotherapy integration.* New York, NY: Plenum Press.

Gold, J. R. (2006). Introduction: An overview of psychotherapy integration. In J. R. Gold & G. Stricker (Eds.), *The casebook of psychotherapy integration* (pp. 3–16). Washington, DC: American Psychological Association Press.

Gold, J. R., & Stricker, G. (2006). *A casebook of psychotherapy integration.* Washington DC: American Psychological Association Press.

Goldfried, M. R. (2001). Conclusion: A perspective on how therapists change. In M. R. Goldfried (Ed.), *How therapists change* (pp. 315–330). Washington, DC: American Psychological Association Press.

Greenberg, L. S. (1986). Research strategies. In L. S. Greenberg and W. M. Pinsof (Eds.), *The psychotherapeutic process: A research handbook* (pp. 707–734). New York, NY: Guilford Press.

Greenberg, L. S., & Pinsof, W. M. (Eds.). (1986). *The psychotherapeutic process: A research handbook.* New York, NY: Guilford Press.

Grencavage, L. M., & Norcross, J. C. (1990). What are the commonalities among the therapeutic common factors? *Professional Psychology: Research and Practice, 21,* 372–378.

Henry, W. P. (1998). Science, politics, and the politics of science: Use and misuse of empirically validated treatment research. *Psychotherapy Research, 8,* 126–140.

Hubble, M. A., Duncan, B. L., & Miller, S. D. (Eds.). (1999). *The heart and soul of change: What works in therapy.* Washington, DC: American Psychological Association Press.

Ivey, A. E. (1980). Counseling 2000: Time to take charge. *Counseling Psychologist, 8,* 12–16.

Kelley, S. D., Bickman, L., & Norwood, E. (2009). Evidence-based treatments and common factors in youth psychotherapy. In B. L. Duncan, S. D. Miller, B. E. Wampold, & M. A. Hubble (Eds.), *The heart and soul of change: Delivering what works in therapy* (2nd ed., pp. 325–356). Washington, DC: American Psychological Association Press.

Kelly, G. A. (1955). *The psychology of personal constructs.* New York, NY: W. W. Norton.

Kelly, G. A. (1963). *A theory of personality: The psychology of personal constructs.* New York, NY: W. W. Norton.

Kelly, G. A. (2003). A brief introduction to personal construct theory. In F. Fransella (Ed.), *International handbook of personal construct psychology* (pp. 320). New York, NY: John Wiley (originally published in 1970).

Kleinman, A. M. (1980). *Patients and healers in the context of culture.* Berkeley, CA: University of California Press.

Kleinman, A. M. (1988). *The illness narratives: Suffering, healing, and the human condition.* New York, NY: Basic Books.

Knoblauch, F. W. (2008). Some disparate thoughts on the idea of a unified psychotherapy. *Journal of Psychotherapy Integration, 18,* 301–309.

Kuhn, T. S. (1973). *The structure of scientific revolution.* Chicago, IL: University of Chicago Press.

Larson, D. (1980). Therapeutic schools, styles, and schoolism: A national survey. *Journal of Humanistic Psychology, 20*(3), 3–20.

Lazarus, A. A. (1971). *Behavior therapy and beyond.* New York, NY: McGraw-Hill.

Lazarus, A. A. (1976). *Multimodal behavior therapy.* New York, NY: Springer.

Lazarus, A. A. (1977). Has behavior therapy outlived its usefulness? *American Psychologist, 32,* 550–554.

Lazarus, A. A. (2006). Multimodal therapy: A seven-point integration. In G. Stricker and J. R. Gold (Eds.), *The casebook of psychotherapy integration* (pp. 17–28). Washington, DC: American Psychological Association Press.

London, P. (1972). The end of ideology in behavior modification. *American Psychologist, 27,* 913–920.

Luborsky, L., Singer, B., & Luborsky, L. (1975). Comparative studies of psychotherapies: Is it true that "Everyone has won and all must have prizes"? *Archives of General Psychiatry, 32,* 995–1008.

Mahoney, M. J. (2008). Power, politics, and psychotherapy: A constructive caution on unification. *Journal of Psychotherapy Integration, 18,* 367–376.

Magnavita, J. J. (2008). Toward unification of clinical science: The next wave in the evolution of psychotherapy? *Journal of Psychotherapy Integration, 18,* 264–291.

Marmor, J. (1971). Dynamic psychotherapy and behavior therapy: Are they irreconcilable? *Archives of General Psychiatry, 24,* 22–28.

Marmor, J. (1976). Common operational factors in diverse approaches to behavior change. In A. Burton (Ed.), *What makes behavior change possible* (pp. 3–12). New York, NY: Brunner/Mazel.

Messer, S. B. (1987). Can the tower of Babel be completed? A critique of the common language proposal. *Journal of Integrative and Eclectic Psychotherapy, 6,* 195–199.

Messer, S. B. (1992). A critical examination of belief structures in integrative and eclectic psychotherapy. In J. C. Norcross & M. R. Goldfried (Eds.), *Handbook of psychotherapy integration* (pp. 130–165). New York, NY: Basic Books.

Messer, S. B. (2001). Introduction to the special issue on assimilative integration. *Journal of Psychotherapy Integration, 8,* 1–4.

Messer, S. B. (2008). Unification in psychotherapy: A commentary. *Journal of Psychotherapy Integration, 18,* 363–366.

Millon, T., & Grossman, S. D. (2008). Psychotherapy unification. *Journal of Psychotherapy Integration, 18,* 359–362.

Norcross, J. C. (1997). Emerging breakthroughs in psychotherapy integration: Three predictions and one fantasy. *Psychotherapy, 34,* 86–90.

Norcross, J. C. (2001). Purposes, processes, and products of the task force on empirically supported therapy relationships. *Psychotherapy, 38,* 345–356.

Norcross, J. C. (2002). *Psychotherapy relationships that work.* New York, NY: Oxford University Press.

Norcross, J. C. (2005). A primer on psychotherapy integration. In J. C. Norcross & M. R. Goldfried (Eds.), *Handbook of psychotherapy integration* (2nd ed., pp. 3–23). New York, NY: Oxford University Press.

Norcross, J. C. (2006). Personal integration: An *n of 1* study. *Journal of Psychotherapy Integration, 16,* 59–72.

Norcross, J. C., Beutler, L. E., & Levant, R. F. (Eds.). (2005). *Evidence-based practices in mental health: Debate and dialogue on the fundamental questions.* Washington, DC: American Psychological Association Press.

Norcross, J. C., & Goldfried, M. R. (Eds.) (2005). *Handbook of psychotherapy integration* (2nd ed.). New York, NY: Oxford University Press.

Norcross, J. C., & Halgin, R. P. (2005). Training in psychotherapy integration. In J. C. Norcross and M. R. Goldfried (Eds.), *Handbook of psychotherapy integration* (2nd ed.; pp. 439–458). New York, NY: Oxford University Press.

Norcross, J. C., & Newman, C. F. (1992). Psychotherapy integration: Setting the context. In J. C. Norcross & M. R. Goldfried (Eds.), *Handbook of psychotherapy integration* (pp. 3–45). New York, NY: Basic Books.

Orlinsky, D. E. (2006). Comments on the state of psychotherapy research (as I see it). *Psychotherapy Bulletin, 41*, 37–41.

Orlinsky, D. E. (2009). Foreword. In B. L. Duncan, S. D. Miller, B. E. Wampold, & M. A. Hubble (Eds.), *The heart and soul of change: Delivering what works in therapy* (2nd ed., pp. 357–392). Washington, DC: American Psychological Association Press.

Patterson, C. H. (1989a). Eclecticism in psychotherapy: Is integration possible? *Psychotherapy, 26*, 157–161.

Patterson, C. H. (1989b). Foundations for a systematic eclectic psychotherapy. *Psychotherapy, 26*, 427–435.

Pinsof, W. M. (1983). Integrative problem-centered therapy: Toward the synthesis of family and individual psychotherapies. *Journal of Marital and Family Therapy, 9*, 19–35.

Pinsof, W. M. (1994). An integrative systems perspective on the therapeutic alliance: Theoretical, clinical, and research perspectives. In A. O. Horvath and L. S. Greenberg (Eds.), *The working alliance: Theory, research, and practice* (pp. 173–198). New York, NY: John Wiley.

Pinsof, W. M. (1995). *Integrative problem-centered therapy: A synthesis of family, individual, and biological therapies.* New York, NY: Basic Books.

Pinsof, W. M., & Lebow, J. L. (Eds.) (2005a). *Family psychology: The art of the science.* New York, NY: Oxford University Press.

Pinsof, W. M., & Lebow, J. L. (2005b). A scientific paradigm for family psychology. In W. M. Pinsof & J. L. Lebow (Eds.), *Family psychology: The art of the science* (pp. 3–22). New York, NY: Oxford University Press.

Polanyi, M. (1964a). *Science, faith, and society: A searching examination of the meaning and nature of scientific inquiry* (rev. ed. with new introduction). London, England: Oxford University Press. (original work published in 1946)

Polanyi, M. (1964b). *Personal knowledge.* New York: Harper & Row.

Prochaska, J. O., & DiClemente, C. C. (1982). Transtheoretical therapy: Toward a more integrative model of change. *Psychotherapy: Theory, Research, & Practice, 19*, 276–288.

Prochaska, J. O., & DiClemente, C. C. (1984). *The transtheoretical approach: Crossing the traditional boundaries of therapy.* Homewood, IL: Dow Jones-Irwin.

Prochaska, J. O., & Norcross, J. C. (2010). *Systems of psychotherapy: A transtheoretical analysis* (7th ed.). Belmont, CA: Brooks/Cole.

Rogers, C. R. (1942). *Counseling and psychotherapy.* Boston, MA: Houghton Mifflin.

Rogers, C. R. (1963). Psychotherapy today, and where do we go from here? *American Journal of Psychotherapy, 17*, 5–16.

Rosenzweig, S. (1936). Some implicit common factors in diverse methods in psychotherapy. *American Journal of Orthopsychiatry, 6*, 422–425.

Safran, J. D., & Messer, S. B. (1997). Psychotherapy integration: A postmodern critique. *Clinical Psychology: Science and Practice, 4*, 140–152.

Saltzman, N., & Norcross, J. C. (1990). *Therapy wars: Contention and convergence in differing clinical approaches.* San Francisco, CA: Jossey Bass.

Sears, R. R. (1944). Experimental analysis of psychoanalytic phenomena. In J. Hunt (Ed.), *Personality and the behavior disorders* (pp. 191–206). New York, NY: Ronald Press.

Smith, D. (1982). Trends in counseling and psychotherapy. *American Psychologist, 37*, 802–809.

Smith, M. L., & Glass, G. V. (1977). Meta-analysis of psychotherapy outcome studies. *American Psychologist, 32*, 752–760.

Smith, M. L., Glass, G. V., & Milton, T. I. (1980). *The benefits of psychotherapy.* Baltimore, MD: Johns Hopkins University Press.

Sparks, J. A., & Duncan, B. L. (2009). Common factors in couple and family therapy: Must all have prizes? In B. L. Duncan, S. D. Miller, B. E. Wampold, & M. A. Hubble (Eds.), *The heart and soul of change: Delivering what works in therapy* (2nd ed., pp. 357–392). Washington, DC: American Psychological Association Press.

Stricker, G., & Gold, J. R. (Eds.). (1993). *Comprehensive handbook of psychotherapy integration.* New York, NY: Plenum.

Stricker, G., & Gold, J. R. (1996). Psychotherapy integration: An assimilative, psychodynamic approach. *Clinical Psychology: Science and Practice, 3*, 47–58.

Stricker, G., & Gold, J. R. (2002). An assimilative approach to integrative psychodynamic psychotherapy. In F. W. Kaslow (Ed. in Chief) and J. Lebow (Vol. Ed.), *Comprehensive handbook of psychotherapy, Volume 4: Integrative/eclectic* (pp. 295–316). Hoboken, NJ: John Wiley.

Stricker, G., & Gold J. R. (2008). Integrative psychotherapies. In J. Lebow (Ed.), *Twenty-first century psychotherapies* (pp. 389–423). New York: Guilford Press.

Strupp, H. H. (1979). A psychodynamicist looks at behavior therapy. *Psychotherapy: Theory, Research, and Practice, 16,* 124–131.

Torrey, E. F. (1986). *Witchdoctors and psychiatrists: The common roots of psychotherapy and its future.* Northvale, NJ: Jason Aronson.

Wachtel, P. L. (1977). *Psychoanalysis and behavior therapy: Toward an integration.* New York, NY: Basic Books.

Wampold, B. E. (1997). Methodological problems in identifying efficacious psychotherapies. *Psychotherapy Research, 7,* 21–43.

Wampold, B. (2001). *The great psychotherapy debate: Models, methods, and findings.* Mahwah, NJ: Erlbaum.

Wampold, B. (2009). The research evidence for the common factors models: A historically situated perspective. In B. L. Duncan, S. D. Miller, B. E. Wampold, & M. A. Hubble (Eds.), *The heart and soul of change: Delivering what works in therapy* (2nd ed., pp. 357–392). Washington, DC: American Psychological Association Press.

Wolfe, B. E. (2001). The integrative experience of psychotherapy integration. In M. R. Goldfried (Ed.), *How therapists change* (pp. 289–312). Washington, DC: American Psychological Association.

# Integrating Play Therapy Theories Into Practice

<table>
<tr><td>2</td></tr>
<tr><td>Chapter</td></tr>
</table>

## *Athena A. Drewes*

## Introduction

The integration of theory, technique, and common factors in psychotherapy has gained prominence since the 1990s. Previously called *eclecticism*, *integration* has now become the preferred term in the blending together of theory, technique, and common factors (Norcross, 2005). Previously, *eclectic* "simply means that you select from different theories and techniques a therapeutic strategy that appears best for a particular client" (Schaefer, 2003, p. 308). However, Norcross (1987) takes eclecticism further into *integration*, whereby various theories are applied to one interactive and coordinated means of treatment.

Because psychological disorders, especially for children and adolescents, are multilayered, complex, and multidetermined, a multifaceted treatment approach is needed (Schaefer, 2003). Many clients come with not one clearly defined diagnosis, but rather several overlapping problems caused by the comorbidity of issues (such as in the case of complex trauma resulting in overlapping anxiety and attention problems, along with phobias and sexualized behaviors). Clinicians trained in one theoretical and treatment approach are finding that one size cannot fit all of the presenting problems they are being faced with today. In addition, no clear research evidence shows that one single theoretical approach (such as Cognitive-Behavioral, Jungian, Rogerian) is able to create therapeutic change across all of the various and multidimensional psychological disorders that exist (Schaefer, 2003; Smith, Glass, & Miller, 1980).

Because of this multidimensional aspect, child/play therapy calls for the unique demand that the therapist wear many different hats and be skillful in changing from one therapeutic stance to that of another in order to meet the needs of the child and the various members in the child's life (Coonerty, 1993). One moment the play therapist is intensely involved in deeply evocative, often very conflicted, play therapy with the child client. At that moment the therapist needs to deal with the child's internal struggles, setting limits, and being an educator or mediator with the child. In the next moment, the therapist needs to engage with a parent or school psychologist or classroom teacher to assess the child's functioning. These often conflicting and rapidly changing roles lead many child/play therapists to adopt an eclectic prescriptive style in which therapeutic interventions are chosen and then changed according to the most pressing external demand (Coonerty, 1993).

In addition, in direct contrast to linear models of psychopathology, integrative theories of psychopathology assume a weaving of various aspects of the client's personal experience, thereby conceptualizing psychopathology from the viewpoint of multicausation. Thus equal weight is given to various aspects of personal functioning, and they are seen in a blended and unified whole (Coonerty, 1993). Such blending implies a circularity as well as the containment of multiple relationships that are seen among cognitive, dynamic, interpersonal, and behavioral aspects of the individual (Coonerty, 1993). Rather than just jumping from one type of treatment to another, the child/play therapist can develop an integrative approach to treatment that broadens the therapist's concept of what is appropriate from the various theoretical points of view and can offer a wider array of tools with which to work. In addition, the prospect of change in one sphere of functioning can potentially lead to broad reverberations and changes throughout all aspects of the client's maladaptive functioning (Coonerty, 1993).

Further adding to the push toward and benefits of an integrative treatment approach is that funding sources (state, federal, and insurance companies) are mandating that clinicians and agencies utilize evidence-based treatment approaches in order to receive continued funding. Consequently, they want to be sure clients are receiving the best treatment, as well as the most effective treatment available. So the selection of treatment interventions should not be ruled by a subjective personal preference or staying within a comfort zone in the way one always works, but rather through the selection of evidence-based practices over personal opinion (Schaefer, 2003).

Finally, the extensive research being done with regard to child sexual abuse and trauma has resulted in evidence-based practices that push for an integrative treatment approach. For example, Stien and Kendall (2004) recommend a three-pronged integrated approach:

> *Although cognitive/behavioral interventions address problematic behaviors and help the child build new skills, psychodynamic interventions are needed to help integrate traumatic memories and emotions along with buried parts of the self. At the same time, the therapist must pay close attention to family interactions— sequences of action and reaction—to root out any that maintain and reinforce symptoms. (p. 139)*

Gil (2006) states:

> *Evidence also suggests that trauma memories are imbedded in the right hemisphere of the brain, and thus those interventions facilitating access to and activity in the*

*right side of the brain may be indicated. The right hemisphere of the brain is most receptive to nonverbal strategies that utilize symbolic language, creativity and pretend play. (p. 68)*

Thus the need for the use of expressive arts, play, and pleasurable activities within therapy have been found to be helpful and needed in helping traumatized and abused children create their trauma narratives (Cohen, Deblinger, Mannarino, & Steer, 2004; Gil, 2006; van der Kolk, 2005). Therefore, it is not surprising then that therapists, and notably play therapists, need to become more flexible in their treatment approaches. The need for flexibility results in changing one's style of working, expanding one's orientation, and seeking out approaches that can best address a particular client's needs or concerns.

Within the past 20 years, integration of theory and treatment has developed into a clearly delineated area of interest for clinicians (Norcross, 2005). Jensen, Bergin, and Greaves (1990) found in a survey of 423 mental health professionals that a majority use an eclectic form of therapy. A recent survey by Norcross, Hedges, and Castle (2002) found that 36% of psychologists responding claim to be eclectic/integrative. Among play therapists, Phillips and Landreth (1995) found that the most common approach reported by respondents was an eclectic and multitheoretical orientation. Such a shift may be a result of the growing dissatisfaction with a single-school or one-size-fits-all treatment approach. No one approach appears to be clinically effective for all clients and situations. Also, there has been a growing desire in the psychotherapy field to find out what can be learned from other theories. All of these factors have made an integrative approach necessary. Finally, Norcross (2005) highlights eight possible reasons for the rapid increase in integrative psychotherapies. Among them are (1) a large increase in therapies, (2) the lack of a single theory or treatment that is adequate, (3) a rise in short-term, problem-focused treatment, (4) the rise in evidence-based treatments resulting from the identification of specific therapy effects, and (5) the recognition that therapeutic commonalities heavily contribute to outcome (Norcross, 2005).

## Basic Concepts, Goals, and Techniques

There are several different avenues toward creating an integrative treatment approach. Norcross (2005) lists them as Technical Eclecticism, Theoretical Integration, Common Factors, and Assimilative Integration.

*Technical Eclecticism* is a prescriptive approach in that it selects the best treatment for the person and the problem. This decision is guided by research on what has worked best for others in the past with similar problems and having similar characteristics (Norcross, 2005).

*Theoretical Integration* takes the best elements of two or more approaches to therapy and blends them with the expectation that the result will be more than the sum of the two separate therapies. The emphasis is on integrating the underlying theories along with integration of therapy techniques. The results lead to a new direction for both practice and research (Norcross, 2005).

The *Common Factors* approach ascertains the underlying core ingredients that the different therapies share in common. The goal is to come up with the simplest and most effective treatment based on those commonalities. Grencavage & Norcross (1990) reviewed 50 publications to discern commonalities among the proposed therapeutic common factors. Factors per publication ranged in number from 1 to 20, with a total of 89 different commonalities noted. Their analyses revealed that 41% of the proposed commonalities had to do with change processes, whereas only 6% were attributed to client characteristics. Consensus across categories were the development of a therapeutic alliance, opportunity for catharsis, acquisition and practice of new behaviors, and the clients' positive expectancies (Grencavage & Norcross, 1990).

With *Assimilative Integration* the clinician is required to have a strong grounding in one theoretical system but a willingness to selectively incorporate or assimilate practices and views from other systems (Messer, 1992; Norcross, 2005). Assimilative Integration thereby "combines the advantages of a single, coherent theoretical system with the flexibility of a broader range of technical interventions from multiple systems" (Norcross, 2005, p. 10). Most clinicians have been and continue to be trained in a single approach. Rather than throw away that foundation as they discover the limitations of their original approach, many rework their approach by gradually incorporating parts and methods from other approaches and molding it into a new form (Norcross, 2005).

Play therapists lag behind mainstream psychotherapy with regard to an integrative treatment approach. Some play therapy articles and chapters have been written regarding an integrative play therapy approach, mostly through case studies, but to date little empirical research has been conducted. Some promising work has been done in coming up with various new approaches and conceptualizations for an integrative approach to treatment that fall under several of Norcross's categories.

*Technical Eclecticism*, utilizing a prescriptive approach, is reported by Kenny and Winick (2000) in a case study of working with an 11-year-old autistic girl with behavioral difficulties. Using a sequential approach, Kenny and Winick chose treatment approaches that would build on one another over time, rather than a blending together within one session. This case is also particularly unique in that fewer than 20% of surveyed play therapists (Phillips & Landreth, 1998) believe that play therapy would help in treating the problems associated with pervasive developmental disorders. The reasoning is that the child's limited cognitive or play skills would inhibit the therapy. Treatment for autistic children has usually included medications for lessening aggressive and self-injurious behaviors, increasing attention span, along with controlling seizures, decreasing agitation, and reducing stereotyped and other maladaptive behaviors (Dawson & Castelloe, 1992). Behavioral techniques are often utilized to lessen self-stimulatory behaviors, and nondirective, child-centered treatment is not utilized at all.

Kenny and Winick utilized the rapport-building component of nondirective play therapy with directive techniques in targeting maladaptive behavior and offering parent education. The rationale for using a flexible integrative approach was because of the multidimensional aspects of the child's behaviors, along with her developmental delays. They combined different treatment approaches into a coherent intervention sequence (Shirk, 1999). They blended nondirective play therapy and directive interventions focused on personal hygiene and social skills, and parent education and support.

During the initial stages (sessions 1–7), child-centered play therapy was utilized as the sole treatment approach to build rapport and establish minimal limit setting. This sequence involved nondirective sessions that allowed for the child to be able to begin to express feelings and offered a needed sense of constancy of the therapist and room. Midway through treatment, the sessions stopped being nondirective and became directive, with the therapist focusing on specific behavioral issues that were presented, such as refusal to brush her teeth and lack of personal hygiene. Although a play-based approach was utilized, the sessions were strictly directive and skill based. As treatment progressed, the therapist brought in parent education and training to help the mother carry over the skill-building components into the home, while also working to lower the mother's frustration level and parent-child conflict. Utilizing this integrative, sequential, and prescriptive approach brief therapy successfully lessened the autistic child's noncompliant behaviors at home and lessened irritable mood, while it increased her basic living skills, social behavior, and compliance at home.

An example of *Theoretical Integration* in play therapy is Ecosystemic Play Therapy (EPT) developed by Kevin O'Connor. The clinician is required to consider the child, his or her problems, and the therapy process within the framework of the child's ecosystem (O'Connor, 2001). EPT is heavily grounded in theory and emphasizes the flexibility of the theory, allowing the play therapist to work with children at any developmental level using a variety of contexts. O'Connor (2001) states that "EPT is an integrative model of play therapy incorporating key elements of the analytic (Freud, 1928; Klein, 1932), child-centered (Axline, 1947; Landreth, 1991), and cognitive-behavioral models (Knell, 1993) of play therapy, as well as elements of Theraplay (Jernberg, 1979; Jernberg & Booth, 1999) and reality therapy (Glasser, 1975)" (p. 33).

Ecosystemic play therapy is theory dependent (rather than technique dependent). The theory is used to match a wide array of techniques and creative activities and interventions, and to utilize them with specific clients and their problems following a well-developed treatment plan. EPT focuses primarily on helping the child client function optimally in the contexts in which he or she lives. EPT was first formally described in 1994 by O'Connor (O'Connor, 1997). Concepts of personality, psychopathology, nested environments that the client is in, treatment goals, and the role of play and techniques are combined into the ecosystemic integrative approach (O'Connor, 1997). These multiple interacting systems are taken into account by the play therapist in conceptualizing the child's presenting problems and formulating the best treatment approach (O'Connor, 1997). EPT is seen as a treatment modality that can be "readily adapted to work with any child or problem because of its developmental and broad systemic approach to the conceptualization of problems" (O'Connor, 1997, p. 245). Consequently, the various components are combined, resulting in an approach and theoretical framework whose sum is far greater than its parts. The play therapist utilizing EPT can develop well-defined treatment goals and design creative interventions geared toward achieving those goals (O'Connor, 2001).

Another example is that of Paris Goodyear-Brown (2010), who has recently developed the Flexibly Sequential Play Therapy (FSPT) model of treatment for traumatized children. She initially takes a variety of treatment techniques to give the child the space to disclose and adjust his or her exposure to the sharing of the trauma content (continuum of disclosure), as well as to restore the child's lost sense of empowerment that occurs as a result of abuse (experiential mastery plan or EMP). These two intertwined processes are grounded in play and expressive mediums and woven in with skill-based work. According to Goodyear-Brown: "The FSPT model delineates specific treatment goals, delivered through a variety of specific play-based technologies and supported by an understanding of the facilitative powers of play and the therapist's use of self in the play space" (2010, p. 3). This model requires the therapist to be flexible in order to integrate directive and nondirective approaches.

In order to utilize FSPT the therapist must have a breadth of knowledge along with the finesse to utilize a variety of treatment technologies. Coping, emotional literacy, and cognitive restructuring require knowledge of cognitive-behavioral theory and therapy for children and teens. In order to soothe the traumatized child's physiology, knowledge of trauma, physiological stress responses, and theoretical components of somatic therapies and mindfulness practices are required as well. In order to work effectively with the parents, the play therapist must also have a good understanding of family systems theory and attachment theory, along with being familiar with the latest dyadic interventions, such as parent-child interaction therapy, Theraplay, child-parent psychotherapy, child-parent relationship therapy, and the Circle of Security Project (Goodyear-Brown, 2010). The therapist is not required to be an expert in every one of the models. However, a working knowledge of their approach and how to conduct dyadic interventions and psychoeducational components in working with parents is needed.

Goodyear-Brown (2010) states that FSPT relies heavily on the therapeutic and facilitative powers of play in order to deliver the developmentally sensitive treatment plan. She delineates how each of the curative factors of play facilitates the treatment process. In particular she notes that counterconditioning of negative affect and the reestablishment of the child's sense of power and control work together in lessening the toxic impact that trauma content and events have on the child. She states that "play becomes the digestive enzyme through which the child is fully able to ingest the therapeutic content that is being conveyed. Play ensures the most potent absorption of conceptual information for children" (Goodyear-Brown, 2010, p. 11).

*Common Factors* as seen in play therapy was utilized by Weir (2008) in working with an adoptive family and their child with Reactive Attachment

Disorder (RAD). The essential components of Structural Family Therapy, Theraplay, and other selected family play therapy models were utilized to target the needs of families and adoptive children with RAD. Numerous treatment approaches exist in order to deal with attachment disorders. Filial therapy (VanFleet, 1994), Theraplay (Booth and Lindaman, 2000), as well as Structural Family Therapy and the work of Daniel Hughes (1997) encourage the use of an integrative model that utilizes a play therapy–based approach within family work with adoptive children where attachment disorders are present.

The commonalities across each of these treatments are play therapy techniques that are utilized within sessions and at home with the parent and child, along with psychoeducational principles of parenting. Consequently, key components of family therapy theories and models and play therapy modalities were extrapolated and utilized to treat a family where an adopted child was diagnosed with RAD. The simplest components of each theory and techniques were utilized, rather than using any one treatment approach in its purest form (Weir, 2008). An amalgam of play, stories, drawings, puppet work, homework assignments, and techniques fostering a balance of structure, engagement, nurture, and challenge dimensions were utilized within the therapeutic context of playfulness that fostered relationship building between child and family. Homework assignments of special time allowed the family to practice what was learned in the session at home, and gave an opportunity for the parents and child to have designated unconditional play time together to further enhance positive interactions. Weir reported success in his case study using this integrated attachment–based model.

A good example of *Assimilative Integration* is seen in a case study within a school setting by Fall (2001), who utilized Integrative Play Therapy as the blending of two or more theoretical foundations into a cohesive treatment approach driven by the child's or family's needs and problems. In a prescriptive way, the child's needs and problems helped direct which theory to use and assist the play therapist in addressing academic, personal, and social issues at any particular time (Fall, 2001). Each theory came with corresponding techniques. Some play therapy research corroborates that differing play therapy interventions are useful in meeting the treatment needs of children and families (Landreth, Homeyer, Glover, & Sweeney, 1996).

Fall (2001) stressed that the integrative approach in a school counseling setting should be guided by the child's problem, a prescriptive approach (Baker, 2000). In addition, she states how the "integrative play therapy approach is both proactive and reactive, two components of a school counselor's job description" (p. 325). As a result, the core theory and approach of child-centered play therapy was blended with Adlerian and cognitive-behavioral play therapy approaches and theory. Fall found that such an integration works well in addressing the variety of problems a school counselor faces.

For example, in helping a child deal with angry feelings, the play therapist may utilize directive cognitive-behavioral techniques to address behaviors and offer alternative strategies that impact on peer interactions (reactive), while also allowing the child the opportunity to master his or her intense affect through an

Adlerian or child-centered approach, which is child-led play and nondirective. Treatment approaches may be blended within one treatment session or independently presented sequentially over a series of sessions.

Another good example of *Assimilative Integration* is Object Relations Play Therapy, which was originated and utilized by Helen Benedict (Benedict, 2006). Object relations play therapy relies primarily on child-responsive, invitational, and highly attuned therapy techniques with specific goals and techniques easily tailored prescriptively to meet each child's specific needs and interpersonal relatedness (Benedict, 2006). This treatment approach is grounded in attachment-based object relations theory, which is a collection of loosely organized models held together by three basic ideas. The first and most important is the prevailing belief that interpersonal relationships are the central driving and motivational force in human development (Benedict, 2006). This is backed by neuroscience research that has been able to show that early brain development requires attuned and interactive events that are experience dependent (Schore, 2003). The second component is that through relating to others over one's initial two to three years of life, a cognitive-affective structure develops, which is not only about the self but also about others, thus forming into object relations. These templates serve as an internal guide to understanding and responding to oneself and others in relationships (Benedict, 2006; Bowlby, 1988). The third assumption is that object relations begin to develop from infancy through the initial relationships between the infant and primary attachment figure. These object relations, which have a neurological and experiential basis, significantly influence the child's (and later adult's) interpersonal relationships, but these templates can be impacted on by ongoing relationships. As a result, the therapist–child relationship becomes the crucible whereby the child's maladaptive internal working models can be modified into a more adaptive object relationship.

The core component of object relations play therapy is the therapist and child relationship (Benedict, 2006). A lengthy part of treatment is the development of a secure-base relationship with the child, who is slow to trust, has negative internal models of self and others, and resists interpersonal connections because of past relational trauma. Therapy with these children is often difficult and time-consuming. In order to do this, the therapist is prescriptive in choosing his or her own activity level and degree of being directive in direct response to cues from the child (Benedict, 2006; Gil, 1991). It is child initiated, rather than directive or nondirective, whereby the therapist creates a safe and protected space (both emotionally and physically) and demonstrates attunement, warmth, acceptance, constancy, developmental appropriateness, and child responsiveness (Benedict, 2006). An invitational approach is taken by the therapist in watching the child's cues and being attuned before moving into any directive work, which the child can freely either accept or reject.

The goal of the therapy is to modify the child's internal working models or object relations. Thematic play becomes pivotal in the healing of traumatic experiences and in turn challenging the child's object relations (Benedict, 2006).

*Play, especially thematic play, is an important avenue to correcting distorted cognitive understandings and resolving both affective reactions and traumatic memories. . . . Thematic play is where the child imagines roles, relationships, and events and enacts these through playful use of objects, role play, and actions . . . . Thematic play serves as a communicative medium to convey their concerns, feelings and ideas. . . . It is often the therapist's understanding of and response to the child's play that facilitates therapeutic change. (Benedict, 2006, pp. 7–8)*

## Therapeutic Powers of Play Underlying the Model

As noted previously, the Common Factors aspects of integrative psychotherapy were assessed by Grencavage and Norcross (1990). In their review they found that almost half of the proposed commonalities had to do specifically with change processes over client characteristics. Consensus across categories were in the development of a therapeutic alliance, opportunity for catharsis, acquisition and practice of new behaviors, and the clients' positive expectancies (Grencavage & Norcross, 1990).

Looking at the variety of integrative approaches in play therapy, the curative powers of play become the change mechanism within play that can help child and adolescent clients overcome psychosocial, behavioral, and emotional difficulties (Drewes, 2009). Consequently, the integrative and prescriptive approach pulls for the play therapist to become skilled in numerous therapeutic powers and differentially apply them to meet the client's individual needs. "This approach is based on the individualized, differential, and focused matching of curative powers to the specific causative forces underlying the client's problem" (Drewes, 2009, p. 1).

Depending on which theoretical frameworks are utilized within the integrative approach, the therapeutic powers of play underlying the models can vary. Aside from those noted previously (using Schaefer's [1999] terms: catharsis, rapport building, behavioral rehearsal, and sense of self), any number of the following factors may also be seen as change agents: self-expression, access to the unconscious, direct/indirect teaching, abreaction, stress inoculation, counterconditioning of negative affect, positive affect, sublimation, attachment and relationship enhancement, moral judgment, empathy, power/control, competence and self-control, accelerated development, creative problem solving, fantasy compensation, and reality testing (Schaefer & Drewes, 2009).

Further research is needed to illuminate which specific therapeutic powers of play are most effective with specific presenting problems and within the blending of different models and treatment approaches. It will be most important for play therapists to understand what "invisible powerful forces resulting from the therapist-client play interactions are successful in helping the client overcome and heal psychosocial difficulties" (Schaefer & Drewes, 2009, pp. 4–5). The greater our understanding of these curative factors and change mechanisms, the more effective the play therapist is in being able to apply them to meet the particular needs of their clients (Schaefer, 1999).

## Role of the Therapist/Role of the Parent

Because each treatment model can vary, the role of the play therapist will vary accordingly. There will be times when the play therapist will need to be non-directive, or child-initiated, allowing the child or adolescent to lead. Other times the therapist will need to take a much more directive and involved stance, offering parent training or introducing treatment components and tasks. Such shifts in approach may happen within the same session or might occur sequentially over the treatment. Consequently, the play therapist needs to be flexible both in thinking and in treatment approach.

The same can be said of the role of the parent. This can vary depending on which theories and style of treatment are utilized. Some integrative play therapy approaches (e.g., filial therapy or child-parent relationship therapy) require the parent to observe the therapist conducting the sessions with their child, thereby learning and rehearsing approaches before actually working with their child together in a dyad. Other approaches may not include the parent in the session at all, until the end, when the child teaches the parent what he or she learned, allowing for solidifying and the generalizing of skill development. Other approaches may work exclusively with the client and only have contact with the parent to obtain information regarding treatment progress and systemic changes.

## Clinical Applications

The integrative play therapy model can be utilized across all disorders and developmental levels. Because it pulls together various theories, along with treatment approaches, the best fit can occur. By its nature, integrative play therapy is also a prescriptive approach in that it seeks out the best treatment for this child's presenting problems at this time and is flexible within and across sessions in achieving the treatment plan. As a result, an integrative play therapy model allows for a broad application in its use over single, fixed theoretical and treatment approaches.

## Case Example

The following is a case example that fits Assimilative Integration, in that several theoretical approaches were utilized, along with a variety of related techniques.

KL was an 8-year-old boy in foster care who presented with behavioral difficulties in school caused by mood dysregulation and struggles with issues related to his father's death, three years before, along with his mother's current wish to surrender parental rights so he could be adopted because she had a reemergence of cancer. Treatment goals were to work on helping KL utilize

(1) child-led play therapy to help build rapport and a therapeutic alliance, along with offering control in selection of materials and tasks and a release from traumatic and stressful material; (2) directive CBT techniques to manage and reduce his strong emotional affect (anger, depression), become aware of the emotional triggers, and develop alternative coping skills; and 3) bereavement work to focus on helping KL deal with unresolved grief and loss of his father and pending loss of his mother. Parent-child dyadic therapy was also utilized to help KL and his mother talk about the past events of his father's death and to better understand his mother's wishes to have him adopted. In addition, this author maintained contact with KL's school setting and foster home parents for information regarding progress and systemic issues.

The various theoretical frameworks used and concomitant techniques included psychodynamic play therapy, sandtray therapy, cognitive-behavioral play therapy, family therapy, and systems theory. KL was seen in individual weekly play therapy sessions over the course of two years for 75 sessions. Our 45-minute sessions were structured and divided into components that allowed for the integrative use of several treatment approaches. Before having KL enter the therapy room, I would meet for 5 to 10 minutes with the foster parent(s) regarding how KL was doing in their home, at school, and on visits with his mother. Then after the foster parent(s) left, KL came into the session. The first 10 to 15 minutes was a check-in period, which facilitated time to talk about how his week was, relaying any information I received from his foster parents that needed to be shared, follow-up on any homework assignments he might have had, and allowed us to work on specific directive techniques. The next 25 to 30 minutes was child-led, which allowed KL to select what he wished to play with and how, and what emotional material he wished to convey. The last 5 to 10 minutes were for cleanup and a closing ritual of using bubbles or deep breathing for affect regulation and transitioning from the session.

In the initial session, I shared with KL what I knew of his history and why he was seeing me, as well as what our time together would be like. Using a balloon to blow in all of his angry and upset feelings, KL was helped to see how the big balloon was like his head and heart, containing so many upset feelings that he felt like he would pop. By letting out some of the air at a time and seeing how much smaller the balloon was getting, KL better understood that this was like our time together in letting out his angry feelings in a safe, slow way with my help. We then looked at what difficulties he felt he needed to work on, and we created a treatment plan together. Using strips of paper to write on, we worked together on selecting three issues/problems each about home, school, and his family for a total of nine items we would work on in therapy. We left one paper blank, which would allow him to spontaneously address something not covered. KL wrote on each strip the goal we selected and decorated an envelope in which the paper strips were placed. Each session when he entered the room, the envelope would be put out and he would get to pick one of the pieces of paper for us to focus on. He could put back the paper and select a different one, only once, before we had to work on it. Then after we talked about the issue or used a directive technique, he would rip off a small piece of the paper and put it back. This way he saw that we were making progress on the goal, but we were still not finished with it.

In this first session, KL then used his child-led, nondirective time to create a sandtray, showing me what his world was like. During other sessions, KL often used the play therapy toys, art materials, and clay to express feelings, but he often preferred to use the sandtray when he was facing deep issues around the death of his father and worries about his mother.

Over the first four sessions I was able to obtain a good sense of KL's developmental level and emotional issues, as well as build rapport and facilitate the creation of a therapeutic relationship. Over the course of treatment, KL began to delve more deeply into his feelings and memories regarding his father's death when he was only 4½ years old. There were missing details to the narrative of his father's death, as well as information lacking as to what happens when someone dies, and even where his father was buried. At this point, once a month, his mother joined KL for dyadic family therapy. His mother was able to discuss with him where his father was buried and details surrounding his illness and death. The foster parents were willing to take KL to the grave, where he was able to leave a letter to his father (that we worked on in sessions) telling him his feelings and that he missed him.

Monthly sessions with KL's mother continued and allowed for discussion about why she wanted him adopted, how she had only one relative available who was not mentally stable, and she wanted to know he was in a good adoptive home. This was her second bout with cancer, and his mother was unsure whether even if she went into remission again that she would not ultimately die from cancer in the near future, leaving KL an orphan with no place to go. His mother also was able to share the unknown fact that she had been in foster care as a child and adopted as well. This was a good experience for her, and she wanted to have KL in a loving home. We were able to work out an open adoption in New York, which allowed for KL and his mother to maintain contact around birthdays and holidays with the consent of the adoptive family.

Through the healing powers of play and the integrative treatment approach, KL learned and applied better coping strategies, gained access to his unconscious issues around his father's death that were previously un-explored, allowed for catharsis in getting out his anger and rage over feeling abandoned, helped him gain power and control, along with competence, self-control, and a greater sense of himself, and through CBT techniques applied creative problem solving, behavioral rehearsal, and counterconditioning of negative affect.

By the end of treatment, an adoptive family was found, and we were able to work toward his successful adoption. He still remains with his adoptive family and has periodic contact with his biological mother. His acting-out behaviors in school significantly diminished, and he is better able to manage his sadness and anger.

## Challenges in Implementing the Model

Although integration is gaining hold in psychotherapy, there are obstacles to its growth in the treatment arena. The most severe obstacle comes from territoriality of the purists, who hold their single-theory views as being the best. As a result, there is inadequate training in eclectic/integrative therapy in university settings (Norcross, 2005). Graduate students may occasionally be taught to look at treatment through the lens of one or two different theoretical frameworks. Therefore, students graduating will call themselves eclectic, but what they are really saying is that they have been taught two different approaches (usually cognitive-behavioral and Rogerian). Consequently, they are not fluid in thinking between the two theories and approaches, and they do not feel well grounded in either approach, resulting in an inability to truly integrate them. Thus the push toward a truly integrative treatment approach is lacking.

In the field of play therapy, there is limited coursework, articles, books, and workshops available to help play therapists in becoming more flexible and integrative. There are still some purists who feel being well grounded in one treatment approach and theoretical framework is satisfactory for the treatment of most clients. However, in recent years there has been a surge in interest, books, and training in blending play therapy with cognitive-behavioral therapy, which has helped move play therapists toward a more integrative direction.

Finally, the lack of a common language and contradictory assumptions about personality development, human nature, and the origins of psychopathology (Messer, 1992) add further roadblocks to its progress (Norcross, 2005). Despite the hurdles, in recent years empirical outcome literature in mainstream psychotherapy has grown considerably (Schottenbauer, Glass, & Arnkoff, 2005). However, little research is being conducted by play therapists specifically looking at the benefits of an integrative treatment approach. It is now time for play therapists to also add to the body of research in studying the effectiveness of integrative treatment approaches. More process research is needed in order to identify which mediators or therapeutic factors produce the desired change in the client's behaviors and presenting problems. Research needs to address which specific change agents in play can be combined to optimize treatment effectiveness (Schaefer & Drewes, 2009). Such knowledge would not only allow the therapist to be able to borrow flexibly from available theoretical positions to tailor treatment to a particular child based on a treatment plan, but also will result in the most cost-effective play interventions.

## Conclusion

Integrative play therapy is a relatively newly developing approach to working with children and adolescents. It offers promise in its flexible use of integrating theory and techniques in order to offer clients the best treatment for their presenting problems. Much work is needed in creating training within university settings on this approach, as well as within the play therapy field through workshops, conference presentations, and publications to help play therapists become flexible in their thinking and approach.

# References

Axline, V. (1947). *Play therapy*. Boston, MA: Houghton Mifflin.

Baker, S. (2000). *School counseling for the twenty-first century* (3rd ed.). Upper Saddle River, NJ: Merrill.

Benedict, H. (2006). Object relations play therapy. Applications to attachment problems and relational trauma. In C. E. Schaefer & H. G. Kaduson, *Contemporary play therapy: Theory, research, and practice* (pp. 3–27). New York, NY: Guilford Press.

Booth, P. B., & Lindaman, S. (2000). Theraplay for enhancing attachment in adopted children. In C. E. Schaefer & H. G. Kaduson (Eds.), *Short-term play therapy for children* (pp. 194–227). New York, NY: Guilford Press.

Bowlby, J. (1988). *A secure-base: Parent-child attachment and healthy human development*. New York, NY: Basic Books.

Cohen, J. A., Deblinger, E., Mannarino, A. P., & Steer, R. A. (2004). A multi-site, randomized controlled trial for sexually abused children with PTSD symptoms. *Journal of the American Academy of Child and Adolescent Psychiatry, 43*, 393–402.

Coonerty, S. (1993). Integrative child therapy. In G. Stricker and J. Gold (Eds.), *Comprehensive handbook of psychotherapy integration* (pp. 413–426). New York, NY: Plenum Press.

Dawson, G., & Castelloe, P. (1992). Autism. In C. E. Walker & M. Roberts (Eds.), *Handbook of clinical child psychology* (2nd ed., pp. 375–398). New York, NY: John Wiley & Sons.

Drewes, A. A. (2009). Rationale for integrating play therapy and CBT. In A. A. Drewes (Ed.), *Blending play therapy with cognitive behavioral therapy: Evidence-based and other effective treatments and techniques* (pp. 1–2). Hoboken, NJ: Wiley.

Fall, M. (2001). An integrative play therapy approach to working with children. In A. A. Drewes, L. J. Carey, & C. E. Schaefer (Eds.), *School-based play therapy* (pp. 315–328). Hoboken, NJ: Wiley.

Freud, A. (1928). *Introduction to the technique of child analysis*. (L. P. Clark, Trans.). New York, NY: Nervous and Mental Disease Publishing.

Gil, E. (1991). *The healing power of play*. New York, NY: Guilford Press.

Gil, E. (2006). *Helping abused and traumatized children. Integrating directive and nondirective approaches*. New York, NY: Guilford Press.

Glasser, W. (1975). *Reality therapy*. New York, NY: Harper & Row.

Goodyear-Brown, P. (2010). *Play therapy with traumatized children. A prescriptive approach*. Hoboken, NJ: Wiley.

Grencavage, L. M., & Norcross, J. C. (1990). Where are the commonalities among the therapeutic common factors? *Professional Psychology: Research and Practice, 21*(5), 372–378.

Hughes, D. (1997). *Facilitating developmental attachment: The road to emotional recovery and behavioral change in foster and adopted children*. Northvale, NJ: Jason Aronson.

Jensen, J. P., Bergin, A. E., & Greaves, D. W. (1990). The meaning of eclecticism: New survey and analysis of components. *Professional Psychology: Research and Practice, 21*(2), 124–130.

Jernberg, A. (1979). *Theraplay*. San Francisco, CA: Jossey-Bass.

Jernberg, A., & Booth, P. (1999). *Theraplay: Helping parents and children build better relationships through attachment based play* (2nd ed.). San Francisco, CA: Jossey-Bass.

Kenny, M. C., & Winick, C. B. (2000). An integrative approach to play therapy with an autistic girl. *International Journal of Play Therapy, 9*(1), 11–33.

Klein, M. (1932). *The psycho-analysis of children*. London, England: Hogarth Press.

Knell, S. (1993). *Cognitive behavioral play therapy*. Northvale, NJ: Jason Aronson.

Landreth, G. (1991). *Play therapy: The art of the relationship*. Muncie, IN: Accelerated Development.

Landreth, G., Homeyer, L., Glover, G., & Sweeney, D. (1996). *Play therapy interventions with children's problems*. Northvale, NJ: Jason Aronson.

Messer, S. B. (1992). A critical examination of belief structures in integrative and eclectic psychotherapy. In J. C. Norcross & M. R. Goldfried (Eds.), *Handbook of psychotherapy integration* (pp. 130–168). New York, NY: Oxford University Press.

Norcross, J. C. (1987). *Casebook of eclectic psychotherapy*. New York, NY: Brunner/Mazel.

Norcross, J. C. (2005). A primer on psychotherapy integration. In J. C. Norcross & M. R. Goldfried (Eds.), *Handbook of psychotherapy integration* (2nd ed., pp. 10–23).

Norcross, J. C., Hedges, M., & Castle, P. H. (2002). Psychologists conducting psychotherapy in 2001: A study of the Division 29 membership. *Psychotherapy, 39,* 97–102.

O'Connor, K. (2001). Ecosystemic play therapy. *International Journal of Play Therapy, 10*(2), 33–44.

O'Connor, K. (1997). Ecosystemic play therapy. In K. O'Connor & M. K. Braverman (Eds.), *Play therapy theory and practice: A comparative presentation* (pp. 234–284). New York, NY: Wiley & Sons.

Phillips, R. D., & Landreth, G. (1995). Play therapists on play therapy: A report of methods, demographics, and professional/practice issues. *International Journal of Play Therapy, 4,* 1–26.

Phillips, R. D., & Landreth, G. (1998). Play therapists on play therapy: II. Clinical issues in play therapy. *International Journal of Play Therapy, 7*(1), 1–20.

Schaefer, C. E. (1999). Curative factors in play therapy. *The Journal for the Professional Counselor, 14*(1), 7–16.

Schaefer, C. E. (2003). Prescriptive play therapy. In C. E. Schaefer (Ed.), *Foundations of play therapy* (pp. 306–320). Hoboken, NJ: Wiley.

Schaefer, C. E., & Drewes, A. A. (2009). The therapeutic powers of play. In A. A. Drewes (Ed.), *Blending play therapy with cognitive behavioral therapy: Evidence-based and other effective treatments and techniques* (pp. 3–15). Hoboken, NJ: Wiley.

Schore, A. N. (2003). Early relational trauma, disorganized attachment, and the development of a predisposition to violence. In M. F. Solomon & D. J. Siegel (Eds.), *Healing trauma: Attachment, mind, body, and brain* (pp. 107–167). New York, NY: Norton.

Schottenbauer, M. A., Glass, C. R., & Arnkoff, D. B. (2005). Outcome research on psychotherapy integration. In J. C. Norcross & M. R. Goldfried (Eds.), *Handbook of psychotherapy integration* (pp. 459–493). New York, NY: Oxford University Press.

Shirk, S. (1999). Integrated child psychotherapy: Treatment ingredients in search of a recipe. In S. Russ & T. Ollendick (Eds.), *Handbook of psychotherapies with children and families* (pp. 369–384). New York, NY: Kluwer Academic/Plenum.

Smith, M. L., Glass, G. V., & Miller, T. I. (1980). *The benefits of psychotherapy*. Baltimore, MD: Johns Hopkins University Press.

Stien, P. T., & Kendall, J. (2004). *Psychological trauma and the developing brain: Neurologically based interventions for troubled children*. New York, NY: Haworth Press.

van der Kolk, B. A. (2005). Developmental trauma disorder: Towards a rational diagnosis for children with complex trauma histories. *Psychiatric Annals, 35*(5), 401–408.

VanFleet, R. (1994). Filial therapy for adoptive children and parents. In K. J. O'Connor & C. E. Schaefer (Eds.), *Handbook of play therapy, Volume 2: Advances and innovations*. New York, NY: Wiley & Sons.

Weir, K. N. (2008). Using integrative play therapy with adoptive families to treat Reactive Attachment Disorder: A case study. *Journal of Family Psychotherapy, 18*(4), 1–16.

# Integrative Play Therapies for Externalizing Disorders of Childhood

# Parent-Child Interaction Therapy for Oppositional Behavior in Children

## Integration of Child-Directed Play Therapy and Behavior Management Training for Parents

*Amanda H. Costello, Karishma Chengappa, Jocelyn O. Stokes, Ashley B. Tempel, and Cheryl B. McNeil*

## Introduction

Parent-Child Interaction Therapy (PCIT) is an integration of play therapy and operant behavioral therapy approaches for managing disruptive behavior problems in preschool and early school-aged children (Eyberg, 1988; McNeil & Hembree-Kigin, 2010). It utilizes key components from both theoretical approaches throughout treatment; these approaches have shown effectiveness in managing child problem behavior (Graziano, 1983; Ryan & Courtney, 2009). As disruptive behavior early in childhood may result in academic, social, and emotional difficulties (Campbell, 1995; Webster-Stratton, 1990), PCIT acts as an early intervention program to help parents learn skills to strengthen their relationship with their child and to learn appropriate ways to manage their child's disruptive behavior. Therapy sessions are structured as a positive and supportive environment, and parents who have received PCIT have reported high levels of treatment satisfaction (Eyberg et al. 2001; Matos, Bauermeister, & Bernal, 2009; Niec, Hemme, Yopp, & Brestan, 2005).

PCIT has been applied primarily to the treatment of externalizing behavior problems associated with oppositional-defiant disorder (Eyberg & Robinson, 1982; Hood & Eyberg, 2003; Schuhmann, Foote, Eyberg, Boggs, & Algina, 1998), conduct disorder (Eyberg & Boggs, 1998), and attention-deficit/hyperactivity disorder (Matos et al., 2009; Wagner & McNeil, 2008). Research supports its efficacy with this population, and PCIT is considered to be a "probably efficacious" treatment of disruptive behavior in children ages 3 through 6 years old (Eyberg, Nelson, & Boggs, 2008). It was designated as a "probably efficacious" treatment by including empirical support from two rigorous research studies showing reduction in disruptive behavior problems as compared to a wait list control. Empirical support from the replication of research studies in independent sites was another important criterion for a "probably efficacious" study (see Silverman & Hinshaw, 2008, for complete criteria of a "probably efficacious" study).

In addition to childhood externalizing behavior problems, PCIT has been applied to parents and children who experience child abuse and neglect (Chaffin et al., 2004; Herschell, Calzada, Eyberg, & McNeil, 2002), intimate partner violence (Borrego, Gutow, Reicher, & Barker, 2008), children who experience separation anxiety disorder (Choate, Pincus, Eyberg, & Barlow, 2005), and children on the autism spectrum (Masse, 2010; Masse, McNeil, Wagner, & Chorney, 2008; Masse, McNeil, & Wagner, 2009; Solomon, Ono, Timmer, & Goodlin-Jones, 2008).

## Rationale for the Integrative Approach

The structure of PCIT was originally modeled after a two-stage treatment developed by Constance Hanf (1969) using operant behavioral principles in the management of disruptive behavior problems in children (Eyberg, 1988). Hanf taught parents the proper use of reinforcement and punishment (Eyberg, 1988). More specifically, parents were taught skills such as consistent discipline, attending to appropriate behavior, and ignoring inappropriate behavior (Eyberg, 1988). Sessions were structured so that the parent and child worked together throughout treatment (Eyberg, 1988). Immediate feedback was provided to parents in-session by the therapist through a listening device (i.e., bug-the-ear device) behind a one-way mirror (Eyberg, 1998; Herschell & McNeil, 2007).

PCIT was also structured as a two-stage model, including a child-directed stage (where the child leads the session) and a parent-directed stage (where the parent leads the session). PCIT differs from Hanf's model in that treatment includes both operant behavioral and play therapy principles (Eyberg, 1988). This was done to target the major goals of strengthening the parent-child relationship and managing disruptive child behavior.

Empirical support has demonstrated the effectiveness of the two-stage structure of PCIT. Eisenstadt and colleagues (1993) showed that including the parent-directed phase in treatment (i.e., teaching parents to manage disruptive behavior) was just as important as including the child-directed phase (i.e., strengthening the parent-child relationship). Mothers attending the parent-directed phase before the child-directed phase were more likely to report less child behavior problems, while therapists observed greater child compliance (Eisenstadt, Eyberg, McNeil, Newcomb, & Funderburk, 1993). These mothers also reported greater treatment satisfaction (Eisenstadt et al., 1993). Support for the inclusion of both phases in PCIT demonstrates the need not only to strengthen the parent-child relationship but also to teach parents appropriate limit-setting strategies.

PCIT therapists teach and coach parents in relationship strengthening and behavior management through the use of observation and coaching. Like Hanf's model, PCIT therapists also observe and coach parents through the bug-in-the-ear device as a way of gathering objective data on parental skills to provide immediate feedback (Herschell et al., 2002). Coaching is an integral part of PCIT because it helps to quickly correct any parental skill deficits or mistakes, and it can be individually tailored to parents based on their treatment progress (Herschell et al., 2002). Additionally, parental skill is coded during each session using a structured and standardized coding system called the Dyadic Parent-Child Interaction Coding System, Third Edition (DPICS-III; Eyberg, McDiarmid Nelson, Duke, & Boggs, 2005). The collected session data are used to develop specific treatment goals for the therapy hour. Throughout treatment, parents are provided with information on their progress toward mastery of the PCIT skills. By including individualized feedback for parents in treatment, PCIT becomes an idiographic treatment for each attending family (Bahl, Spaulding, & McNeil, 1999).

## Child-Directed Interaction

The first phase of PCIT, Child-Directed Interaction (CDI), is conducted to strengthen the parent-child relationship and make the relationship rewarding to both the parent and child (Eyberg & Robinson, 1982; Hembree-Kigin & McNeil, 1995; McNeil, Capage, Bahl, & Blanc, 1999). Early work by Sheila Eyberg, the developer of PCIT, demonstrated that strengthening the parent-child relationship was important, because many young children referred to the clinic for disruptive behavior disorders were engaging in negative interactions with their parents (Eyberg, 2004).

These negative interactions can be effectively described by Gerald Patterson's (1976) *coercion hypothesis*, based on social learning theory. According to Patterson's hypothesis, as a child is continually noncompliant with a presented demand, the parent may eventually remove the demand, thus providing negative reinforcement for the child's defiant behavior (Patterson, 1976, 1982). In this cycle, parents may develop punitive or aversive disciplinary practices in order to achieve child compliance. If the child eventually complies, then the parent's aggressive tactics become negatively reinforced (e.g., the parent escapes undesirable child behavior by increasing aversive disciplinary practices) (Urquiza & McNeil, 1996). As the negative behavior of both individuals is continuously negatively reinforced, the cycle continues, and the parent and child develop a coercive interaction pattern (Urquiza & McNeil, 1996).

To decrease the coercive interaction pattern with oppositional children, PCIT values an authoritative parenting style as described by Baumrind (1966). In this approach, parents learn to set and enforce rules, but they pair the ability to set limits with the parenting practices of providing nurturance, support, and a sense of autonomy to children. PCIT therapists teach and coach parents to use a specific combination of play therapy and behavioral skills. Play therapy skills are based primarily on Virginia Axline's play therapy principles (1947). A main goal of play therapy is to create a strong, positive therapeutic relationship that fosters a sense of safety in the child by letting the child take the lead in session to be the primary problem solver (Axline, 1947; Kranz & Lund, 1993). In play therapy, by letting the child lead the session, the therapist is able to observe and reflect on the child's behaviors (Axline, 1947; Kranz & Lund, 1993; Ryan & Courtney, 2009).

PCIT utilizes the play therapy setting as an environment in which the parent and child can form a strong bond early in treatment (Eyberg, 2004). During this phase, parents are instructed to be nondirective and let the child lead the session (Eyberg & Robinson, 1982), so they can observe and comment on the child's behavior. In CDI sessions, parents are taught to use play therapy skills behaviorally with their children to increase appropriate behavior. Parents are taught to *positively reinforce* (e.g., add something to increase behavior) desired child behavior through the use of praise, reflecting the child's verbalizations, using imitation, describing the child's behaviors, and using enthusiasm (Eyberg & Robinson, 1982; McNeil et al., 1999).

Parents are also taught operant behavioral principles to decrease the child's inappropriate behavior. PCIT therapists teach and coach parents to *negatively punish* (e.g., remove something to decrease behavior) child behavior that is maladaptive but not harmful (e.g., whining, playing rough with the toys) through *removal of attention* (e.g., not providing any attention to the child's inappropriate behavior; see Martin & Pear, 2007, for a more detailed description of behavioral terms). When a child engages in negative attention-seeking behavior, parents are taught to briefly remove verbal and physical attention (usually lasts 2 to 30 seconds) until the child engages in a neutral or positive behavior for just a few seconds. Then, the parent returns the attention, providing enthusiastic positive responses to the child's appropriate behaviors.

To maintain a positive parent-child relationship, parents are taught and coached to avoid using verbalizations that may be harmful to the relationship. Parents are instructed to avoid using critical comments, as these may reduce the quality of the interaction and may induce frustration or anger within the child (Eyberg, 1988). Commanding the child is avoided as it may take away the child's lead from the play and may result in oppositional behavior or child frustration (Eyberg, 1988). Asking the child questions is also taught to be avoided because, along with commands, these may take away the child's lead from the session (Eyberg & Robinson, 1982). This practice also teaches parents to only use questions when necessary, which may increase the likelihood that the child responds appropriately to future commands or questions. The strengthened parent-child relationship built in CDI is an important foundation for effectively changing child behavior throughout the continuation of treatment (Eyberg, 1988). Table 3.1 gives examples of the skills taught during CDI.

Another important aspect of CDI is that parents are instructed to schedule 5 minutes of special playtime each day to spend with their child

Table 3.1  **Skills Taught to Parents During Child-Directed Interaction (CDI)**

|  | Description | Example |
|---|---|---|
| **Behaviors to Increase** | | |
| Labeled Praise | Praise child for the exact behavior he/she is doing. | Parent says: "I love the way you are cleaning up all of the blocks!" |
| Reflections | Repeat child's verbalizations. | Child says: "The cow goes Moo"; Parent says "The cow does go Moo." |
| Behavioral Descriptions | Describe the behavior the child is engaging in. | Parent says: "Now you are stacking the red block on top of the blue block." |
| Enthusiasm | Show excitement for the child's behaviors. | Parent uses varying vocal tones and inflections. |
| Imitation | Mimic the child's behaviors. | Child is drawing a flower, so the parent draws a flower. |
| **Behaviors to Decrease** | | |
| Criticisms | Negatively commenting on child's behavior | Parent says: "This picture would be better if you wouldn't color outside of the lines." |
| Questions | Asking child about his/her behavior or for a favor | Parent says: "What do you want to play with?" |
| Commands | Telling the child to engage in certain behaviors | Parent says: "Put the cars and trucks into the bin." |

*Note.* For more information, reference PCIT treatment manual (Eyberg, 1999); DPICS training manual (Eyberg et al., 2004); *Parent-Child Interaction Therapy*, 1st and 2nd editions (Hembree-Kigin & McNeil, 1995; McNeil & Hembree-Kigin, 2010).

(McNeil et al., 1999). During this time, parents are instructed to practice using CDI skills (e.g., praise, reflections, imitation, descriptions, and enthusiasm) and refrain from negative verbalizations (e.g., criticisms, commands, questions). Special playtime is encouraged as a means of decreasing the amount of negative parent-child interactions and building up the child's self-esteem (McNeil & Hembree-Kigin, 2010). The incorporation of special playtime into PCIT was influenced by the work of Bernard Guerney (1964), who emphasized expanding play therapy principles to the home.

## Parent-Directed Interaction

The second phase of PCIT, Parent-Directed Interaction (PDI), is used to teach parents consistent limit-setting and the application of direct consequences to shape child compliance and listening skills (Eyberg & Boggs, 1998; Hembree-Kigin & McNeil, 1995; McNeil et al., 1999). This phase continues to incorporate play therapy principles from CDI (e.g., reflection, behavioral descriptions) and maintains the play therapy setting. In PDI, however, PCIT therapists also teach and coach parents in operant behavioral skills to form a contingency management program to decrease inappropriate behavior and increase low-occurring, alternative appropriate behavior (McNeil, Eyberg, Eisenstadt, Newcomb, & Funderburk, 1991). PDI is important because many children with disruptive behavior problems engage in oppositional behavior at an extremely high rate (e.g., disobeying 80% of parental commands) while also displaying aggressive and destructive behaviors when the parent attempts to provide supervision (Brestan, Eyberg, Boggs, & Algina, 1997).

In PDI, parents are coached to continue with brief removal of attention for disruptive, nonharmful behaviors (Eyberg, 1988; Eyberg & Robinson, 1982). Child compliance and listening skills are learned through teaching parents to use appropriate commands (Eyberg & Boggs, 1998). Child compliance is further shaped by first practicing listening with play commands and moving toward more challenging instructions that involve real-life situations. Parents reinforce each incidence of child compliance with positive attention, particularly labeled praise for listening. In addition to rewarding child compliance, parents are taught to provide a negative consequence for child noncompliance. The use of time-out in a chair is taught to parents as a safe way to decrease noncompliant and harmful child behavior (Eyberg & Boggs, 1998). The typical length of the time-out procedure is 3 minutes, but longer time-outs sometimes are needed as termination of time-out is contingent on the child's compliance with the presented demand. In that way, time-out cannot be used to escape demands. The procedure always ends with child compliance (Eyberg & Boggs, 1998), thereby increasing the probability of the child complying with future parental requests.

The time-out procedure is structured, done in a safe setting, and clearly explained to the child and parent. This is done to ensure the best chance for child compliance and success. In this procedure, the child is able to clearly and predictably learn the direct consequences of noncompliance and is offered a choice at each step to comply with the command and receive reinforcement (Eyberg, 1988). Parents are continuously supported by PCIT therapists during the time-out procedure, and child compliance to subsequent commands is followed by positive attention (e.g., labeled praise, following the child's play) to increase the probability of this behavior occurring in the future (Eyberg & Boggs, 1998). The procedure is practiced multiple times across sessions in PDI as a way for the child to incorporate the new rules and overpractice compliance until it becomes a routine response to parental directions (McNeil & Hembree-Kigin, 2010).

## Research Findings

Although there is extensive empirical support for PCIT, this chapter highlights a few foundational studies as an illustration. Additional research studies are available through the PCIT website (www.pcit.org), which adds further support to treatment outcomes. The studies highlighted have demonstrated positive treatment outcomes in parent-child relationships and behavior management with children with disruptive behavior problems as parents learn and practice play therapy and behavioral skills in CDI and PDI.

In an early treatment outcome study (Eyberg & Robinson, 1982), PCIT was shown to significantly improve the behavior of the target child. Therapist observation of parent behaviors revealed that (a) mothers used significantly more praise during PDI than they had at pretreatment; (b) mothers and fathers used significantly more praise during CDI; (c) mothers and fathers used significantly more direct commands than at pretreatment; and (d) target children were significantly more compliant. Additionally, use of all prosocial skills (e.g., labeled praise, reflection, imitation, behavioral description, and enthusiasm) was significantly higher, and use of potentially negative skills (e.g., commands, questions, criticisms) was significantly lower at post-treatment. Also, mothers showed general improvement in functioning, such as less anxiety and greater involvement with others.

Schuhmann and colleagues (1998) examined the efficacy of PCIT with preschool-aged children with Oppositional Defiant Disorder (ODD) compared to a wait list control group. Parents were given the DSM-III-R Structured Interview for Disruptive Behavior Disorders (McNeil et al., 1991), the Eyberg Child Behavior Inventory (ECBI; Eyberg & Pincus, 1999), and the Parenting Stress Index (PSI; Abidin, 1995). Additionally, parent-child interactions were coded using the DPICS-II. At post-treatment, scores on the ECBI and PSI for the PCIT group were no longer in the clinical range, whereas scores remained relatively constant for the control group. Specifically, parents felt more confident in their ability to handle their child's behavior problems and felt less distress in their relationship with their child. Children in the PCIT group no longer met criteria for ODD. Mothers and fathers in the immediate treatment group used significantly more praise and less criticism. Despite some limitations (e.g., higher IQ of parents in PCIT group; lower treatment attrition in PCIT group), this study provided further support for the efficacy of PCIT in the treatment of externalizing behavior problems associated with ODD compared to a wait list control.

Given its strong emphasis on building the parent-child relationship and teaching parents appropriate behavior management strategies, PCIT has demonstrated empirical support for parent skill generalization to untreated siblings (Brestan et al., 1997). In this study, parent-report of child behavior was collected for both the target child and the sibling. Following treatment, parents reported that the sibling's behavior was less problematic and easier to manage. The frequency of sibling behavior problems did not decrease significantly; however, the majority of siblings did not have clinically significant frequency of behavior problems.

PCIT has also demonstrated generalization of skills to other settings, a key component of behavioral therapy. McNeil and colleagues (1991) assessed the classroom behavior of children between the ages of 2 and 7 who presented with disruptive behavior in both the home and at school. Classroom behavior was assessed at pretreatment and post-treatment. Teacher-report of child behavior was collected, and the child behaviors of appropriate vs. oppositional behavior, compliance vs. noncompliance, and on-task vs. off-task were coded during a classroom observation. All measures of oppositional behavior revealed significant reductions and improvement to within normal limits for the children in the intervention group. This study supports the generalization of treatment gains to the school setting in the area of oppositional behavior. Additionally, at follow-up assessments conducted 12 months and 18 months post-treatment, treatment gains in compliance were maintained, but most other behaviors had declined to pretreatment levels (Funderburk et al., 1998).

Finally, as PCIT therapists continuously coach parents to overpractice skills learned in CDI and PDI, treatment outcomes have been shown to maintain from three to six years post-treatment completion (Hood and Eyberg, 2003). Results indicated that child behavior problems at follow-up were significantly less frequent and problematic than at pretreatment, as measured by the ECBI. Additionally, examination of clinical significance of behavior change showed that three-quarters of children who had made clinically significant improvement at post-treatment maintained this improvement at follow-up. Table 3.2 describes empirical evidence of the effectiveness of PCIT with oppositional children.

## Practical Implementation of the Integrative Approach

### Assessment

PCIT therapists engage in a pretreatment intake session to learn the developmental, social, medical, and psychological history of the parent and child, while also using this time to begin rapport building with each person (Eyberg, 1999). As PCIT is a data-driven approach, therapists also use multiple assessment measures to assess parent-child interactions and child behavior across multiple contexts (Herschell & McNeil, 2007). Key assessment measures used in treatment are described as follows.

*Dyadic Parent-Child Interaction Coding System, Third Edition* (DPICS-III; Eyberg et al., 2005). The DPICS-III is a behavioral coding system designed to assess the quality of parent-child interactions. Each parent and child dyad is observed interacting and is coded in three separate analog settings: Child-Directed Interaction (CDI), Parent-Directed Interaction (PDI), and Child Cleanup (without parental assistance; CU). Parents and children are coded in each of the three situations for a period of 5 minutes. Examples of coded parent behaviors include labeled praise, unlabeled praise, negative talk, questions, commands, behavioral descriptions, and reflections. In addition to parent behavior, children's compliance with parental commands is coded in these situations and can be compared to norms.

*Eyberg Child Behavior Inventory* (ECBI; Eyberg & Pincus, 1999). The ECBI is a self-report measure completed by parents to identify externalizing behavior problems and the need for treatment in preschool and school-aged children. To identify clinically significant symptoms, therapists use a *t*-score of 60 on the ECBI scales (e.g., whether or not a behavior is a problem; the intensity of the problem) as a cutoff for disruptive behavior problems.

*Sutter-Eyberg Student Behavior Inventory – Revised* (SESBI-R; Eyberg & Pincus, 1999). The SESBI-R is a brief teacher rating scale that is designed to measure

**Table 3.2** Treatment Outcomes of PCIT Used With Oppositional Children

| Investigators (Year) | Sample | Outcome Measures | Therapist | Treatment Conditions | Results |
|---|---|---|---|---|---|
| Eyberg & Robinson (1982) | seven 2- to 7-year-olds with behavior problems at home; at least one sibling age 2 to 10 | Clinician Observation: DPICS; Parent (self): MMPI (scales 2, 4, and 8) and Taylor Manifest Anxiety; Parent (on child): ECBI and Becker Bipolar Adjective Checklist | Clinical psychology interns and clinic residents | Pre/Post | Improvement in parent-reported child problem behavior, observed parental use of praise, effective commands and follow-through, child compliance, and parental attitude toward the child |
| Brestan, Eyberg, Boggs, and Algina (1997) | 30 2- to 16-year-olds untreated siblings of 3- to 6-year-old children diagnosed with ODD treated with PCIT | Parent (on child): ECBI | Graduate student therapists | Pre/Post; Between: Treatment group, wait list control group | Improvement in mother- and father-reported perceived problem and frequency of disruptive behavior of untreated siblings |
| Schuhmann, Foote, Eyberg, Boggs, & Algina (1998) | 64 3- to 6-year-old children diagnosed with ODD | Clinician Observation: DPICS; Parent (self): PSI, PLOC, DAS; Parent (on child): ECBI | Graduate student therapists | Pre/Post; Between: Immediate treatment, wait list control group | Increase in observed positive parent-child interactions and child compliance; Improvements in parent-reported child behavior at home, parent-reported internal locus of control; Reduction in parenting stress; Maintenance of treatment gains at 4-month follow-up *(continued)* |

47

Table 3.2 *(Continued)*

| Investigators (Year) | Sample | Outcome Measures | Therapist | Treatment Conditions | Results |
|---|---|---|---|---|---|
| Hood & Eyberg (2003) | 23 mothers who had completed a PCIT outcome study 32 to 76 months prior; at pretreatment, mothers had 3- to 6-year-old children with a diagnosis of ODD | Parent (self): PLOC-SF, BDI<br><br>Parent (on child): ECBI | Not applicable because it is a follow-up study; Original therapists not reported | Pre/Post/32- to 76-month follow-up | Maintenance of treatment gains in child disruptive behavior and parenting stress; 75% maintained clinically significant behavioral improvement at follow-up, 25% of children who had clinically significant improvement at post-treatment did not maintain these gains at follow-up |
| McNeil, Eyberg, Eisenstadt, Newcomb, & Funderburk (1991) | 10 2- to 7-year-old children with high parent-reported behavior problems, low observed compliance rate, and teacher-reported behavior problems; 10 normal classroom controls; 10 deviant classroom controls | Clinician Observation: DPICS<br><br>Parent (on child): ECBI<br><br>Teacher (on child): RCTRS, SESBI, Walker-McConnell Test of Children's Social Skills | Clinical psychology doctoral students | Pre/Post<br><br>Between: Treatment group, normal classroom controls, untreated deviant classroom controls | Significant improvement in parent-reported child problem behavior at home and observed child compliance in clinic; significant improvement in teacher-reported and observed compliance and disruptive behavior at school |

*Note.* ODD = Oppositional Defiant Disorder; DPICS = Dyadic Parent-child Interaction Coding System; MMPI = Minnesota Multiphasic Personality Inventory; ECBI = Eyberg Child Behavior Inventory; PSI = Parenting Stress Index; PLOC = Parent Locus of Control; PLOC-SF = Parent Locus of Control–Short Form; BDI = Beck Depression Inventory; DAS = Dyadic Adjustment Scale; RCTRS = Revised Conner's Teacher Rating Scale; SESBI = Sutter-Eyberg Student Behavior Inventory disruptive behavior in the school. It is given to achieve a comprehensive assessment of children across multiple contexts to assess the consistency of behavior problems.

In some cases, parents may also be given additional self-report measures (e.g., Parenting Stress Index [PSI; Abidin, 1995]; Child Abuse Potential Inventory [CAPI; Milner, 1986]) to assess for parental functioning (Eyberg & Boggs, 1998; Herschell & McNeil, 2007). Parents may also be given the *DSM-IV* rating scale to broadly assess for internalizing and externalizing behavior problems (Eyberg & Boggs, 1998). If it is suspected that the child may have an intellectual disability, then the child may be administered an intelligence test (Eyberg & Boggs, 1998). In some cases, therapists will also conduct home and school observations to gather observational data across these settings.

## Child-Directed Interaction

The first CDI session involves the parents and therapist meeting without the child. During this session, the therapist provides the rationale for CDI (Eyberg, 1999). The therapist also teaches parents CDI skills based on play therapy principles. These include the PRIDE skills (e.g., labeled Praise, Reflections, Imitation, behavioral Descriptions, and Enthusiasm) (see Eyberg, 1999). At this time parents are also taught to avoid questions, commands, and critical statements (Eyberg & Boggs, 1998). At the end of the session, parents are instructed to start the 5 minutes of special playtime at home, and to continue this practice throughout treatment (Herschell & McNeil, 2007).

The remaining CDI sessions involve the parent and child working together in-session (Herschell & McNeil, 2007). During these sessions, therapist coaching is introduced. To shape parental skills, the therapist gives parents labeled praise for their use of PRIDE skills while not providing social reinforcement for their use of questions, commands, and criticisms (Eyberg, 1999). Parents are also shaped to use removal of attention for disruptive, nonharmful behavior (Eyberg & Boggs, 1998). For example, if a child was to start banging the blocks together, the parent would be instructed to turn away and pretend like he or she was playing by him or herself until the child would become interested in what the parent was doing. Parents would then be coached to give the child labeled praise for appropriate behaviors (e.g., coming back to the play carpet) that would help the child learn the difference in their responses to positive and negative behaviors.

The criteria for mastery of CDI skills that would allow the progression to the PDI phase include 10 behavior descriptions, 10 reflections, and 10 labeled praises with no more than three questions, commands, or criticisms in a 5-minute coding interval using the DPICS-III (Eyberg, 1999). CDI usually lasts between six to seven sessions (Herschell & McNeil, 2007).

## Parent-Directed Interaction

In the first PDI session, therapists present parents with the rationale of using consistency, predictability, and follow-through with commands (Herschell &

McNeil, 2007). In the remaining sessions (about five to six sessions), therapists teach and coach parents in the specific skills needed to achieve the goals of PDI. The first skill taught is the use of effective commands. Effective commands are described as being clear and direct, and to be stated in age-appropriate language (Eyberg & Robinson, 1982; McNeil et al., 1999). Direct commands are encouraged so that the child is provided with a clear instruction to engage in a specific behavior (Patterson, 1982; Reid, 1978). Therapists provide parents with examples of direct commands (e.g., "Please pick up Mr. Potato Head") for the parents to model (see Eyberg, 1999, for direct command examples). In addition to teaching parents direct commands, therapists also teach parents to give reasons for their demands. Parents may give a reason either before the command is stated or after the child complies.

Parents are also taught to provide commands addressing one behavior at a time, and to tell the child what to do, not to focus on what the child should not be doing (Eyberg & Robinson, 1982). Parents are coached to say commands in an even tone of voice, beginning with the word "Please" to be respectful and to help make them direct rather than indirect. For example, the command "Clean up your room" could be broken down into two separate commands such as "Please put the blue block into the box" (parent provides a praise for compliance) and then "Please put the red block into the box" (parent provides a praise for compliance to the second command as well) (see Eyberg, 1999, for rules of effective commands).

The second skill of PDI involves the application of the time-out sequence. PCIT therapists provide a thorough rationale for the time-out procedure and then role-play each step in the sequence with the parent. This procedure is usually role-played with the child as well so the child has a basic idea of what will happen (Eyberg, 1999). When parents are first learning the time-out sequence, they are instructed by the therapist to refrain from using the sequence at home until they have practiced it enough times in-session to do it correctly (Eyberg, 1999).

In the time-out sequence, parents are instructed to present the child with a specific command (Eyberg & Boggs, 1998). If the child does not comply with the command, the therapist instructs the parent to start the sequence (Eyberg & Boggs, 1998). For each instruction, the child is presented with a choice to comply with the command or sit on the chair. This warning statement is a developmentally appropriate way to provide inattentive children with another opportunity to comply. The warning also provides parents with a way to be consistent and follow through with consequences, rather than escalating into a coercive interaction with numerous repetitions of commands and idle threats.

The time-out sequence includes specific procedures for escorting the child to the chair, managing the 3-minute time-out in the chair, and a backup plan for refusal to stay in time-out (Eyberg & Boggs, 1998). If the child does not comply with the command, then the parent is coached to lead the child safely to the time-out chair. Therapists then coach parents to wait until the child has sat in the chair for approximately 3 minutes plus 5 seconds of quiet (McNeil & Hembree-Kigin, 2010). At the end of this time period, the child is presented with the choice to comply with the original command. If the child agrees to comply with the demand, the parent is coached to gently lead the child back to the play area and acknowledge the compliance. The parent then presents an additional command; if the child complies with this request, the parent is coached to give an enthusiastic praise to increase compliance in the future (Eyberg & Boggs, 1998).

If the child refuses to remain in time-out or engages in potentially dangerous behavior while on the time-out chair (e.g., standing on the chair), then the final step in the procedure is to follow through with a predetermined backup plan. This plan usually consists of finding a safe room or area that can be used as a safe alternative for harmful or dangerous behavior. The time-out room is a setting where the child receives little attention and positive reinforcement. Once the child is in the time-out room, parents are coached to wait for 1 minute plus 5 seconds of silence (Eyberg, 1999; McNeil & Hembree-Kigin, 2010). At this point, the child is presented with the choice to comply with sitting on the chair. If the child refuses to sit on the chair, the child is placed in the backup area for another 1 minute plus 5 seconds of silence. If the child complies with sitting on the chair, then the original sequence is continued. Throughout the time-out sequence, parents are reminded to be predictable and calm and to maintain this consistency at home.

Mastery criteria for PDI skills include at least four commands, with 75% being effective commands (e.g., direct commands stated clearly), 75% correct follow-through of effective commands, and correct follow-through with the time-out procedure if needed (Eyberg, 1999). Once parents reach mastery criteria in the playroom, therapists encourage the practice of skills in progressively more difficult situations at home (Herschell & McNeil, 2007). PDI usually lasts between six to seven sessions. Once parents master the skills taught in PDI, feel confident in their ability to manage their child's behavior, and report that the child's disruptive behavior has improved to within normal limits, a graduation session is scheduled and treatment ends (Eyberg, 1999; Herschell & McNeil, 2007).

# Case Example

## Presenting Problem

Sam was 4 years old when he was brought for therapy by his parents, Mr. and Mrs. Gardner, after complaints from his preschool teacher on two different occasions that he had punched children in his class. His teacher had complained that Sam did not follow directions well and that he liked to draw the attention of other children while they were engaged in other classroom activities (e.g., circle time). Although his problems at school appeared to be emerging recently, his mother reported that her main concerns were related to him not complying with parent requests and "aggression" toward his younger sisters. Mrs. Gardner felt that she was "neither a good mother nor a good teacher" because she was unable to manage Sam's behavior.

Sam's mother reported that Sam had a low frustration tolerance, was sassy, and talked back to his parents. She described what she called "monster melt-downs" in which Sam would whine loudly, stomp on the ground, slam doors, and throw himself on the ground when he was either frustrated or did not get his way. Mrs. Gardner had such difficulty getting Sam dressed for school that she made him go to bed wearing the clothes he was supposed to wear to school the next day. Sam did not get along with his two sisters and did not have other friends because of his "bossy" behavior. Sam's father reported that Sam "hated following directions" and "could not accept authority." His parents felt that there was no marital discord but did report their relationship was at times strained as a result of Sam's oppositional behavior.

## Assessment

Assessment focused on measuring the extent of disruptive behaviors and the quality of the parent-child interactions that could be related to Sam's behaviors. Data collected would also help track the progress of treatment. Assessment included the use of a behavioral observation coding system and parental report of child behavior. Additionally, a teacher report was included to track disruptive behavior at preschool. The DPICS-III was used as the objective, observational measure to assess the quality of parent-child interactions. The Gardners both showed a lack of prosocial interactional skills (e.g., labeled praises, behavioral descriptions, reflections) and an abundance of less prosocial interactional skills (e.g., questions, commands). Sam was observed to comply with approximately 25% of his parents' commands during the structured observations, a compliance rate that is significantly lower than norms for the DPICS-III (i.e., approximately 60% to 70% in the same situations). After the intake session, therapists coded parent-child interactions using the DPICS-III at each weekly session.

Both parents were also administered the ECBI to determine the extent of Sam's externalizing behavior problems. The Gardners reported elevated levels on the problem and intensity scores on the ECBI; these scores demonstrated significant impairment and suggested the presence of a disruptive behavior disorder. After the intake session, the Gardners were administered the ECBI at each treatment session to track changes in their perception of Sam's disruptive behavior.

Additionally, Sam's preschool teacher was given the SESBI to assess for disruptive behavior at school. The SESBI was an important measure for tracking Sam's behavior over multiple contexts to look for consistency. Sam's teacher's scores on the SESBI were clinically elevated, suggesting the presence of clinically significant disruptive behaviors in the classroom as well as the home.

In addition to the data gathered in the clinic and from the school, the therapist and co-therapist made a home visit. Both therapists observed Sam to be very domineering and pushy with his sisters. His mother appeared considerably hypervigilant and was constantly worried that Sam was engaging in disruptive behavior. She constantly told Sam to stop taking things from his sisters, such as crayons or candy, but Sam was noncompliant with her requests. After repeatedly telling him to share his toys with his sisters, and after he had been noncompliant with many of her requests, Mrs. Gardner gave Sam a "time-out." She put him on a comfortable chair and sat with him for 5 minutes while holding him. He kept joking and playing with his mother to make her giggle at his behavior. During the home visit, Mrs. Gardner reported that she felt guilty about not spending enough time with Sam as she spent more time taking care of his younger sisters. She also reported feeling guilty about her hesitancy to discipline her son.

## Treatment

### Child-Directed Interaction (CDI)

Sam's parents attended the first CDI didactic session without Sam; during this session the therapist and co-therapist explained the rationale of PCIT and provided an outline of the treatment components. When both parents reported concern with being able to consistently schedule special playtime every day, the therapist and co-therapist emphasized the importance of this practice and problem-solved with both parents to help structure their time. The Gardners were instructed to let Sam lead during special playtime and avoid using questions, commands, and criticisms for the 5 minutes as it would take the lead away from the child, bring a negative atmosphere to the interaction, and possibly increase some of the problem behaviors.

In subsequent sessions, skills taught to Mr. and Mrs. Gardner included the use of labeled praise, reflections of Sam's verbalizations, descriptions of his behaviors, imitation, and enthusiasm. The therapist explained that these skills would add warmth to the interaction, increase Sam's desirable behaviors, and keep him on task. Mr. Gardner was skeptical that playing with Sam for 5 minutes every day would improve his behaviors and was reassured that CDI was not just playtime but was a special therapeutic time that would also set him up for success during the second phase, PDI.

During CDI, the therapist and co-therapist modeled the CDI skills and the selective ignoring of undesirable behaviors, after which CDI was role-played with Sam's parents. During the CDI coaching sessions, both parents usually took turns to be coached while the other parent watched and learned how to code CDI skills on the DPICS-III. Sam's parents reported that they disagreed with each other on parenting issues and were inconsistent when disciplining their children. Mrs. Gardner felt Mr. Gardner shouted more than he spoke to his children, and she complained about his lack of involvement in treatment. His inability to separate time for special playtime for Sam further exacerbated their conflict. Mr. and Mrs. Gardner also reported an inability to spend time with each other, as the majority of their time was spent taking care of the three children, putting more stress on their relationship. Although the need to work on their marital conflict was emphasized during CDI, the focus of therapy sessions remained to improve Sam's behaviors.

It took six sessions for Mrs. Gardner to achieve mastery of DPICS-III skills, and seven sessions for Mr. Gardner to achieve mastery. Mrs. Gardner was able to easily learn and use labeled praises, but she found difficulty in learning and using reflections and decreasing the amount of questions she asked. Mr. Gardner was able to master reflections and behavioral descriptions, but he had difficulty in using labeled praises and decreasing his use of commands. With individual coaching, the Gardners were able to effectively use the PRIDE skills and decrease the use of questions, commands, and critical statements by the time they started PDI. Although the therapist and co-therapist noticed weekly ECBI scores dropping from pretreatment, the problem and intensity scales still remained in the clinical range, identifying the need to teach the Gardners effective ways to manage Sam's disruptive behavior in PDI.

*Parent-Directed Interaction (PDI)*
To teach Sam to comply with commands, the Gardners were taught to give effective commands that increased the likelihood of this behavior. Both parents were encouraged to be direct and specific about what they wanted Sam to do. For instance, to help with Sam's hyperactive behavior, Mr. and Mrs. Gardner were instructed to use commands such as "Keep your hands to yourself" and "Please use walking feet" instead of "Calm down" and "Be careful." "Calm down" and "Be careful" were identified as vague commands, as they did not specifically address the problematic behavior. Mr. Gardner was also encouraged to tell Sam to do behaviors that were incompatible with his current inappropriate behaviors so that it was clear to Sam how he was expected to behave.

During PDI, the time-out procedure was explained, modeled by the therapist and co-therapist, and then role-played with Mr. and Mrs. Gardner. To ensure that the sequence was predictable and consistent so that it was effective, the time-out procedure was also role-played with Sam using a toy bear named Mr. Bear. In the procedure, a time-out chair was used to remove Mr. Bear from any source of attention if he did not comply with the presented task within 5 seconds.

The Gardners were instructed to give Sam only one warning for the time-out chair (e.g., "If you do not put the blue Lego into the box, you will have to sit on the chair."). They were then instructed to take him to the chair if he had not complied with the command after 5 seconds of the chair warning. The therapists also engaged in problem solving with Mr. and Mrs. Gardner to identify and prepare a backup room, as they were sure that Sam would get off the chair. The backup room would be a safe environment in which all parental attention would be removed, and it would shape Sam's sitting on the time-out chair.

In the play situation, with the help of the bug-in-the-ear device, Mr. and Mrs. Gardner were coached to give effective play commands and to give Sam labeled praise for complying. Although both parents had memorized the time-out sequence, the entire sequence was carried out with constant guidance of the therapists. Mrs. Gardner had given Sam a reason and then a command, saying, "Sam, we need to clean up the Legos as we are not using them right now. Please put the blue Lego into the toy box." Immediately after the command, she was instructed to silently count for 5 seconds while pointing to the blue Lego and the toy box. Sam ignored his mother's request, and at the end of 5 seconds, he had not complied with her command. Mrs. Gardner was then coached to give Sam a warning only once, saying, "If you don't put the blue Lego in the toy box, you're going to have to sit on the chair." In this manner, Mrs. Gardner was coached to take Sam to the chair, give him the time-out warning when he got off, and later put him in the time-out room when he got off the chair again. The therapist and co-therapist encouraged Mrs. Gardner to stay calm and praised her for her correct follow-through statements while she waited for Sam to be quiet. The first time-out sequence ended when Sam put the blue Lego into the toy box. The time-out sequence lasted 8 minutes (including two trips to the back-up room).

During the middle of PDI (the fourth session), the therapist and co-therapist reviewed the ECBI graphs with Mr. and Mrs. Gardner and concluded that although Sam's scores appeared to reduce gradually, the scores were still in the clinical range and were similar to scores at the end of CDI. Neither Mr. nor Mrs. Gardner admitted that they were straying away from the prescribed time-out procedure at home. Yet, the therapists encouraged the parents to problem-solve how they could be consistent when using PDI at home. In subsequent sessions, both parents reported they were able to consistently and effectively use the time-out procedure to decrease Sam's disruptive behavior at home.

The difficulty of the tasks given to Sam was gradually increased as his parents successfully progressed through the PDI sessions. For instance, initial homework consisted of a daily 5- to 10-minute PDI practice session after special playtime, in which Sam was required to engage in a cleanup session. Mr. and Mrs. Gardner were also asked to use two to four extra commands in their daily lives to increase generalization and to follow each incidence of compliance with enthusiastic labeled praise. Both parents observed that the length of the time-out sequences kept reducing and the rate of compliance was increasing. This was reassuring to them as they seldom needed to use the backup room, because Sam had learned to stay in the time-out chair.

To ensure hurting behaviors would not be reinforced, Mr. and Mrs. Gardner set the house rule of "no hurting," which entailed putting Sam in time-out without a warning every time he broke the house rule. Additionally, the Gardners reported they had a difficult time taking Sam to public places and were encouraged to set expectations for Sam before an outing to set him up for success. Both therapists accompanied the Gardners on one of their regular trips to the grocery store and discovered that the parents took all three children on a 3-hour shopping trip without doing anything fun or giving their children rewards for good behaviors. The parents were coached to use CDI skills to reinforce positive behaviors while shopping, such as holding onto the shopping cart and staying close to the parent. Other tangible or activity rewards were also discussed, such as allowing Sam to pick out a small, inexpensive toy or get a 5-minute trip to the playground.

## Skills Generalization Session and Termination

One session was assigned to include both of Sam's sisters in treatment to generalize the therapeutic skills. Mr. and Mrs. Gardner were encouraged to use CDI and PDI skills not only with Sam, but with all the children in the home to increase positive interactions with all family members.

After reviewing the DPICS-III Summary sheets and the weekly progression of the ECBIs, it was determined that Mr. and Mrs. Gardner had reached mastery in both CDI and PDI and that Sam's scores on the ECBI no longer fell within the clinical range. The last session consisted of a graduation to celebrate the progress made by the family. Mr. and Mrs. Gardner were congratulated and given certificates, while Sam was given a blue ribbon for good behavior. The booster session was scheduled for two months post-treatment.

## Conclusion

Parent-Child Interaction Therapy (PCIT) involves the integration of play therapy principles with an operant behavioral approach. The overall goals of PCIT are twofold: (1) to help parents develop a positive, nurturing relationship with their children to increase the overall relationship quality, and (2) to teach parents appropriate discipline skills in managing disruptive behavior. Both stages of treatment, CDI and PDI, are important to use with children with disruptive and oppositional behavior. CDI is important given the strong impact parents have on their child's life at an early age. For preschoolers, parents and immediate family are the most influential individuals for the child (Hart & Risley, 1995). Therefore, PCIT aims to target and strengthen the parent-child relationship by intervening early in the child's life and including the parents as the co-therapists for the treatment.

In addition to the importance of enhancing the parent-child bond, empirical evidence has also demonstrated that parents can benefit greatly from learning how to manage disruptive behavior problems (Eisenstadt et al., 1993). In fact, as parents become consistent and children's behavior improves, the child's self-esteem and parent-child relationship has been found to improve as well (Eisenstadt et al., 1993). Studies of PCIT have shown the following: (a) increases in child compliance, (b) decreases in child disruptive behavior, (c) increases in parental use of praise, (d) decreases in parental use of criticism, and (e) improvements in parental ability to set limits and follow through consistently with consequences for defiant and aggressive behavior. These treatment gains have been shown to maintain for at least three to six years following treatment (Hood & Eyberg, 2003).

In addition to alleviating child disruptive behavior, PCIT also has been found successful with children who are experiencing child maltreatment and anxiety disorders. And, improvements in parenting behaviors have been shown to be robust in that they result in positive changes in the behavior of non-targeted siblings, as well as more cooperative behavior in the classroom setting.

With mounting evidence from programmatic research conducted in the United States and abroad, PCIT has earned a reputation as one of the most powerful early intervention programs available. Therapists should consider PCIT as a promising mental health option when developing treatment plans for young children and their families.

## References

Abidin, R. R. (1995). *Parenting stress index* (3rd ed.). Lutz, FL: Psychological Assessment Resources.

Axline, V. (1947). *Play therapy.* Cambridge, MA: Houghton Mifflin.

Bahl, A. B., Spaulding, S. A., & McNeil, C. B. (1999). Treatment of noncompliance using Parent-Child Interaction Therapy: A data-driven approach. *Education and Treatment of Children, 22,* 146–156.

Baumrind, D. (1966). Effects of authoritative parental control on child behavior. *Child Development, 37*(4), 887–907.

Borrego, J., Gutow, M. R., Reicher, S., & Barker, C. H. (2008). Parent-child interaction therapy with domestic violence populations. *Journal of Family Violence, 23,* 495–505.

Brestan, E. V., Eyberg, S. M., Boggs, S. R., & Algina, J. (1997). Parent-child interaction therapy: Parents' perceptions of untreated siblings. *Child and Family Behavior Therapy, 19,* 13–28.

Campbell, S. B. (1995). Behavior problems in preschool children: A review of recent research. *Journal of Child Psychology and Psychiatry, 36,* 113–149.

Chaffin, M., Silovsky, J. F., Funderburk, B., Valle, L. A., Brestan, E. V., Balachova, T., et al. (2004). Parent-child interaction therapy with physically abusive parents: Efficacy of reducing future abuse reports. *Journal of Consulting and Clinical Psychology, 72*(3), 500–510.

Choate, M. L., Pincus, D. B., Eyberg, S. M., & Barlow, D. H. (2005). Parent-child interaction therapy for treatment of separation anxiety disorder in young children: A pilot study. *Cognitive and Behavioral Therapy, 12,* 126–135.

Eisenstadt, T. H., Eyberg, S., McNeil, C. B., Newcomb, K., & Funderburk, B. (1993). Parent-child interaction therapy with behavior problem children: Relative effectiveness of two stages and overall treatment outcome.

*Journal of Clinical Child Psychology, 22*(1), 42–51.

Eyberg, S. M. (1988). Parent-child interaction therapy: Integration of traditional and behavioral concerns. *Child and Family Behavior Therapy, 10*(1), 33–46.

Eyberg, S. M. (1999). *PCIT treatment manual: Session outlines.* Unpublished manuscript, University of Florida.

Eyberg, S. M. (2004). The PCIT story: Conceptual foundation. *PCIT Pages: Parent-Child Interaction Therapy Newsletter, 1,* 1–2.

Eyberg, S. M., & Boggs, S. R. (1998). Parent-child interaction therapy: A psychosocial intervention for the treatment of young conduct-disordered children. In J. M. Briemeister & C. E. Schaefer (Eds.), *Handbook of parent training* (2nd ed., pp. 61–97). Hoboken, NJ: Wiley.

Eyberg, S. M., Funderburk, B. W., Hembree-Kigin, T. L., McNeil, C. B., Querido, J. G., & Hood, K. K. (2001). Parent-child interaction therapy with behavior problem children: One- and two-year maintenance of treatment effects in the family. *Child & Family Behavior Therapy, 23*(4), 1–20.

Eyberg, S. M., McDiarmid Nelson, M., Duke, M., & Boggs, S. R. (2005). *Manual for the dyadic parent-child interaction therapy coding system* (3rd ed.). Unpublished manuscript, University of Florida.

Eyberg, S. M., Nelson, M. M., & Boggs, S. R. (2008). Evidence-based psychosocial treatments for children and adolescents with disruptive behavior. *Journal of Clinical Child and Adolescent Psychology, 37,* 215–237.

Eyberg, S. M., & Pincus, D. (1999). *Eyberg Child Behavior Inventory and Sutter-Eyberg Student Behavior Inventory—Revised: Professional Manual.* Odessa, FL: Psychological Assessment Resources.

Eyberg, S. M., & Robinson, E. A. (1982). Parent-child interaction training: Effects on family functioning. *Journal of Clinical Child Psychology, 11,* 130–137.

Funderburk, B. W., Eyberg, S. M., Newcomb, K., McNeil, C. B., Hembree-Kigin, T., & Capage, L. (1998). Parent-child interaction therapy with behavior problem children: Maintenance of treatment effects in the school setting. *Child and Family Behavior Therapy, 20,* 17–38.

Graziano, A. M. (1983). Behavioral approaches to child and family systems. *The Counseling Psychologist, 11*(3), 47–56.

Guerney, B. (1964). Filial therapy: Description and rationale. *Journal of Consulting Psychology, 28*(4), 304–310.

Hanf, C. (1969). *A two-stage program for modifying maternal controlling during mother-child (M-C) interaction.* Paper presented at the meeting of the Western Psychological Association, Vancouver, British Columbia, Canada.

Hart, B., & Risley, T. R. (1995). *Meaningful differences in the everyday experience of young children.* Baltimore, MD: Paul H. Brookes.

Hembree-Kigin, T. L., & McNeil, C. B. (1995). *Parent-child interaction therapy.* New York, NY: Plenum Press.

Herschell, A. D., Calzada, E. J., Eyberg, S. M., & McNeil, C. B. (2002). Clinical issues in parent-child interaction therapy. *Cognitive and Behavioral Practice, 9,* 16–27.

Herschell, A. D., & McNeil, C. B. (2007). Parent-child interaction therapy with physically abusive families. In J. M. Briesmeister & C. E. Schaefer (Eds.), *Handbook of parent training* (3rd ed., pp. 234–267). Hoboken, NJ: Wiley.

Hood, K. K., & Eyberg, S. M. (2003). Outcomes of parent-child interaction therapy: Mothers' reports of maintenance three to six years after treatment. *Journal of Clinical Child and Adolescent Psychology, 32,* 419–429.

Kranz, P. L., & Lund, N. L. (1993). Axline's eight principles of play therapy revisited. *International Journal of Play Therapy, 2*(2), 53–60.

Martin, G., & Pear, J. (2007). *Behavior modification: What it is and how to do it* (8th ed.). Upper Saddle River, NJ: Pearson Education.

Masse, J. J. (2010). Autism spectrum disorders. In C. B. McNeil & T. Hembree-Kigin (Eds.), *Parent-child interaction therapy* (2nd ed., pp. 237–254). New York: Springer.

Masse, J. J., McNeil, C. B., Wagner, S. M., & Chorney, D. B. (2008). Parent-child interaction therapy and high-functioning autism: A conceptual overview. *Journal of Early and Intensive Behavior Intervention, 4,* 714–735.

Masse, J. J., McNeil, C. B., & Wagner, S. M. (2009). *Examining the efficacy of parent-child interaction therapy with high-functioning autism.* Manuscript in preparation.

Matos, M., Bauermeister, J. J., & Bernal, G. (2009). Parent-child interaction therapy for Puerto Rican preschool children with ADHD and behavior problems: A pilot efficacy study. *Family Process, 48*(2), 232–252.

McNeil, C. B., Capage, L. C., Bahl, A., & Blanc, H. (1999). Importance of early intervention for disruptive behavior problems: Comparison of treatment and waitlist-control groups. *Early Education & Development, 10*(4), 445–454.

McNeil, C. B., Eyberg, S. M., Eisenstadt, T. H., Newcomb, K., & Funderburk, B. (1991). Parent-child interaction therapy with behavior problem children: Generalization of treatment effects to the school setting. *Journal of Clinical Child Psychology, 20,* 140–151.

McNeil, C. B., & Hembree-Kigin, T. L. (2010). *Parent-child interaction therapy* (2nd ed.). New York, NY: Springer Science & Business Media.

Milner, J. S. (1986). *CAP inventory manual: An interpretive manual for the CAP inventory* (2nd ed.). Lutz, FL: Psychological Assessment Resources.

Niec, L. N., Hemme, J. M., Yopp, J. M., Brestan, E. V. (2005). *Parent-child interaction therapy: The rewards and challenges of a group format. Cognitive and Behavioral Practice, 12,* 113–125.

Patterson, G. R. (1976). The aggressive child: Victim and architect of a coercive system. In E. J. Mash, L. A. Hamerlynck, & L. C. Handy (Eds.), *Behavior modification and families.* New York, NY: Bruner/Mazel.

Patterson, G. R. (1982). *Coercive family process.* Eugene, OR: Castalia.

Reid, J. B. (Ed.). (1978). *A social learning approach to family intervention: Observation in home settings.* Eugene, OR: Castalia.

Ryan, V., & Courtney, A. (2009). Therapists' use of congruence in nondirective play therapy and filial therapy. *International Journal of Play Therapy, 18*(2), 114–128.

Schuhmann, E. M., Foote, R. C., Eyberg, S. M., Boggs, S. R., & Algina, J. (1998). Efficacy of parent-child interaction therapy: Interim report of a randomized trial with short-term maintenance. *Journal of Clinical Child Psychology, 27,* 34–45.

Silverman, W. K., & Hinshaw, S. P. (2008). The second special issue on evidence-based psychosocial treatments for children and adolescents: A 10-year update. *Journal of Clinical Child and Adolescent Psychology, 37*(1), 1–7.

Solomon, M., Ono, M., Timmer, S., & Goodlin-Jones, B. (2008). The effectiveness of parent-child interaction therapy for families with children on the autism spectrum. *Journal of Autism and Developmental Disorders, 38*(9), 1767–1776.

Urquiza, A. J., & McNeil, C. B. (1996). Parent-child interaction therapy: An intensive dyadic intervention for physically abusive families. *Child Maltreatment, 1*(2), 134–144.

Wagner, S. M., & McNeil, C. B. (2008). Parent-child interaction therapy for ADHD: A conceptual overview and critical literature review. *Child & Family Behavior Therapy, 30*(3), 231–256.

Webster-Stratton, C. (1990). Long-term follow-up of families with young conduct problem children: From preschool to grade school. *Journal of Clinical Child Psychology, 19,* 144–149.

# Integration of Sandtray Therapy and Solution-Focused Techniques for Treating Noncompliant Youth

| 4 |
|---|
| Chapter |

## *Daniel S. Sweeney*

Sandtray therapy is one of several expressive therapies that have the unique quality of being adaptive with a variety of theoretical and technical psychotherapeutic approaches. When dealing with the challenge of noncompliant youth, it is helpful to combine the benefits of cognitive and solution-focused techniques with an expressive therapeutic approach that honors developmental variances and the safety that crisis- or trauma-generated noncompliance call for in therapy. Sweeney and Homeyer (2009) assert that sandtray therapy "can be used with clients of all ages, it can be nondirective and directive, and can be fully nonverbal and projective while also being cognitive and solution-focused" (p. 297). This complements the observation made by Taylor (2009): "Solution-focused and sandtray therapists share several underlying principles that might generate potential for their convergence into theoretical applications that stress resiliencies, strengths, and possibilities without the limitations that primarily verbal approaches often demand" (p. 58).

Noncompliance is one of the most common presentation issues for children and youth (Johnston, Murray, & Ng, 2007; Kalb & Loeber, 2003; McMahon & Kotler, 2008; Wilder, Harris, Reagan, & Rasey, 2007). The importance of family therapy and parent training with these youth is obvious. Equally important is the need for these youth to find a place for individual expression and processing. This is where sandtray therapy can be an effective intervention.

## Introduction

There is a history for the integration of solution-focused therapy (SFT) and work with children. Selekman (1997) in fact discusses the combination of SFT and play therapy, even noting: "Young children inject spontaneity and playfulness into family sessions" (p. 2) and "a good grasp of developmental theory can aid us in determining how best to communicate with the child and with designing and selecting therapeutic tasks that he or she is capable of understanding and performing" (p. 22). Although not extensive, there is reference in the literature regarding the combination SFT with sandtray therapy (Nims, 2007; Homeyer & Sweeney, 2010; Sweeney & Homeyer, 2009; Taylor, 2009).

Children and families dealing with noncompliance and oppositional behavior often need an expressive medium because of the inherent communication challenges with these families and children. Research demonstrates that in terms of social problem solving, aggressive children tend to have more diminished ability to generate verbal assertion and negotiate solutions than do nonaggressive children (Lochman, Powell, Whidby, & Fitzgerald, 2006). Lochman et al. also note that aggressive children are deficient in their ability to resolve interpersonal problems. Provision of a therapeutic intervention that is not limited to verbalization would seem to be an appropriate fit for these clients.

There is a history of solution-focused brief therapy being successfully used with children presenting with behavior problems and noncompliance (Berg & Steiner, 2003; Gingerich & Wabeke, 2001; Selekman, 1997, 2000, 2005; Stringer & Mall, 1999). This integrates well with the demonstrated success in sandtray therapy research (Homeyer & Sweeney, 2010).

Another connection between sandtray therapy and SFT is worth noting. Sandtray therapists, while process-focused, are also goal-directed (Bainum, Schneider, & Stone, 2006; Homeyer & Sweeney, 2010; Sweeney & Homeyer, 2009)—which fits well with the goal-directed nature of SFT (De Jong & Berg, 2008; de Shazer, 1988; Selekman, 2005).

## Rationale and Foci for Sandtray Therapy and SFT

Homeyer and Sweeney (2010) define sandtray therapy as "an expressive and projective mode of psychotherapy involving the unfolding and processing of intra- and interpersonal issues through the use of specific sandtray materials as a nonverbal medium of communication, led by the client(s) and facilitated by a trained therapist" (p. 4). It is an intervention that promotes therapeutic safety and client control, involving use of a tray of sand, a deliberate collection of miniature toys and items, and a specified process in the treatment milieu. The requisite elements for sandtray therapy are fundamental across theoretical approaches. Sweeney and Homeyer (2009) assert:

> The tools of the sandtray therapist are simple. First, there is sand and water, which are basic elements of the earth, naturally and kinesthetically appealing. Then there is a tray, a container for not only the sand and play media, but also a container of the client's psyche. Finally, there is the collection of miniatures, which serves as a universe of symbols and images and more specifically the "words" that the client can present in therapy without having to directly verbalize painful issues. It is important to note that these are tools for the therapist; however, it is the sandtray process and product that create a milieu in which clients can approach and work through turmoil and trauma. (p. 297)

There are multiple rationale and foci detailed for the use of sandtray therapy (Homeyer & Sweeney, 2010; Sweeney & Homeyer, 2009). These include:

- *Sandtray therapy gives expression to nonverbalized emotional issues.* Play is not only the language of childhood; it is also a valuable language for any client who is unable or unwilling to verbalize. Because the sandtray process is the language, the miniatures are the words. Clients need no creative or artistic ability to participate in sandtray therapy.

- *Sandtray therapy has a unique kinesthetic quality.* Sandtray therapy provides a sensory and kinesthetic experience, which serves as an extension of foundational attachment needs. The very tactile experience of touching and manipulating the sand is a therapeutic experience in and of itself. Some nonverbal clients have simply run their fingers through the sand and then begin to talk—seeming like the sensory experience with the sand causes a loosening of the tongue.

- *Sandtray therapy creates a necessary therapeutic distance for clients.* Clients who have a psychological and/or neurobiological difficulty expressing pain through verbalization often find expression through a projective medium such as sandtray therapy. It is often easier for traumatized clients to speak through one or more of the sandtray therapy miniatures than to directly verbalize their pain. Sandtray clients often experience emotional release through symbolization and sublimation, through the projection onto the tray and miniatures.

- *The therapeutic distance that sandtray therapy provides creates a safe place for abreaction to occur.* Clients who have experienced chaos and trauma need a therapeutic setting in which to abreact. This is a place where unexpressed issues can emerge and be safely relived, including an opportunity to experience the associated negative emotions. Abreaction finds facilitated expression through the sandtray therapy process.

- *Sandtray therapy with families is a truly inclusive experience.* Many family therapy experiences are based upon a typical adult talk therapy approach, which is fundamentally exclusive, because it fails to recognize and honor the developmental level of all participants in the family therapy process. Sandtray therapy recognizes the need to address the lowest developmental denominator and creates a level playing field for all family members, by giving everyone the opportunity to express him or herself.

- *Sandtray therapy naturally provides boundaries and limits, which promote safety for clients.* All relationships, particularly therapeutic relationships, are defined by boundaries and limits. The sandtray therapy process involves a prescribed structure and deliberately selected tools, which provides boundaries for clients that creates a sense of safety needed for growth. This includes the size and shape of the tray, the size and selection of miniatures, and the facilitation of the therapist. Such limits are both important and intentional but also promote freedom for expression.

- *Sandtray therapy provides a unique setting for the emergence of therapeutic metaphors.* Metaphors, particularly those generated directly by clients, can certainly be therapeutically powerful. Sandtray therapy creates a unique setting for this to occur, as the process is ideal for clients to express their own therapeutic metaphors.

  A side note is crucial on a related issue. Therapists are often tempted to provide a therapeutic interpretation in response to emergence of therapeutic metaphors. Therapists should be cautioned against this focus, with the recognition that the client's own interpretation is the most pertinent and therapeutic. The therapist's interpretation of trays is not necessarily essential to the healing process, as this comes with bias.

- *Sandtray therapy is effective in overcoming client resistance.* Sandtray therapy is inherently engaging and nonthreatening, which can often captivate the involuntary client and draw in the reticent family member. For family members who are resistant or have a fear of verbal conflict, sandtray therapy can provide a safer means of communicating. The identification of client resistance may be discovered and overcome through the sandtray therapy process.

- *Sandtray therapy provides a needed and effective communication medium for the client with poor verbal skills.* In addition to the importance of providing clients with developmentally appropriate therapeutic interventions, some clients may have poor verbal skills. This can include clients who experience language delays or deficits, social or relational difficulties, and physiological challenges. Because sandtray therapy does not depend on verbalization, clients with poor verbal skills, regardless of the etiology, find a place of relief.

- *Conversely, sandtray therapy cuts through verbalization used as a defense.* For clients who project pseudo-maturity, who are verbally astute yet developmentally delayed, or who use verbalization as a means to defend or manipulate—sandtray therapy provides a means of genuine communication. For clients who use intellectualization and rationalization as a defense, sandtray therapy can cut through these defenses. Sandtray therapy can identify these dynamics and provide a nonverbal and expressive manner of addressing them.

- *Sandtray therapy creates a place for the child client or family to experience control.* Individuals and families in crisis frequently contend with the frustration and fear of having lost control. The sandtray therapy process, even when structured, provides client-directed opportunities for a renewed sense of control. For clients needing the attainment and retention of responsibility and self-control, sandtray therapy promotes the autonomy for this to occur. For clients attempting to avoid responsibility, the sandtray therapy process places the responsibility for and control of the process on clients.

- *The challenge of transference may be effectively addressed through sandtray therapy.* Regardless of theoretical perspective on transference, sandtray therapy provides a means for transference issues to be safely identified and addressed. Most therapeutic interventions involving an expressive medium help create an alternative object of transference. With sandtray therapy, the tray and miniatures usually become the objects of transference or the means by which transference issues are safely addressed.

- *Finally, deeper intrapsychic issues are arguably accessed more thoroughly and more rapidly through sandtray therapy.* The collective rationale and benefit for sandtray therapy noted earlier creates a therapeutic atmosphere where deep and complex intrapsychic issues can be safely approached. Recognizing that many clients are defensive when confronting challenges to their injured egos, the safety of sandtray therapy can decrease ego controls and other defenses and foster increased levels of disclosure. This in turn creates an increased capacity to consider interpersonal and intrapersonal alternatives.

These rationale and benefits of sandtray therapy fit well with SFT, which is considered to be a competency-based model that deemphasizes problems and prior failures and focuses on clients' strengths and prior success. There is a focus on the clients' perspective and the clients' desire to change (De Jong & Berg, 2008; de Shazer, 1988; Selekman, 2005). Some basic tenets of SFT include the following:

- The focus is on strengths and solution-building as opposed to problem-solving.
- The focus is on the clients' desired future as opposed to past failures or current conflicts.
- Clients are encouraged to increase the frequency of useful emotions and behaviors.
- Recognition is given that no problematic situations constantly occur; there are times when the problem could have occurred or have been worse. These exceptions can be used in therapy to co-construct solutions.
- Therapy helps clients explore alternatives to current undesired behaviors, thoughts, emotions, and interactions, which are within the clients' capabilities or can be co-constructed.
- The model assumes that solutions already exist for clients, as opposed to approaches focused on building skills and/or behavioral interventions.
- It is assumed that small incremental change leads to large incremental change.
- It is not assumed that client solutions are directly connected to the identified problem.
- Therapist skills should be more focused on partnering with clients to build solutions as opposed to traditional diagnosis and treatment (De Jong & Berg, 2008; de Shazer & Dolan, 2007).

Selekman (2000) discusses five solution-focused assumptions that should guide the therapist and therapeutic process of SFT. These are arguably cross-theoretical and certainly apply to the sandtray therapy process. These assumptions include: (1) Change is inevitable; (2) Cooperation is inevitable; (3) All children have the strengths and resources to change; (4) Clients succeed when their goals drive therapy; and (5) There are many ways to look at a problem (pp. 2–4).

## Integration of Sandtray Therapy and SFT

Although the SFT literature discusses use of SFT with children and youth (e.g., Berg & Steiner, 2003; Gingerich & Wabeke, 2001; Selekman, 1997, 2000, 2005; Stringer & Mall, 1999), there is little discussion of SFT in a play therapy context. Selekman (2000) states that he presents "an integrative solution-oriented brief family therapy approach that combines the best elements of modified traditional play and art therapy techniques with other compatible competency-based family therapy approaches" (p. 1). There are rich opportunities for further integration, particularly within the context of sandtray therapy.

Nims (2007) makes the argument for integration of SFT with play therapy, asserting that SFT "is relevant for working with young children. Expressive play therapy techniques are effective in facilitating this process. Adjustments need to be made according to the child's developmental level" (p. 65). Taylor adds to the call for integration, focused on sandtray therapy: "The use of SF theory and techniques with sandtray therapy offers a positive and empowering approach to working with clients" (p. 67). Homeyer and Sweeney (2010) discuss specific ways of employing SFT techniques in the sandtray therapy process, which will be discussed as follows.

There are many theoretical approaches to sandtray therapy. This cross-theoretical element makes the application of SFT a natural fit for most sandtray therapy approaches.

## Practical Implementation for Integration

A summary discussion of sandtray therapy is important before looking at integration. However, it is not possible to fully discuss the theory and process of sandtray therapy in this chapter. The following is a brief summary, taken from Homeyer and Sweeney (2010).

The basic materials needed are one or more sandtrays, water (if possible—if only one tray is available, it should be a dry tray), and a selection of miniatures. There is no need to have an elaborate set of media. In fact, an expansive and elaborate collection may be overwhelming for some clients and may meet the needs and desires of therapists rather than clients.

The standard sand trays are usually 20 inches by 30 inches by 3 inches, painted blue on the inside to simulate sky and water, and are half filled with quality sand. Playground sand, while inexpensive, may be problematic because it usually contains small pebbles, which some clients object to. Sand that is very fine may also be problematic, as it can result in clouds of dust, which can be an allergen. The size of the tray is important, as it naturally provides boundaries and limits for clients, and so the product of a sandtray session can be viewed in a single glance. It is preferable to have two waterproof trays, so that one can be used with dry sand and the other with wet sand. It is suggested that the tray(s) be set at an average desktop height surface, with some surface space around the base of the tray. Some clients like to place miniatures outside of the tray, perhaps to represent intra- or interpersonal issues that are not ready to be approached and processed.

A selection of miniatures (averaging 2 to 4 inches in height) should be made available for use in the sandtray. They should be purposively selected (not collected) exclusively for the sandtray therapy process. On average, a collection of 300 to 400 miniatures is adequate. Thousands of miniatures are not necessary (and may in fact be emotionally flooding for some clients). It is important to offer a wide assortment of miniature toys and objects. Some basic categories include the following:

- Buildings (houses, castles, factories, schools, churches, stores)
- People (various racial/ethnic groups, military, cowboys, sports figures, fantasy, mythological, various occupations)
- Vehicles (cars, trucks, planes, boats, emergency vehicles, farm equipment, military vehicles)
- Animals (domestic, farm, zoo, wild, marine, prehistoric)
- Vegetation (trees, shrubs, plants)
- Deities (both western and eastern religions)
- Structures (fences, bridges, gates, highway signs)
- Natural objects (rocks, shells, driftwood, feathers)
- Miscellaneous (jewelry, wishing well, treasure chest)

Deliberate and careful sensitivity to issues of diversity should be a priority in the selection of miniatures. Miniatures should be grouped together by category, and preferably displayed on open shelves. Other means of display are possible, but clients are simply less likely to rummage through drawers or bins than they are to select objects from a shelf.

Homeyer and Sweeney (2010) describe six basic phases of the sandtray therapy process, including (1) preparation of the sandtray setting; (2) introduction of the process to the client; (3) creation of the sandtray; (4) post-creation phase; (5) sandtray cleanup; and (6) documentation of the session. For the sake of brevity, these phases will not be discussed in this chapter. Integration of SFT interventions would occur during phases 2, 3, and 4. SFT interventions can be integrated well with the sandtray therapy process (Homeyer & Sweeney, 2010; Nims, 2007; Taylor, 2009). There are multiple examples, some of which will be discussed.

A specific directive technique that can be used in the sandtray is similar to the solution-focused "miracle question" (de Shazer, 1988), which facilitates clients conceptualizing options, as well as a world beyond their current pain. Traditionally, this might look like: If you woke up tomorrow, and sometime during the night a miracle happened and the problem that brought you here today was solved just like that, how would you know it happened? What would it look like? These are fabulous questions, which focus not only on the absence of the presenting problem, but also imagining a future that is positive and ideal. Like many structure techniques, however, the miracle question calls for considerable abstract thinking, which may be challenging to verbalize.

Homeyer and Sweeney (2010) suggest a simple adaption: If you woke up tomorrow, and sometime during the night a miracle happened and the problem that brought you here today was solved just like that, I wonder what that might look like? Could you make a sandtray of this? I wonder what your tray would be like, knowing this had happened? (p. 59).

Several other solution-focused questions (de Shazer & Dolan, 2007) can be adapted for use in the sandtray. Rather than asking for a verbal response, therapists can ask clients to create sandtrays that depict the answers. Homeyer and Sweeney (2010) suggest some possibilities:

- Could you make a tray that shows the last time this was not a problem?
- This challenge could be a lot bigger: Could you make a tray about how you've kept this from getting to be a bigger problem?
- If someone were making a movie about you, having resolved this problem, could you make a tray of what hitting the pause button on this movie would look like?
- Can you make a tray showing what you see down the road for yourself after this is resolved?
- How will you even know that this is resolved? Can you make a tray on what this looks like?
- This past week, when you chose not to [argue, get depressed, act out], what was it like? Can you make a tray about this?
- This past week, when you chose to [argue, get depressed, act out], what was it like? Could you make a tray about how you'd like to do it differently?
- Can you make a tray on what you might be doing, if you were to "act as if" there was no problem? What would it look like?
- When you were dealing with this challenge a little better than you are right now, what did that look like? Could you make a tray of that? Could you make a tray on what you might need to do in order to get back there?
- If someone threw you a victory parade after you've journeyed though this, could you make a tray on what the parade would be like?
- If your partner/friend/family member was here and making a tray about you, what would it look like? Can you make this tray?

- If I were making a sandtray to describe you, what kind of a tray would I make about you? Can you make this one?
- If you picked a miniature to represent you and another to represent the challenge that brought you into counseling, what would these be? If you picked one or more miniatures to represent what it would take to subdue the one you chose to represent the challenge, what would these be?
- When things are moving in the right direction, what will that look like? Can you make a tray on this? Who will be the first to notice? What miniature would you select for this person?
- Can you make a tray on what is happening right now that you'd like to continue happening? What might you add to the tray to make this happen more? (p. 59)

There are many other possible questions, which are commonly questions that clients may be expected to or are able to answer verbally. For those clients who struggle to respond or for those clients whose answers are quick, brief, or shallow, sandtray therapy provides an alternative forum for response and process.

Another SFT adaption for the sandtray therapy process involves the use of scaling questions (Homeyer & Sweeney, 2010; Selekman, 2000). Scaling questions are commonly used in SFT as well as other therapeutic approaches, and they generally call for a verbal response. They can be therapeutically helpful in the assessment of client self-perception and therapeutic progress, because some clients may be challenged in verbally expressing a rating number or may have a cognitive view of themselves that may not match their intrapsychic or interpersonal reality (Homeyer & Sweeney, 2010).

Some examples of adaption for the sandtray therapy process, suggested by Homeyer and Sweeney (2010), include the following:

- *For example, the client may be asked*: Some people rate their level of depression using a scale from 1 to 10. You might be able to come up with a number, but I am wondering if you could make a sandtray that would depict how depressed you feel today.
- *Another example would be to assess how far clients see themselves as having come in the therapy journey*: I'd be interested in your assessment of how far we've come in therapy. One way to do this is to rate it on a scale—with 10 being the solution you've been looking for, and 1 being the place you were at when you came in for counseling. Instead of this, I'm wondering if you could make a sandtray that depicts where you see yourself today.
- *An adaption of this could be*: Today, I'd like to ask you to do two sandtrays. The first would be a scene of how you were when you first came in for counseling, and the second would be a scene of where you see yourself now. This could be further adapted by showing the client a picture taken of an earlier sandtray: This is a picture of one of the trays you did when you

first came in for counseling. It seems like you've come a long way. Looking at this, I wonder if you could make a tray that shows where you feel you're at today.

- Another way scaling questions are used in therapy is to ask clients to rate how others might perceive their current functioning. This can be nicely adapted to the sandtray, by asking clients to create trays instead. For example: If your partner/employer/friend was here, and I ask them to make a tray about you, I wonder what that would look like. It might be tough to do this, but could you make the tray you think they'd make? (pp. 60–61).

Hackett and Shennan (2007) discuss an effective integrative SFT technique, which they refer to as "Show Me":

> A wonderful technique with younger children, whether asking about the desired future or about progress toward it, is to ask them to show rather than tell you about constructive behavior (constructive in this context tending to mean behavior desired by significant adults in their lives) they can imagine themselves doing or have done already. Children love to respond to the injunction, "Show me!" Showing is a useful activity because it is both a clear example of the ability to behave in a certain way and a rehearsal for future behavior of this kind.

This technique would have increased attraction for children and could potentially have greater effect if used within the context of sandtray therapy. The use of a wide variety of miniatures provides a wide palette for creative expression. Using the injunction "Show Me" has greater potential expression if the client is not limited to a verbal response.

These are a few brief examples of integrating SFT and sandtray therapy. There are as many possibilities as the creative abilities of trained sandtray therapists using SFT in the therapeutic process.

## Case Example

This case example involves a 12-year-old boy, Matt, who was referred for counseling by his parents. The first session involved a meeting with his parents only, which is preferable for child referrals. This first session often involves parents unloading their emotions about the referred child, which often includes multiple complaints and pejorative remarks. It is preferable that children are not included in this negative experience, as well as avoiding their initial contact with the therapist possibly being seen as an alignment with the parents' negative perspective. Matt was reportedly noncompliant with parental directives, fighting with his peers and siblings, and arguing with teachers at school. It is worth noting that the parents were experiencing couple conflict, to which Matt's behavior might be attributed. The parents were offered a counseling referral, which was declined.

Matt had some knowledge of play therapy and quickly told the counselor that he was far too mature for such an activity. It is not uncommon for preadolescents and adolescents to have this perspective. In these cases, such clients are offered a "way of counseling that is used with adults" (sandtray therapy) and are told that they are viewed as being "mature enough for this." This tends to hook them, as they are motivated to participate in an adult activity.

Initially, Matt was invited to create a sandtray with no directions. He seemed to enjoy the activity, but little metaphorical material emerged. Following this, a solution-focused intervention, the "miracle question," was employed as described earlier. A point should be made that with preadolescents and adolescents, the wording is often changed from "miracle" to "magic"—while most do understand the word "miracle," they seem to have a better response to "magic":

> *I'd like to ask you to do something specific in the sandtray today, Matt. I've got a question for you to consider, and then make a scene in the tray. If something magical were to happen tonight, while you were sleeping, and tomorrow morning you woke up, and all this stuff we've been talking about was gone—pretty nice if we had that kind of magic, huh?—what would it look like in the morning? Could you make a scene in the tray about what this would look like?*

Matt quickly went to work dividing the tray in half, using fences and trees to separate the sides. On his own he created a scene about how he saw things in his world at present and how he would like things to be if something magical could happen. Although these instructions were not given, this does illustrate a nice SFT intervention strategy in sandtray therapy. Individuals, couples, and families can be asked to essentially create two scenes, for example: (a) one scene being how they view life now and the other how they would like to see their life; (b) one scene being how life was like before the presenting problem existed and the other how life is with the presenting problem; (c) one scene being how they view the presenting problem and the other how someone else might view it; and (d) as many variations as the therapist might develop.

On the side of the tray that depicted how Matt currently viewed the problem, there were multiple scenes of conflict, each one involving himself. These included conflicts at school and at home. Interestingly, Matt chose only animals on this side of the tray. This may be a reflection of the benefit of the therapeutic distance that can be created in sandtray therapy, because it was not easy for Matt to identify with his problematic behavior. He was, however, able to take some responsibility for his disruptive behavior, as this was the first tray in which he identified himself as a "trouble maker."

The other side of the tray essentially represented the focus of the solution-focused miracle question, where Matt was able to initially identify a future apart from the presenting problem. Interestingly, he did not include himself on this side of the tray but only included his parents. In this case, he selected human figures (one male and one female), in a setting that Matt identified as "paradise." He verbalized some sadness about how much his parents argued and how he wished they could find a "magic place where there were no fights."

Matt recognized that a large part of the etiology of his problems related to his parents' conflict. He wasn't blaming his parents, and he did not attribute his own disruptive behavior to them—at least not at a verbal or conscious level. When asked about why he did not include himself on the "paradise" side of the tray, he said that he did not want his problems to get in the way of their happiness. This tray represented a turning point in the therapeutic process. Matt's challenging behaviors began to decrease, but more importantly, his parents agreed to seek couples counseling. After this began (with positive results), Matt's noncompliance diminished considerably.

## Conclusion

There is significant potential for adaptation and integration of solution-focused and other cognitive interventions to the process of sandtray therapy, keeping in mind the important issue of developmental fit. Grave and Blissett (2004) suggest that "young children can demonstrate the cognitive capacity to benefit from creatively delivered forms" of cognitive-behavioral interventions, and that "the challenge is to continue to integrate cognitive, social, and emotional developmental theories into cognitive behavioral theory, and creative methodologies, such as the use of narrative and analogy" (p. 417).

As sandtray therapists look to integrate solution-focused or other techniques, Sweeney (2011) provides an essential reminder:

> An important reminder is necessary about therapeutic techniques. Theory is important, but theory without technique is merely philosophy. Techniques are valuable, but techniques without theory are reckless, and potentially damaging. . . . Play therapists, as well as all therapists are encouraged to ponder some questions regarding employing techniques: (1) Is the technique developmentally appropriate? [which presupposes that developmental capabilities are a key therapeutic consideration]; (2) What theory underlies the technique? [which presupposes that techniques should be theory-based]; and (3) What is the therapeutic intent in employing a given technique? [which presupposes that having specific therapeutic intent is clinically and ethically important]. (p. 236)

With these things in mind, sandtray therapists are encouraged to use the creativity that led them to use sandtray to creatively integrate effective techniques into the wonderful expressive medium of sandtray therapy. There are no limits to the imagination.

## References

Bainum, C., Schneider, M., & Stone, M. (2006). An Adlerian model for sandtray therapy. *The Journal of Individual Psychology*, 62(1), 36–46.

Berg, I. K., & Steiner, T. (2003). *Children's solution work*. New York, NY: W. W. Norton.

De Jong, P., & Berg, I. K. (2008). *Interviewing for solutions* (3rd ed.). Belmont, CA: Brooks/Cole.

de Shazer, S. (1988). *Clues: Investigating solutions in brief therapy.* New York, NY: W. W. Norton.

de Shazer, S., & Dolan, Y. (2007). *More than miracles: The state of the art of solution-focused brief therapy.* New York, NY: Routledge.

Gingerich, W., & Wabeke, T. (2001). A solution-focused approach to mental health intervention in school settings. *Children and Schools, 25,* 33–47.

Grave, J., & Blissett, J. (2004). Is cognitive behavior therapy developmentally appropriate for young children? A critical review of the evidence. *Clinical Psychology Review, 24,* 399–420.

Hackett, P., & Shennan, G. (2007). Solution-focused work with children and young people. In T. Nelson & F. Thomas (Eds.), *Handbook of solution-focused brief therapy: Clinical applications* (pp. 191–212). New York, NY: Haworth Press.

Homeyer, L., & Sweeney, D. (2010). *Sandtray therapy: A practical manual* (2nd ed.). New York, NY: Routledge.

Johnston, C., Murray, C., & Ng, L. (2007). Types of noncompliance in boys with attention-deficit/hyperactivity disorder with and without oppositional behavior. *Child & Family Behavior Therapy, 29*(1), 1–20.

Kalb, L., & Loeber, R. (2003). Child disobedience and noncompliance: A review. *Pediatrics, 111*(3), 641–653.

Lochman, J., Powell, N., Whidby, J., & Fitzgerald, D. (2006). Aggressive children: Cognitive-behavioral assessment and treatment. In P. Kendall (Ed.), *Child and adolescent therapy: Cognitive-behavioral procedures* (3rd ed., pp. 33–81). New York, NY: Guilford Press.

McMahon, R., & Kotler, J. (2008). Evidence-based therapies for oppositional behavior in young children. In R. Steele, T. D. Elkin, & M. Roberts (Eds.), *Handbook of evidence-based therapies for children and adolescents: Bridging science and practice* (pp. 221–240). New York, NY: Springer.

Nims, D. (2007). Integrating play therapy techniques into solution-focused brief therapy. *International Journal of Play Therapy, 16*(1), 54–68.

Selekman, M. (1997). *Solution-focused therapy with children: Harnessing family strengths for systemic change.* New York, NY: Guilford Press.

Selekman, M. (2000). Solution-oriented brief family therapy with children. In C. E. Bailey (Ed.), *Children in therapy: Using the family as a resource* (pp. 1–19). New York, NY: W. W. Norton.

Selekman, M. (2005). *Pathways to change: Brief therapy solutions with difficult adolescents* (2nd ed.). New York, NY: Guilford Press.

Stringer, B., & Mall, M. (1999). *A solution-focused approach to anger management with children.* Birmingham, England: Questions.

Sweeney, D. (2011). Group play therapy. In C. Schaefer (Ed.), *Foundations of play therapy* (2nd ed., pp. 227–252). Hoboken, NJ: Wiley.

Sweeney, D., & Homeyer, L. (2009). Sandtray therapy. In A. Drewes (Ed.), *Effectively blending play therapy and cognitive behavioral therapy: A convergent approach* (pp. 297–318). Hoboken, NJ: Wiley.

Taylor, E. (2009). Sandtray and solution-focused therapy. *International Journal of Play Therapy, 18*(1), 56–68.

Wilder, D., Harris, C., Reagan, R., & Rasey, A. (2007). Functional analysis and treatment of noncompliance by preschool children. *Journal of Applied Behavior Analysis, 40*(1), 173–177.

# Holistic Expressive Play Therapy

## An Integrative Approach to Helping Maltreated Children

### *Marie-José Dhaese*

## Introduction

When I speak of maltreated children, I am referring to children who have been given no personal sense of value, whose basic needs have been ignored, and who have been consistently attacked and misused emotionally, physically, and/or sexually. This maltreatment often occurs at the very hands of those who should have been taking care of the child. Typically, the caregivers are unavailable, unpredictable, and/or out of control, creating a chaotic environment. These caregivers are often reenacting their own history of abuse that has come from multigenerational dysfunction. Chronic mistreatment is likely compounded by further incidents of trauma, given that the caregivers are not available to protect the child from other potentially dangerous situations.

By the time these children are referred to therapy, they are often in foster care, having been through several placements, while others are in adoptive homes. Many children continue to live in an unsafe environment in the context of a society where indiscriminate exposure to media increasingly promotes fear and violence. In addition, we are often working within a larger helping system that wants quick, convenient fixes for this overwhelming picture. How do we help such children come to a point where they can begin to heal their wounds and live more healthily, while they are still frequently living in a grim reality that often cannot be changed? How can we begin to stop the cycle of abuse? How, within the limits of a 50-minute therapy session once a week, can we stay hopeful and continue to help?

These concerns and questions were the impetus for developing my approach to working with this population of children. Holistic Expressive Play Therapy is an integration of the components that I have found necessary to create a safe place where the child can begin to heal: creative play and self-expression, caregiver involvement, relationship, and milieu. This is not meant to be yet another model of therapy, but rather, a sharing of insights gleaned through my own journey of self-healing and the journey of those I have accompanied for more than 35 years. It is a distillation and integration of what I have learned and *know* to be helpful to my clients and the clients of the professionals I have taught.

## My Journey Toward An Integrated Model of Play Therapy

My search for self-knowledge and self-healing took me from the farm in France of my childhood to a life of teaching at various universities in England, the United States, and finally Canada. I became increasingly disenchanted and developed a yearning for meaning in life that could not be found while secluded in an ivory tower.

My first encounter with satisfying answers came when I started reading Rudolf Steiner's *Anthroposophy* which, in its holistic approach, takes into account the reality of a spiritual world that lies behind physical reality and manifests itself to the inner eye in the form of images. Having found enough meaning in these ideas, I pursued my search for healing, switched professions, and thus began my journey as a therapist in the early 1970's (Steiner, 1923).

While working in a treatment center for severely disturbed adolescents, I was exposed to the various theories of counseling for individuals, groups, and families that were available at the time. I soon experienced the limitations of verbal counseling and began a search for more effective modes of treatment. Inspired by my reading of *Anthroposophy*, I sought to combine the profound power of imagery as a healing tool along with counseling, so I subsequently became an art therapist. I went on to run a therapeutic day program offering individual counseling for adolescents and children in foster care, who had been severely abused, neglected, or traumatized, and had attachment issues. Most of them were not interested in drawing or other kinds of art making. Still convinced of the healing power of imagery, I began to experiment with other materials that might engage my clients in the process of strengthening themselves and safely expressing the painful feelings that plagued them.

In 1980, my first co-therapist, Monseigneur, a black standard poodle, joined me. He was loved by all, whether a tough youth with tattoos or a shy, fearful young child. He assisted me whether I used art, crafts, sewing, knitting, music, movement, dress-up, masks, dollhouse play, storytelling, going for nature walks, creating a garden, or playing in the outdoor sandbox. The outdoor sandbox proved to be particularly both healing and grounding for my young clients. One rainy day, a child suggested we bring the sand indoors. A small tray filled with sand was the solution. The objects we had collected on our nature outings, such as seashells, feathers, stones, acorns, chestnuts, and pine cones, found their way into the sandbox and images were created—stories evolved. All along, I recorded the images that were created, as well as the activities we engaged in, through photography. At the end of therapy, the children got an album, a record of their memories.

Thus, I started developing a wide variety of body-centered expressive methods that simultaneously allowed for strengthening, nurturing experiences and safe expression and transformation of emotional blocks. I continued to hone my therapeutic skills, as my capacity to hold this process was being continuously tested both by the severity of the children's presenting issues and by the dysfunctional aspects of the system the children lived in. My approach evolved as I began to integrate my experiences with clients with my own personal journey for self-knowledge and self-healing, as I continued my search to find new ways of helping my most difficult clients.

## My Holistic Expressive Play Therapy Approach

At the heart of my approach is a memory I carry from my childhood. At harvest time, after the men gathered in the crops, my mother and I would glean the fields and collect the wheat sheaves. When it got too hot, we would sit in the shade of a tree. This was one of those special times with my mother, when she was at rest, and I could finally ask one of the many questions that whirled about in my 6-year-old mind. I asked her my most puzzling question: Where is God? Her answer was to pull out one of the sheaves of wheat, take out one of the grains, and point to the little white dot on the grain. At my questioning look, she explained that the grain was the seed and the little white dot was the germ that allowed the seed to grow and become the tall sheaf of wheat again. That germ was, she said, where God was. I liked that explanation better than any I had been given before or since.

As I accompany people of all ages on their journeys, I consistently come back to the belief that all human beings hold within themselves an innate kernel of wisdom. Just as every seed has within it a germ that holds the capacity and drive to grow toward the light and to become whatever plant is coded within its genes, it is my view that all human beings are born with the possibility and drive to grow into their potential. I call this potential the person's "true nature."

This true nature holds within it a capacity for self-healing—an immune system that flows through and guides each part of our organism: physical, emotional, cognitive, and spiritual, with each level influencing, interacting, and communicating with all the others. This innate wisdom has been called many different names: the spirit, the self, or God, among others. As a helper, I feel it is crucial to remember that all clients, no matter how wounded, hold within themselves that innate wisdom. When I acknowledge their true nature and their drive not only to survive but also to grow, flourish, and be whole, then I can help them reconnect to it and awaken their strength and capacity to heal.

Not all seeds germinate and not all plants survive. Much will depend on whether they have been lovingly tended to, according to their unique needs. In the same way, children need someone with whom they can form a secure and nurturing attachment in which their true nature is recognized, protected, and nurtured according to their unique qualities, so that they can grow into their potential as they face life's challenges.

Attachment is thus integral to our survival, growth, and development. Healthy attachment starts from the moment the fertilized egg attaches to the mother's uterus. The mother lends the embryo her physical body and provides nurturance and protection so it can grow and be born. During pregnancy, mother and child are one, and growth depends on this all-encompassing fusion. These crucial nine months will continue to have an influence on the rest of the child's development. The long-lasting effects of abuse and neglect can start this far back.

After birth, although the child is no longer within the mother's physical womb, he continues to be surrounded by what I call her emotional womb. Ideally, the mother will now provide the kind of physical and emotional nurturance and protection that will allow the child's developing self to grow and eventually form an emotional body of his own.

Inside that protected space, from the flexible inner wall of this emotional egg, love and unconditional acceptance shines and wraps the child in its warm and gentle light. In this ideal scenario, the mother mirrors the child's true nature, reflecting his intrinsic beauty and value; what is reflected in the mother's eyes becomes the child's self-image.

This mirroring is balanced with the containment and protection of consistent and age-appropriate limits. The child gradually develops the skin of his own emotional body, at first fused with the mother's and then increasingly becoming more separate. This boundary will become as clear, strong, and flexible as the mother's. The mother's protective eggshell acts like a sieve that only allows exposure to age-appropriate stimulation, while keeping out whatever might be unhealthy or dangerous for the child.

An essential quality the mother brings to this process is her capacity for attunement to the child—her capacity to clearly sense and *know* what the child needs and to respond accordingly. This is when the flexibility of her eggshell-boundary comes into play: ideally, it allows her to step back as the child matures, giving him room to move and explore while maintaining the reassurance that is needed. As the mother steps back, she remains available for support and encouragement. She is ready to move closer again if needed. Ideally, the mother's sun shines consistently, giving the child the message that he is just as lovable whether he is having a tantrum or smiling, whether he manages to do something right away or struggles with it. He will trust, know, and feel that, no matter what, he is valuable and his mother's unconditional love and acceptance continues to shine on him.

It is within this nurturing and protected space that the child will begin to explore the world and be given the opportunity to play and use his imagination. One of the many benefits of imaginative play is that it allows him to play out how he thinks, feels, and what he can do about what he has experienced and thus make sense of it, integrate it, and learn from it. Imaginative play is therefore essential to the child's emotional, cognitive, and behavioral development.

Within this ideal atmosphere, the child will build self-confidence, self-esteem, and self-validation with a realistic sense of his own strengths and limitations. He will have clear and flexible boundaries and show a healthy balance between dependence and independence. He will develop the ability to give, receive, learn, and focus. He will learn self-discipline, self-soothing, and self-regulation. He will thus emerge as a mature human being, equipped to meet the challenges that life will bring him.

In contrast, let us now consider the situation of maltreated children. Instead of the warm, egglike protection of healthy bonding, the emotional womb is inconsistent, if it even exists at all. Sometimes the sun shines and sometimes it disappears with total unpredictability. Sometimes, out of nowhere and without warning, the child is hit by a tornado. Not only is there no sieve to sift out what is not appropriate and no shell providing protection from the outside world, but the primary attachment may become a place of danger where the child is attacked, rejected, and abandoned. Whether it is physical, emotional, and/or sexual abuse, the attack comes from within the emotional womb, the place that should be a source of protection. The child has no safe place to be comforted.

What the maltreated child sees in his parent's face is not a mirror reflecting his true nature with unconditional love, but a mirror that is cracked and distorted. He sees badness and ugliness. This is only heightened when he expresses his needs. The sun might show up momentarily when the child meets the parent's narcissistic needs, but the storm soon returns.

Within this atmosphere of unpredictability, limits are inconsistent, expectations are unrealistic, and the child is left with destructive messages, such as that he is not good enough, or if he were perfect there would be no problem and he would be safe. Sometimes the child is left entirely alone. He is expected to know how to do things without guidance. Fear of punishment will constrain his ability to play. On the one hand, he is bombarded with age-inappropriate images and traumatic experiences, and on the other hand, he has no safe place where he can make sense of these experiences and integrate them. Unresolved traumas create emotional blocks that are so large and intricate they cannot be expressed and transformed without expert help. Blocked from resolution, the child's experiences go around in circles. The mass of blocks continues to grow and becomes a driving force, making the child compulsively reenact the trauma inwardly or outwardly. Unassimilated traumas create layer upon layer of repression, denial, and defenses that prevent him from connecting with his innate wisdom and its guidance when he most needs it.

Such children are no longer able to play creatively, and their imagination, which is unused and underdeveloped, becomes atrophied. If they play at all, it mostly consists of either compensatory or repetitive reenactment of their experiences. Such play will often compensate for their sense of helplessness but will not offer release, nor will it offer the true sense of power or learning that is found in healthy play. Instead, their play only reinforces their traumatic behaviors. Some children, overwhelmed by painful experiences, implode through dissociation or somatization and withdraw into themselves. Others will explode outwardly through destructive behaviors, in an attempt to play out and reenact their trauma.

As the blocks take over, they develop into what might be diagnosed as a disorder of one kind or another, with the many labels we have now acquired for different types of inner and outer reenactment. The disorder now takes the place of the child's true nature and pushes him from behind, rather than guiding him forward. This profound disconnection from his true nature interferes with his emotional growth and with evolution through appropriate developmental stages. All of this results in what might be called the discarded self, without impulse control or capacity for self-regulation, leaving the child with no sense of self, personal worth, or personal boundaries.

Let us now consider what will be needed for these children to heal from such profound wounds. First and foremost, I provide for them the safe and protected space of the emotional womb they never got in order to give them a reparative experience of the mother-child bond.

Although he longs for this bond, it has been fraught with danger and trauma and has brought him the most dangerous and difficult experiences of his life. Therefore, he experiences closeness as a source of danger, and this injury might take years to heal. In addition to consistently mirroring his true self with unconditional acceptance, the restorative relationship provides consistent limits, a healthy new container. The child slowly develops a new skin that solidifies and eventually becomes his boundary: strong, flexible, and so different from the brittle defenses he first brought to therapy.

Rather than deal immediately with overwhelming traumatic memories, I create the opportunity to make positive memories. I provide nurturing and ego-strengthening activities that will be remembered, stored, and internalized in the form of images that are life giving. Simultaneously, I give the child a safe environment to learn to play and to regain the innate faculty of imagination and creativity. Positive memories, together with the experience of relationship, will help the child internalize a safe place within, to which he can go when needed. Because many of these children are still subjected to a toxic, neglectful environment, this is often as far as one will be able to help. However, we should not underestimate the value of their experience, just because we're not delving into trauma.

For emotional health to be recovered, the expression, transformation, and eventually the resolution of his traumas still need to occur. This next step will not be taken until the child's ego has been strengthened and nurtured enough to face the release of his painful images and the energy held in each of these blocks. When the child is able to play, use his imagination, and have access to images other than his own painful memories, it is time to bring out each block, one by one. This is done in the language of symbols, which the child now has recovered.

As each block is removed, the child is more connected to his innate wisdom. The expression of painful images brings with it a release of energy that the child's psyche must be ready to incorporate. One must release this energy so that the flow can irrigate the child's inner world rather than flooding it. When released without flooding, the energy then becomes available for the child to deal with his daily life.

With the safe and gentle transformation of each block, the child begins to catch up to his developmental stage of growth. The ego can now regain its age-appropriate functioning, as he learns to observe and take charge of his impulses rather than be blindly driven by his traumas. This helps the child gain a sense of true power and helps repair his damaged self-esteem. *I have noticed that at this stage, a spurt of physical growth often occurs.*

As the child gains the strength to address his traumas directly, he now needs the opportunity to voice his views and ask the questions he may have regarding what actually took place with regard to the abuse and traumas. This will help him understand and repair some of his mistaken views, thereby dispelling his sense of badness, guilt, and shame. He is now able to understand his experiences from a more mature and realistic point of view, and to incorporate the recovered memories as part of the whole picture of himself and the world he lives in. The older the child is, the more verbalizing of memory there will be.

In situations where the traumas have controlled the child's thinking, feeling, impulses, and behaviors for a long time, release alone is not sufficient. One must be able to help the child channel this new energy into constructive patterns, while retraining old habitual destructive and/or self-destructive ways of being. It is important at this stage to engage the ego, to strengthen it, and to allow it to grow in a healthy way. This is akin to an arm that needs physiotherapy and exercise after the cast is taken off. The child needs to be given practical alternatives that he can practice in the playroom and then eventually transfer into his daily life. Thus, the child's energy, which had been used in a self-destructive groove expressed in misbehaviors and symptoms, is now trained to flow in a constructive, contained, alive, and helpful way.

Emotional healing can be compared to physical healing. One needs to clean a wound and, if infected, drain the pus. This is healing from inside-out. The inside-out process takes place when the child releases inner tensions and repressed feelings related to traumatic experiences, giving expression to them in a creative way, using a variety of expressive media such as art, sand play therapy, music, and so forth.

Once cleansed, the wound needs ointment and a dressing, protecting it from further hurt. This is healing from outside-in. Outside-in healing originates in the environment. For this I have created a playroom that soothes and delights the senses: sight, smell, sound, and touch. The link between these two processes, inside-out and outside-in, is the therapeutic relationship, just as the relationship between nurse and patient plays a major role in the experience and success of any medical procedure.

However, even with the most excellent care, skilled interventions, and miraculous medicines, if the wound is constantly being reopened and reinfected, it will not heal. This is where family therapy is critical to the outcome. Once cleansed and disinfected, covered with ointment, and bandaged, the wound needs to be left alone to mend. The emotional immune system of the child will take over and do the healing, but that takes time and cannot be forced.

## Practical Application of Holistic Expressive Play Therapy

Holistic Expressive Play Therapy is an integration of all the components that are brought together to create a safe place, a safe emotional womb where the child can connect to his true nature and access its wisdom and guidance in order to heal. All of the modes of creative play and self-expression, along with caregiver involvement, relationship, and milieu, are woven together to make that safe place and thus facilitate that connection. Each layer has the function and basic quality of the mother's emotional womb: attunement, protection, and nurturing, with flexible boundaries to create the vessel where the resiliency of the seed will be awakened, healing will take place, and growth will resume.

Such healing needs to take place on all levels, as each level, at all times, influences the other. The physical level is body centered and provides soothing and healing for the senses. The emotional level provides repair of attachment and the recovery of the whole range of feelings with the ability to express them creatively. On the cognitive level, the child repairs the mistaken views and faulty understanding that have so far interfered with his healing process. He becomes able to make sense of his life situation and gain a more realistic view of the world. On the spiritual level, he gains a sense of being intact, no matter what, as he remains connected to his true nature and has access to its wisdom and guidance.

We must always start from where the client is, with his primary need. A hungry child will not be interested in drawing. When one starts from where the client is, there are no clear-cut, well-defined, step-by-step procedures to follow. No formula guarantees a successful outcome. Instead, Holistic Expressive Play Therapy demands that the therapist has the ability to attune herself to both the client's and her own wisdom in order to create the methods needed for this particular client, at that particular moment.

The wonder and challenge is that no two children will deal with the combination of nature, nurture, and trauma in the same way, and the therapy will need to be reinvented for each client. In this way, the work is purely child centered, whether I follow or guide, whether I am nondirective or use structured interventions. Throughout this process, the therapist helps the child to stand his pain without dissociating, numbing, distracting, or acting it out at his own or another's expense. He will gradually learn to build a place of safety within himself and then begin to give his pain a shape, a voice, a sound, and an image, so that it can be expressed, transformed, and integrated. I will now describe how I do this in more concrete terms by considering the major components of the methods I use.

### Caregiver Involvement

When working with a child, much will depend on my ability to maintain the engagement with the child's primary caregiver, as I depend on her commitment to continue bringing the child to therapy, especially since it is long term and it will take time for progress to show. As much as possible, I want to prevent premature and sudden removal from therapy. It is antitherapeutic and destructive to start therapy, especially with a child with attachment issues, to bring him to a place where he finally feels safe enough to let go of his defenses, and then to suddenly rupture the process without proper closure. This is the first layer of safety and is essential for any work to begin.

When a committed caregiver is available, I will meet with her on a regular basis and coach her in forming a reparative relationship with the child. Often, a new caregiver will need help in understanding the seriousness of the problems she is dealing with and how to cope with them on a daily basis. She will need to learn to neither invade nor abandon the child when his behaviors trigger his personal issues. The caregiver is made aware of the child's struggles and the current stage of the therapy process in order to support what is being done.

When both are ready, I will have joint sessions to facilitate their developing relationship. Thus the child can rely more and more on not being invaded or abandoned whether in the playroom or in his home situation. I may also suggest ego strengthening, grounding, and physically releasing activities (horseback riding, swimming, martial arts) or activities that, when shared, provide an opportunity both for self-soothing and bonding (knitting, gardening, walking in nature, and bird-watching). I might also recommend massage and other forms of healing touch, as appropriate.

Even with a committed caregiver in a new home, maltreated children often need the full-time services of a treatment center that is not usually available. I therefore use my influence to create as much therapeutic support as possible within the system in which the child lives. I position myself so that I am able to influence and affect the child's life in larger and larger circles. This might also mean being in touch with teachers and school counselors.

When the system is less supportive or not capable of change, I focus more on the therapeutic relationship to provide a reparative experience and work to build positive memories. I also look for someone who might be able to be a source of nurturance and to keep an eye on the child, especially when there are protection issues involved. This might be a teacher, a school counselor, or a social worker.

## The Relationship

Just as the quality of the emotional womb of the mother and her capacity for attunement and responding to her child's needs is essential to the child's development, the therapist's capacity for attunement to the needs of each child is essential to the effectiveness of the therapeutic process. The therapist provides and constantly adjusts the amount of containment and freedom the child needs to safely explore his inner and outer world. We all know the challenges of attunement to such emotional distress, allowing ourselves to come close enough to it that the child feels our soothing presence, yet not so close that we get caught in their pain, thereby activating our own emotional issues and impeding our capacity to retain our autonomy in our response to his needs. We need to stay firm in the unique balance of nurturance, mirroring, and consistent limits that each child and each situation calls for. We must stay firm and true to our commitment to providing what is best for the child, even in the face of extreme rage and projections, at times both from the child and often from the system he lives in. Such challenges, in my experience, can only be met with an equal commitment to one's own self-knowledge and self-care.

From a grounded place, starting from the child's primary need, I will position myself at a physical and emotional distance that is comfortable for the child and create an emotional egg that provides physical, emotional, cognitive, and spiritual safety, including the following agreements:

- *Physical*: No one gets hurt here.
- *Emotional*: All feelings expressed here are accepted; no matter what you do, say, or play out, you will not be invaded or rejected.
- *Cognitive*: As best as I can, I will help you make sense of, understand, find, and speak the truth of your situation.
- *Spiritual*: I remember and see who you are, the power and sacredness of your true nature, and I am here to help you reconnect with it.

Such messages will be given in my attitude, mostly nonverbally, and they will be continuously tested as the child learns to trust in them.

## The Milieu

My goal in setting up a playroom is to create a safe and protected space that will facilitate the self-healing process and reflect its sacredness. I try to create a milieu where the child who has been bombarded with chaotic, harsh, painful, and age-inappropriate sense impressions can be exposed to a soothing and harmonious environment. The walls are painted white with a warm rosy tinge. The room is well lit with windows that look onto a garden where the child can see flowers grow and birds feeding. A small door opens out onto the garden, which can also be used as an extension of the therapy room. While setting up the elements that will be used to create this image of safety, I am conscious of appealing to as many senses as possible. When coming into the playroom, we are welcomed by the scent of lavender and lemon, the sound of the rain on the skylights, the light filtering through filmy curtains.

There is a sense that this building, which is surrounded by trees, bushes, and flowers, is a cosy, protected space and is a part of the natural world. Whether with a few items on a nature table, a large planter at my entrance, or a whole garden that is part of the play area with all the creatures that come and visit, I have found nothing as powerful as the beauty of nature to soothe and heal the senses and help connect with body and spirit.

Touch is an essential part of providing a soothing, comforting, calming experience. Yet, for most of these children, touch has been abused and distorted and, often, is a source of pain. The repair of such an experience is crucial and must be approached in the most careful, nonthreatening way. For children with whom it is appropriate and who are comfortable with dogs, my co-therapist standard poodles have been the greatest source of soothing, healing touch as they wrap themselves around the child, sit close by, intuitively finding just the right distance and amount of touch the child is comfortable with. This is something they learn to do from the time they are puppies. When a client walks in the door, the dogs are experts at showing that they are pleased to see him, letting him know clearly that his presence is important to them.

I recall a child looking at me and saying with a mixture of wonder and pleasant surprise: "He really likes me, you know." Their barking at the sound of outside noises has helped reassure many children, whose lives had been threatened, that they are safe in the playroom because no one will be allowed in. Of course the dogs are close by, whatever the child may be involved in, providing that calm, relaxed, and reassuring presence. For children who are uncomfortable with dogs, or if my co-therapists are not available that day, I have a warm water bottle inside a soft bear or a large soft stuffed animal or puppet.

I also have a large basket filled with colorful pieces of silk and colorful mohair blankets I have knitted as another helpful tool for soothing tactile experiences. I have found these particularly useful with hyperactive children, as they wrap themselves in the different colors and textures, which will slow them down enough to start relaxing. I might also give a child a small piece of silk, either of his favorite color or the color of the playroom, to take home and use for self-soothing. Baskets filled with small pieces of cloth are also wonderful for cloth fights; as the child throws the cloths with all his force, they are received as a shower of soft colors.

Nurturance, protection, and flexibility are essential elements that recapitulate the ideal qualities of the mother's emotional womb. The layout of the room is versatile. It allows freedom of movement and imagination and encourages creativity. It can be spacious and at the same time offer many enclosed cozy spaces. It can be used in a variety of ways. For example, a stage was designed in such a way that it can be used to play dress-up, build a fort, play house, or put on a concert or puppet show.

## Expressive Activities

My room is set up to accommodate choices and offers a wide variety of modes of expression, such as painting, sand-play therapy, movement, drama, and so forth. I am careful to not give children too much stimulation. I keep most of my materials behind curtains, which we lift at the pace of the client. Lifting the veils of the inner world too soon can be dangerous. Each expressive therapy has its own area that can be gradually opened or closed, so it can be adjusted to the child's needs and the level of stimulation that suits him. Each expressive therapy is one of my tools. How useful my tools will be depends on my familiarity with them and my knowing when and how to use them skillfully. It is essential that I acquire an intimate knowledge and firsthand experience of the gift and power of each expressive therapy before using it with a vulnerable and fragile child.

Some expressive therapies, such as art, sand play, dollhouse, and puppets, are used for expression and transformation of the whole range of feelings, which I refer to as healing from the inside-out. Each mode can also be used for soothing purposes, to create and provide healing imagery; this is what I refer to as healing from the outside-in. *The ratio is one inside-out intervention to three healing from the outside-in interventions.* Both are constantly woven together as I follow and guide the child's expression in whatever mode he may choose.

Other expressive activities, such as sewing, felting, knitting, cooking, and gardening, still allow for some expression but offer increased opportunity for ego strengthening, nurturing, and grounding. Each expressive therapy has its unique gift and contribution to an aspect of the healing process, at different stages of the therapy process. Some are more opening than others. My choice and the way I use each expressive therapy always involves starting from where the child is at and is informed by the child's primary need. It is essential to find the pace of release and expression the child can integrate.

Whether art, sand play, music, puppets, movement, storytelling, sewing and talking, felting, candle making, knitting and talking, cooking, gardening, walking and singing, walking and balancing on logs, walking and talking, or walking and storytelling, all of these modes are part of the play session and all are used with body-centered intention. Some of the most effective activities are those that are rhythmical and involve the use of hands and feet combined with an expressive mode, as it helps a child to be grounded and stay in his body as he voices his powerful feelings.

With all of the expressive modes available to the children, I use a person-centered approach, not in the traditional sense of being nondirective, but by being focused on the needs of each individual, according to his physical and emotional age, history, strengths, wounds, and present living situation.

## Closure

Each session has a beginning, middle, and end. The closing ritual provides the final layer that envelops the whole experience. This ritual is something the child can count on and is adapted to what feels comfortable for each client. I put a lot of emphasis on providing closure, never assuming that I will see the child again, as he may be removed without an opportunity to say goodbye. We may read a story while having a snack, then light a candle and make a wish, providing nurturance and closure. As he eats his snack out of an abalone shell, we might reflect on what he has done during the session. As he eats, sitting by the nature table where I keep crystals and seasonal flowers, he might notice the crystals and ask where they come from. We then talk about how they come from inside the earth, under the ground, thus giving him a sense that the earth holds beauty and is safe to stand on. It creates a sense that the earth is filled with light and beautiful colors and that it can support him. The more wounded a child is, the more stressful and demanding a life he goes back to, the more crucial it is to give time to close a session in a healing way, providing images of a beautiful and secure place.

## Case Study

This is a case study about Nadia, an 8-year-old child who lived with her mother, a single parent of three children who was struggling with drug addiction. A social worker was involved because of concerns from Nadia's teacher. Nadia was unusually withdrawn and lethargic. She did not respond when her teacher spoke to her, apparently always "seeming to be elsewhere." She functioned far below her age level and had few friends. She seemed generally depressed but occasionally had extreme fits of rage that were very difficult to manage.

When her mother came to the first appointment, she described her daughter as being very shy around people but also as a child who loved animals, especially cats and dogs. We arranged with the social worker for the child to be brought to therapy on a weekly basis. This was 1984, and I was working in a small basement room where children could touch the ceiling. This room had access to a kitchen and a garden.

Nadia responded with a slightly amused expression in her eyes to the enthusiastic greeting from my co-therapists Monseigneur and Dauphine. Dauphine was then a puppy; she soon curled up inside Nadia's coat. Nadia acknowledged their presence as I greeted her and introduced the three of us. We spent some time outside in the garden entrance before I invited her to follow me into the playroom. I wanted to give her time to get more comfortable with me before going inside in an enclosed space. Most of the session was spent on the floor, interacting with the dogs. She showed absolutely no interest in the toys or other media I had available. The idea of playing seemed foreign to her.

Now and again, her eyes went to the shelf where I kept the snacks. Although it was not yet the end of the session, I invited her to have some of the corn chips that she had been eyeing while we petted the dogs. It was soon apparent to me that Nadia was hungry and, as I found out in a later session, was not getting proper sleep either. Her favorite food turned out to be pancakes. I used the kitchen upstairs, and we made pancakes. At first she did a lot of watching as I stirred the ingredients. She remained standing by the stove and talked about her experiences at school and with her peers. I tended not to look directly at her, as she was uncomfortable with eye contact. I reflected her comments, gently guiding the conversation toward her home life as I continued to stir. Sometimes I encouraged her to breathe in the smell of her favorite food. Taking deep breaths helped her to relax, as I had noticed a visible tension in her shoulders and a glaze over her eyes whenever we approached anything remotely related to her home life. We occasionally interrupted the cooking to admire a bird feeding in the kitchen window.

When it was time to eat, I placed Nadia's special plate and cup on the table, along with flowers. It was spring, and I had hyacinths in a pot that week. I always tried to find flowers with strong scents, which we could later plant in her spot in the garden. She was encouraged to smell the flowers and inhale their sweet, strong scent, again breathing deeply. Nadia enjoyed the ritual and consistency of our meals together. She knew she could count on me to keep her special plate and cup in a place where no one else would touch them, for they were for her and her alone. Through our weekly meals, she was repeatedly given the experience of being cared for and prized.

When we finished eating, we washed her dishes with peppermint and eucalyptus castile soap. We cleaned the table together with warm, soapy water. This gave her an opportunity to learn how to care for things she valued. With a little encouragement, she began to enjoy squishing the soapy water with her hands while making funny sounds and giggling. She was thus given the opportunity for a reparative early childhood experience that was not too regressive, as she stood tall behind the sink. After she dried her hands carefully with a soft towel, she was encouraged to smell them, now perfumed by the cleansing scent of peppermint and eucalyptus.

She liked to have her picture taken and asked that I take a picture of her, proudly stirring the flour. Later serving her first pancake, she posed, looking straight into the camera with a big smile. These pictures would be put into her album. The photo album is a tool I use to hold and facilitate access to the positive memories created in the sessions. It is reviewed periodically and given to the child during the last session.

Nadia shared much of herself while cooking, as she felt safe, valued, and cared for. The sessions progressed, and as the cooking and eating gradually took up less of our time, I engaged Nadia in some drawing exercises. We made scribbling pictures together, taking turns as we passed the paper back and forth. This is often a favorite game of children 8 years old and older who feel they cannot draw. Each scribble represented part of the activity we had just engaged in, thus further anchoring the memory of her experience and encouraging her to find a medium of self-expression. This process evolved into making up stories about the scribbles that were increasingly expanded upon. As we continued taking turns, she was playfully encouraged to use her imagination.

Because I was eventually able to engage the social worker in helping bring about some changes in her living situation, Nadia was now eating regularly and was no longer hungry. We could then shift from stirring the milk and flour to make pancakes to stirring flour, salt, and food coloring to make play-dough. We then used the play-dough to make figures and shapes, thus moving into an art therapy process.

As Nadia stirred the flour and colors, she proceeded to share parts of herself. It should be noted that as we worked in the kitchen, we stood rather than sat. When standing, the child's feet are firmly planted on the ground; this helped Nadia feel less vulnerable while she explored difficult intrapsychic material as it began to surface. If I sense that the child is becoming triggered or flooded, going into the past, I encourage awareness of hands and feet as well as breathing, so the child can be safely grounded in the body before going any further. Any effective expression and transformation of trauma needs to be done from a grounded place to be a healing experience, or otherwise the child will be retraumatized.

Nadia proceeded to tell me that she felt like she had monsters inside of her. I asked what the monsters looked like. I sensed a door opening, an emotional block coming to the surface ready to be externalized and conversed with. I asked her what color and shape they were. I then asked if she would like to make the monsters out of the play-dough she had just finished making. As Nadia used the red play-dough to mold two red monsters, she was now giving her fears and emotions a shape, the shape of two monsters, small enough that she could hold them in her hands. Her painful feelings no longer took the form of large, frightening figures floating inside her, overwhelming her, and running the show. They were now small and manageable, and she was large and in charge of them. She was now able to be with them, observe them, reflect on them, as together we continued to get to know them and befriend them while she continued to give them a more definite shape. She was now having the experience of being with her painful feelings in a creative way, thus expressing, releasing, and transforming them as they became an owned and integrated part of her whole experience.

She said the two red monsters were like large snails that lived underwater, but that they had never grown a protective shell to go into when they were in danger. Nadia described how, because the snails did not have a protective shell, their backs were very sensitive and could easily get hurt, so they had to grow spikes on their backs to protect themselves. The spikes started appearing when they were touched on that sensitive spot by creatures that sometimes came into the water where they lived. Each time this happened, the spikes grew bigger, tougher, and the monsters became more dangerous. If they were left alone and no one bothered them, they were quite peaceful.

We continued our conversation in this symbolic language, speaking about the monsters and their painful feelings and experiences. Occasionally I offered open-ended questions to continue amplification of the image, thus allowing the image to speak without interference, only guidance. As I sensed her readiness and capacity to continue this process, I went a step further and asked if there was anything we could do to help the monsters. She said that the monsters would really like to have a blanket on their backs—something soft, shiny, and beautiful.

We looked into one of my baskets of colorful cloths, and she found some bright red satin with white stars. As Nadia searched through the colors and handled the different pieces, she had a pleasurable tactile soothing experience while simultaneously developing ego strength as she made deliberate, conscious choices as to what shape and color of fabric to choose. This intervention, along with the sound of my voice as I continued to reflect, contributed to helping her contain and slow down her feelings, yet allowed the flow of imagery that was now pouring out. The monsters with spiky backs, which I understand as healing inside-out imagery, were now being soothed and taken care of, the healing from the outside-in imagery of the blanket with stars. I gave Nadia scissors to cut the piece of cloth into two little blankets, which she put carefully on each of the monsters' spiky backs. She looked at them and sighed deeply; spontaneous sighs are always such a good sign.

Nadia then decided to create a body of water where the monsters would be safe to swim freely without fear of creatures touching them. To represent the blue water, she chose a large bright-blue piece of cloth, and to show the waves, a large piece of blue, curly uncarded wool. She noted how beautiful the monsters were as they now swam in the blue water. I asked if there was anything else they would like, and she decided to give them some of her favorite seashells to play with.

Nadia stood back to view the whole image with an expression of contentment. She was viewing her inner world, and she liked what she saw in the mirror. Her whole body was relaxed, her shoulders back, she had rosy cheeks, and her eyes shone. She asked me to take a picture of her with her image to add to her album. We agreed that I would put her image in a box for her so it could stay intact and she could look at it again the following week. This was a good place to stop the process. She was ready for us to light a candle and make a wish.

During the following session, the first thing she wanted to do was to open the box and look at the image. At my suggestion, she decided to decorate the box, as she wanted it to be as beautiful on the outside as it was on the inside. We made a colorful scribbling picture together, which we could later tape all around the box. It was then, as we took turns drawing, that I mentioned I had noticed that the monsters had been touched in a way that made them feel very uncomfortable, and I wondered if that had also happened to her. She said no, it had not happened to her. Then I told her that if that was ever the case, she could tell me, and together we could speak with her social worker. She had the small pocket calendar I had given her where her appointments were written with my card in it if she needed to call. We also added the number of her social worker. This information was not new to her, as children are told from the beginning that part of my role is, as much as possible, to help children be safe. Although she had not openly disclosed, I continued to be in regular contact with her social worker and her mother, with the focus of providing her with a safer place to live.

The next session, Nadia seemed more closed and restless and complained of having had to sit inside at school all day. It was spring and the cherry blossoms were in bloom in the neighborhood streets. I suggested that we go for a walk. Each of us had a dog on a leash as we walked under the blossoms. I asked her, on a scale of 1 to 10, how things were, starting from the least threatening topic. When talking about a situation that was too much for her, we stopped to look at and smell the blossoms.

Walking and talking, then drawing a picture before our regular closure became our weekly routine. We thus continued the healing from outside-in and ego-strengthening activities, opening up difficult topics just a little, safely, as she walked, feeling the strength of her feet on the ground. We would sometimes concentrate on one foot and then the other and experiment with different ways of stepping. While doing this, Nadia was surrounded by soothing and harmonious sensory experiences, continuing to create positive memories. It is important to stay tentative in the verbal exploration, to make sure that the child can handle such exploration. I maintained focus on her strength and her ability to cope and survive, while acknowledging but not opening her pain more than she was able to manage.

Walking side by side as we talked allowed for grounding and for energy to be released and continue to flow as we addressed a variety of topics. Walking is less threatening, especially for those who might be self-conscious and uncomfortable with eye contact, than sitting in a chair across from each other; in this way, walking facilitates verbal expression and communication. Looking at the flowers, engaging in a little obedience dog training, and offering the dogs a lot of praise as they sat by our sides before crossing a street—all of this gave safe interruptions when topics became too difficult.

We went for nature walks, talking about her feelings and struggles more openly and directly, finding solutions, making up stories, singing, using our walking sticks, and howling with Monseigneur and Dauphine—a wonderful, safe, and joyful way of expressing and releasing the feelings she had no words for. We walked and sang and made up songs and stories about her life, each taking a turn, as we had taken turns making scribbling pictures.

After a child draws a picture, I encourage the telling of a story. Being their secretary, I write down, in their favorite color on another sheet of paper, word for word what they tell me. At first the story might consist of simple sentences that describe what is in the picture; the picture is still like a tableau. However, little by little, mostly through reflecting and the odd open-ended question, the image is amplified and comes to life. Not only does this encourage the child's imagination, but it also gives further opportunity for expression and communication of the child's inner world. My part is to facilitate that communication and allow a direct interaction between the client and her own image, without imposing my interpretations that could very well be projections.

Up to that point, Nadia had drawn stick figures to represent people, but after this particular walk she drew a picture of the two of us walking in the forest. She drew us as two full-bodied people wearing similar sweaters, Monseigneur and Dauphine as two black shapes with four legs and a tail. In the background, Nadia had drawn an owl sitting in a large tree. This is what she dictated: "Nadia, Marie-José, Monseigneur, and Dauphine are walking in the woods. They are having fun. An owl lives in the tree and is sitting and watching. The owl sees everything, especially at night, even things she does not tell. The end."

She was then invited to sign her name at the bottom of the story and write the date; this helps close and come back to the present, moving back from her inner to outer world. I sensed that this was as much as she could do that day, so I did not say: "I noticed that the owl sees a lot at night that she does not tell. I wonder if that might also be the case for you." Instead, we had our closing ritual. She picked up one of the large crystals on the nature table and quietly admired it. She opened her calendar and put a star on the day of her next appointment, and as we had routinely done, we respectfully shook hands and said *Au revoir*.

During the following session, Nadia decided that she wanted to use modeling clay to make a butterfly, and she asked me to make a flower for it to land on. As we each made our own image, I reflected what she was doing and we talked. When I asked about what the owl saw, Nadia disclosed that at times some of the night visitors—friends of her mother's who did not want to go home after a party—had come to the living-room couch where Nadia was sleeping and touched her on her private parts in the middle of the night, while she pretended to sleep. She said she did not say anything because she thought it was her fault because some of it felt good. With my support, Nadia told the social worker what had happened. While Nadia was not removed from her home, as far as we knew, her mother stopped having her night visitors.

We continued our walks between sessions, where she processed more directly the trauma of the abuse through drawing and talking, addressing the issues of guilt and shame that plagued her. Nadia was later able to express and release her anger and voice it clearly, as we went walking and stomping and letting the abusers know what she thought of them. Then we would walk back to the playroom, singing: "We are the stompers, we are not afraid." We continued to make up songs that went with the stomping. I also taught her an aboriginal song I had found very helpful: "O Great Spirit, Sun, Sky and Sea, you are inside and all around me," which she learned to sing at the top of her lungs. She also practiced imagining singing it aloud and experienced that it was also very reassuring. In that way she could use it anytime, anywhere, whether she was in a position to make sounds or not.

A year had gone by, and I was told by the school counselor, who was now involved, that although she was still shy with adults and reserved with her peers, Nadia was generally more present, she took part in school activities, and she was now part of a friendship group. Her mother was rarely available to meet, but I heard from her mother's therapist that, despite her good intentions, the mother's addictions came and went and that she missed a lot of her sessions before terminating without warning or closure. The chaos and neglect in Nadia's home, although less extreme, apparently continued.

Nadia's therapy ended abruptly as her mother suddenly moved. I was told by the social worker that, wherever they had moved, she would make sure another social worker would be involved. We never said good-bye. I was never able to locate her and give her her album. I never heard from her again.

Many years later, after I also had moved away, a therapist I had mentored called me and told me that a young woman had come to her office with her little child; she had referred herself, saying that her child needed play therapy. When she came in for her appointment, she looked around the room as if in amazement, her face lit up, and she exclaimed: "You have all the same things as Marie-José!" and proceeded to tell of her time in the playroom. I gathered that her life had continued, both as a child and later as a young adult, to be difficult and chaotic. She was also now a single mother, but she had voluntarily looked for help for herself and for her child, for whom she strongly believed that play therapy would be helpful—and it was.

## Conclusion

One needs to be realistic and understand that, for maltreated children, coming to terms with their relationship to their family of origin and the multiple traumas they were subjected to is a lifelong journey that involves healing the consequences of distorted attachment and multiple forms of abuse and neglect. These issues will reappear at different developmental stages and will need to be dealt with repeatedly. However, the reparative experience of another reality—the experience of having been witnessed and valued—can, even if we are unable to change their living situation, make a difference and affect the future course of children's lives.

I have witnessed that, despite all of the obstacles, the drive to form strong affectional bonds, to love and be loved, and for growth and healing is as tenacious as the child who keeps on falling and getting up until she can walk. It is as powerful as the drive of the plant that grows through concrete to reach the sunlight and as compelling as the instinct of migrating birds to come home. We can facilitate the awakening and reconnection to this drive, so that our clients will discover the power of their resiliency. They can count on this power to guide them as they learn to live with their pain more healthily and learn to find and maintain the strength and resolve to gradually transform their painful and traumatic beginnings. The goal of the journey is to transform the poison into medicine.

# Reference

Steiner, R. (1923). *Knowledge of higher worlds and its attainment*. London, England: Anthroposophical Publishing Company.

# Social Skills Play Groups for Children With Disruptive Behavior Disorders

|  |
| --- |
| *6* |
| Chapter |

## Integrating Play and Group Therapy Approaches

### *Julie Blundon Nash and Charles E. Schaefer*

## Introduction

As Hartup (1992) aptly stated, "the single best predictor of adult adaptation is not I.Q., not school grades, and not classroom behavior, but rather the adequacy with which the child gets along with other children." The quality of peer relations in childhood predicts children's adjustment across academic, emotional, and social domains, and can also predict the quality of later friendships and adult intimate relationships (e.g., Kupersmidt & Coie, 1990; Masten & Coatsworth, 1995; Parker & Asher, 1987). Social competence can be defined as the capacity to initiate, develop, and maintain satisfying relationships with others, especially peers. Social skills are the specific skills or proficiencies that are needed to develop and maintain social competence. Among these skills are behaviors that increase positive social interactions, such as cooperation and initiating conversations, and behaviors that decrease negative interactions, such as conflict resolution and social problem solving.

Social skills are typically taught in a group setting, so children can receive immediate reinforcement for appropriate modeling. Within a play therapy framework, therapists often use games, metaphors, stories, and role-plays to foster positive emotions and enhance skill-building and learning. This chapter outlines the therapeutic factors inherent in both group and play therapies, and describes a coaching model of social skills training utilizing play group therapy that has been effective in teaching social skills to children with disruptive behavior disorders.

# Integrating the Therapeutic Powers of Group and Play Therapy

## Group Therapy

The field of group therapy has greatly expanded since its inception in the 1940s to provide treatment for a wide range of psychological and medical disorders (Yalom & Leszcz, 2005). The particular benefit of group therapy is the component of interpersonal interaction. When people are encouraged to meet others with similar concerns and discuss these issues in a supportive and constructive environment, they have structured opportunities to interact with their peers. Through these interactions, people are given the ability to examine their own maladaptive patterns. This facilitation of introspection and support of the process of personal change creates effective group therapy (Yalom & Leszcz, 2005).

Group therapy can be provided using any number of theoretical approaches, such as cognitive-behavioral, psychodynamic, and play-based approaches. Underneath each of these approaches lies specific therapeutic factors. Yalom and Leszcz (2005) outlined the following 10 therapeutic powers or change mechanisms inherent in group therapy: instillation of hope, universality, imparting information, altruism, the corrective recapitulation of the primary family group, vicarious learning, interpersonal learning, group cohesiveness, catharsis, and existential factors.

### Instillation of Hope

Instillation of hope means awakening in clients not only their ability to change but also their expectation that the therapeutic process will be successful. Group members are often at different points along the continuum of change. By interacting with peers who have developed a larger skill set, group members can see possibilities for their own future, which is a strong encouragement to begin and continue therapy.

### Universality

The concept of universality means that group members come to realize that they are not alone in their problems or concerns. Group therapy is particularly suited to introducing clients to others who are going through similar situations or experiencing comparable symptoms. While some cultures encourage the idea of uniqueness, this can be a very lonely concept for people with psychological distress.

### Imparting Information

Group therapy allows clients to receive information from both peers and group leaders about their symptoms, diagnoses, and coping skills. Group leaders may choose to give direct information through didactic teaching methods and/or group members may give specific advice to peers. Clients are then able to alleviate their irrational fears, replace misconceptions with appropriate knowledge, or learn new skills.

### Altruism
The process of giving help and support while receiving the same is important to the therapeutic impact of group therapy. While this concept is specifically outlined in some group therapy settings (i.e., Alcoholics Anonymous, where group members who maintain sobriety are encouraged to give support to new members), many groups encourage altruism through the simple interactions of group members.

### The Corrective Recapitulation of the Primary Family Group
The group therapy model includes group leaders/therapists and group members. This structure encourages many of the interactions inherent in the primary family group, which, for many clients, has not been the most supportive environment. Therapists are often seen as parental figures while peers can take the roles of siblings or other relatives. Within the group setting, many relationship dynamics can play out in a corrective manner, such as parent-child interactions, sibling conflict, the expression of intimate feelings in a supportive environment, and so on.

### Vicarious Learning
By observing and then imitating the behavior of others and therapists in a group, clients can improve their own social skills. Clients can observe others in dealing with a similar problem and learn a new way to solve the issue, or they may benefit from watching similar peers be successful. Imitative behavior also allows a person to try a variety of approaches to life and determine both what does and does not work for them personally.

### Interpersonal Learning
Clients usually play out their typical patterns of interpersonal interactions within the group setting. This allows other group members to give feedback as to problematic patterns of interaction. The client can then learn and practice new skills in the moment.

### Group Cohesiveness
The close relationships that develop among group members are similar to that of a therapist and client in individual therapy. The therapeutic bonds among group members help ensure that the members maintain motivation to persevere in the hard work of psychotherapy.

### Catharsis
Group therapy allows for the release of negative emotions within a supportive setting. Members can learn how to talk freely about things that are bothering them and generally let go of feelings that are bothersome and often counterproductive to treatment.

*Existential Factors*
Acknowledging existential factors refers to the process of recognizing that there are some things over which a person does not have complete control. For example, clients will have to deal with issues like death, significant responsibility, and the uncontrollable actions of others at some point in their lives. Having a group in which others are dealing with similar factors and learning that one has the ability to take ultimate responsibility for his or her own life and situations can be very powerful.

## Play Therapy

The field of play therapy has grown substantially since Freud first worked with Little Hans (Freud, 1909). From the early roots in psychoanalytic traditions, to the use of miniatures in sandtrays (e.g., Klein, 1955; Lowenfeld, 1939), to humanistic approaches (Axline, 1947), play therapists have expanded the field to include numerous theoretical orientations. There are also multiple formats in which to provide play therapy, including individual, family, and group work. Play therapy can be utilized with any age group throughout the life span, with a particular focus on children between the ages of 3 and 12. The use of play therapy suggests that a clinician believes in the multiple healing powers of play.

The eight major therapeutic powers of play that have been described by Schaefer (1993) and Schaefer and Drewes (2009) are as follows: communication, emotional regulation, relationship enhancement, moral judgment, stress management, ego boosting, preparation for life, and self-actualization.

*Communication*
Verbal communication is difficult for young children, because they have limited vocabulary and lack abstract thinking ability. Play, on the other hand, is one of the most natural forms of communication for a child and is universal. A child from Japan will be able to interact with a child from the Netherlands without speaking, if they play together. Because play is such an innate and basic method of sharing internal needs, conflicts, and masteries, it is an effective way for people across ages to communicate (i.e., a therapist and a child). Children can also use play to gain some emotional distance from the issue at hand and deal with both conscious and unconscious issues.

*Emotional Regulation*
Play allows clients to alleviate the intensity of negative feelings (Schaefer, 1999). A child can use play to cathartically release emotions that have been bottled up or to reenact and master reactions to traumatic situations through abreaction (Terr, 1990). These processes allow a child to gain control over his or her emotional responses to stressful events, thus regulating internal states. In addition, the many positive emotions arising in play can effectively counteract such negative feelings, such as boredom, depression, and anxiety (Schaefer, 1999).

*Relationship Enhancement*
Play creates a positive emotional bond between the players. Thus, play can be used to foster and improve the relationship between child and parent. Studies have shown that involving parents or caregivers in play interactions with their children (often through structured or coached sessions) can improve parental empathy, the family climate, and children's self-concept (Rennie & Landreth, 2000).

*Moral Judgment*
The development of moral judgment is fostered when children develop rules for interacting with others. Piaget (1932) noted that the formation of these rules allowed a child to learn the skills necessary for future morality. By mutually creating rules with peers during game play, children move past the belief that all rules are imposed by authority figures.

*Stress Management*
When children face new experiences, they often experience anticipatory anxiety. These anxieties can lead to considerable distress. Play allows a child to overcome fear of an upcoming event by playing it out in advance using miniature toys. In this way they can safely practice coping skills and make the strange more familiar by repeated practice.

*Ego Boosting*
In free play, children have complete power and control. They are in charge of the play and are physically larger than the objects they are controlling. This power enhances the child's inner locus of control and overcomes personal vulnerabilities and feelings of helplessness.

*Preparation for Life*
People are constantly learning or practicing new ways to approach previously unknown situations. For example, the high school student who needs to give an oral report may practice in front of a mirror, or a person preparing for a job interview may think of possible questions that may be asked by an interviewer to prepare answers. Children are faced with many new experiences on a routine basis and often do not have the time or opportunity to practice these experiences in the moment. Using play to practice and try out multiple approaches will help them overcome fears, promote mastery, and find appropriate solutions to the task.

*Self-Actualization*
Play is the one arena where children have the freedom to be completely themselves. Play allows a child to think for himself or herself; learn about his or her limits, desires, and needs; and develop self-understanding and self-confidence. In nondirective play therapy, therapists accept children as they are without judgment or conditions.

The following is a description of an intervention that integrates a number of the therapeutic powers of play and group therapy to resolve the social difficulties of disruptive children.

## Play Group Therapy for Social Skills Deficits in Disruptive Children

When utilizing the therapeutic factors of a theory, it is important for the clinician to recognize how they can be tailored to particular problems and settings. Social skills training is best performed in a group format, as suggested by a number of Yalom's therapeutic factors of group therapy (Yalom & Leszcz, 2005). For example, installation of hope, universality, imparting information, vicarious learning, and interpersonal learning are change agents specifically applied in group training of social skills. In regard to the therapeutic factors of play, the ones most often used for social skills training include direct instruction, emotional regulation, moral judgment, stress management, and preparation for life.

Children with disruptive behavior disorders often need support from each of these curative factors of both group and play therapy theories. For the purposes of this chapter, "disruptive behavior disorders" will refer to a range of difficulties that include oppositional defiant disorder, attention deficit/hyperactivity disorder, and social anxieties that are manifest in negative behaviors in social settings. Children with these difficulties often are social isolates or are rejected by their peers because of their antisocial behaviors.

Children referred for social skills training exhibit a variety of social deficits, including shyness, bossiness, and social aggression (e.g., Bullis, Walker, & Sprague, 2001; DeRosier, 2004; Lane et al., 2003; Lo, Loe, & Cartledge, 2002). Training groups may include both socially inhibited and aggressive children. By mixing children with different presenting problems, it is hoped that the shy children will become more assertive and the disruptive children less aggressive. Other groups target a single disorder, such as attention deficit/ hyperactivity disorder (e.g., Antshel & Remer, 2003; Gol & Jarus, 2005), conduct disorder (e.g., Ison, 2001; Webster-Stratton & Hammond, 1997), Asperger's syndrome (e.g., Barry, Klinger, & Lee, 2003; Weiss & Harris, 2001), and social anxiety (e.g., Beidel, Turner, Young, & Paulson, 2005; Spence, Donovan, & Brechman-Toussaint, 1999). The advantage of these single-symptom groups (such as for disruptive behaviors) is that specific social deficits can be targeted more directly.

By imparting information to these children about social skills in a peer group setting that involves fun and play, children are using a more naturalistic environment than individual talk-based therapy to develop socialization techniques. They practice the skills and prepare to use the skills in daily life through imitative behavior and interpersonal learning, and the play encourages reduction of social anxieties, or emotional regulation. Children see that other children struggle with similar difficulties, thus engaging the concept of universality, which instills hope. They are naturally able to communicate with each other and the therapists, and they learn ways to change their own behaviors to improve their acceptance by peers.

Within group sessions, instruction and practice of new behaviors typically occurs through games, role-plays, use of metaphors, and other play activities. The positive emotions that result encourage optimal learning conditions for children, thus maintaining interest and motivation as well as enhancing the retention of information. Linking social skills instruction with positive emotions has been shown to help children remember the new material, especially for elementary school-aged children (Hartmann & Rollett, 1994).

Oden and Asher (1977) were among the first to present the coaching model of group social skills training that has become the most widely used training model in the field. As opposed to individual training or educational groups without immediate practice of skills, the coaching model consists of (a) education to teach new skills, (b) practice to increase skill performance, and (c) performance review with therapists. This training model involves both individual and group instruction and practice to give children more opportunities to fully learn and practice the skills. To generalize skills to daily life, outside practice must occur, which is promoted by homework assignments.

A meta-analysis of research on social skills groups (Lösel & Beelmann, 2003) found that the majority of training models consist of 10 sessions or less (41.5%), while 11 to 30 sessions is the next most common duration (33.3%). Group leaders are usually mental health professionals (25.9%), teachers (23%), or supervised students (22.2%). Cognitive-behavioral and behavioral models are the most common theoretical modalities (39.3% and 28.9%).

## Case Example

A review of the literature indicated that social skills training models typically involve instruction in four general domains of social skills: communication, interaction, self-control, and feelings (Blundon & Schaefer, 2006). Communication includes such skills as initiating and maintaining conversations, making and maintaining appropriate eye contact, and recognizing and understanding interpersonal cues. Interaction skills include taking turns, being assertive instead of aggressive or passive, sharing and cooperating, and showing empathy. Impulsivity control and solving social problems appropriately are examples of self-control skills. Skills associated with feelings include identifying and naming emotions, and expressing and regulating emotions appropriately.

Based on this literature review, a manualized 10-week psychoeducational model of social skills training that involves coaching, modeling, operant conditioning, and reinforcement techniques was developed (Blundon & Schaefer, 2007). This curriculum is play-based in that the training is conducted through the use of games, role-plays, metaphors, storytelling, and art activities. The skills are presented in a group format to best utilize peer interactions and the resulting therapeutic factors of group therapy.

A basic assumption of the program is that children best learn skills when therapists present strategies in a playful manner that is fun and interactive (Hartmann & Rollett, 1994). Children are introduced to specific skills to be practiced through a three-phase modeling procedure: therapist-to-therapist, therapist-to-child, and child-to-child. The 10 social skills covered in this curriculum are starting and joining conversations, group entry, handling rejection, assertiveness, social problem solving, cooperation, complimenting, awareness of feelings in the self, awareness of feelings in others, and good sportsmanship.

During each of the 10 sessions, children are introduced to one of these topics. Group leaders verbally explain the skill and steps involved before beginning practice. For example, when children are learning about assertiveness, a leader describes passivity, assertiveness, and aggression, and then acts out examples of each as a way to solve a social problem. Two leaders then model how to be assertive in an imaginary interaction. Children practice this skill with leaders in front of the group and separately in dyads. Once the learning portion is completed, children continue to practice through games. They enjoy watching leaders demonstrate a problem-solving technique and telling the leaders if passive, assertive, or aggressive methods were being used. The children then act out how the leaders should have solved the problem, using the appropriate assertiveness skills they just learned.

When learning about an awareness of feelings in the self, children create a word bank with a large variety of feelings words. They play Feelings Charades with the group and leaders to demonstrate an understanding of each emotion (Blundon & Schaefer, 2007). Once they have practiced with several other games and interactions, children learn about empathy. A leader places five cards around the group room that indicate various emotions (e.g., happy, sad, scared, confused, and angry). The leader begins to tell an imaginary story about herself, stopping when she would likely experience an emotion. The children run to the various cards to indicate how the leader is likely feeling. For example, the leader might say, "I was out walking my dog, and it was a beautiful day!" followed by "Then it started to rain, and I stepped in a puddle." The children explain their choices and often begin to discuss the ability to feel more than one emotion in reaction to a situation.

This training program was evaluated using a quasi-experimental design in which 46 children participated in social skills play group therapy (Nash, 2008). Although the original research was intended to evaluate the differences in effectiveness among various training models, the data were also analyzed to view children's progress regardless of treatment condition. Treatment conditions included child training alone and variations of parent involvement in the training. All children received the same training regardless of treatment condition. Results indicated that children showed significant improvements in their social behaviors when specific social skills were measured by both parents and therapists in all models of training ($p < 0.001$). Overall, no treatment model was shown to be more effective than another. Children's results were stable across conditions, showing that this play group therapy program was effective in improving children's social skills regardless of parents' treatment programs.

Anecdotally, children tend to report that they enjoyed this social skills play group program. They start the program by showing their typical inappropriate patterns of interactions, but soon these patterns are modified or outright rejected by their peers. Over time, children take ownership of the group rules and norms, and they encourage their peers to appropriately participate in activities. Teachers have told therapists about children who have gone into school and told their peers about what they have learned and about the fun games they played. Children come to sessions and ask to teach their parents the skills. Parents have noticed changes in their children's behaviors at home, school, and in peer interactions. Overall, very positive reports have been made regarding this intervention, and the data reflect the program's effectiveness.

## Conclusion

The research regarding this play group therapy intervention provides further empirical support for the effectiveness of a coaching model of social skills training for children. Following this coaching model, therapists explain and model specific social skills to children and have the children practice the skills in session through group game play, role-plays, and use of metaphor. The fun and excitement of playing games together keeps the children interested and motivated to practice the skills until they are mastered. This integrated therapy approach combines the therapeutic powers of play therapy and group therapy, and the results suggest that the combination is useful and effective.

## References

Antshel, K. M., & Remer, R. (2003). Social skills training in children with attention deficit hyperactivity disorder: A randomized-controlled clinical trial. *Journal of Clinical Child and Adolescent Psychology, 32,* 153–165.

Axline, V. M. (1947). *Play therapy.* New York, NY: Ballantine Books.

Barry, T. D., Klinger, L. G., & Lee, J. M. (2003). Examining the effectiveness of an outpatient clinic-based social skills group for high-functioning children with autism. *Journal of Autism and Developmental Disorders, 33,* 685–701.

Beidel, D. C., Turner, S. M., Young, B., & Paulson, A. (2005). Social effectiveness therapy for children: Three-year follow-up. *Journal of Consulting and Clinical Psychology, 73,* 721–725.

Blundon, J., & Schaefer, C. (2006). The use of play group therapy for children with social skills deficits. In H. Kaduson & C. Schaefer

(Eds.), *Short-term play therapy for children* (2nd ed., pp. 336–375). New York, NY: Guilford Press.

Blundon, J., & Schaefer, C. (2007). *Play group therapy for social skills deficits in children (ages 4-12 years): A ten session training manual.* (Available from C. Schaefer, Department of Psychology, Fairleigh Dickinson University, T-WH01-1, 1000 River Road, Teaneck, NJ, 07666).

Bullis, M., Walker, H. M., & Sprague, J. R. (2001). A promise unfulfilled: Social skills training with at-risk and antisocial children and youth. *Exceptionality, 9,* 67–90.

DeRosier, M. E. (2004). Building relationships and combating bullying: Effectiveness of a school-based social skills group intervention. *Journal of Clinical Child and Adolescent Psychology, 33,* 196–201.

Freud, S. (1909). *Analysis of a phobia in a five-year old boy.* London, England: Hogarth Press.

Gol, D., & Jarus, T. (2005). Effect of a social skills training group on everyday activities of children with attention deficit hyperactivity disorder. *Developmental Medicine & Child Neurology, 47,* 539–545.

Hartmann, W., & Rollett, B. (1994). Play: Positive intervention in the elementary school curriculum. In J. Hellendoorn, R. van der Kooij, and B. Sutton-Smith (Eds.), *Play and intervention* (pp. 195–202). Albany: State University of New York Press.

Hartup, W. W. (1992). *Having friends, making friends, and keeping friends: Relationships as educational contexts* (Report No. EDO-PS-92-4). Urbana, IL: ERIC Clearinghouse on Elementary and Early Childhood Education. (ERIC Document Reproduction Service No. ED345845.)

Klein, M. (1955). The psychoanalytic play technique. In C. E. Schaefer (Ed.), *The therapeutic use of child's play* (pp. 125–140). Northvale, NJ: Jason Aronson. (Reprinted from *American Journal of Orthopsychiatry, 25,* 223–237.)

Ison, M. S. (2001). Training in social skills: An alternative technique for handling disruptive child behavior. *Psychological Reports, 88,* 903–911.

Kupersmidt, J. B., & Coie, J. D. (1990). Preadolescent peer status, aggression, and school adjustment as predictors of externalizing problems in adolescence. *Child Development, 61,* 1350–1362.

Lane, K. L., Wehby, J., Menzies, H. M., Doukas, G. L., Munton, S. M., & Gregg, R. M. (2003). Social skills instruction for students at risk for antisocial behavior: The effects of small-group instruction. *Behavioral Disorders, 28,* 229–248.

Lo, Y., Loe, S. A., & Cartledge, G. (2002). The effects of social skills instruction on the social behaviors of students at risk for emotional or behavioral disorders. *Behavioral Disorders, 27,* 37–38.

Lösel, F., & Beelmann, A. (2003). Effects of child skills training in preventing antisocial behavior: A systematic review of randomized evaluations. *Annals of the American Academy of Political and Social Science, 587,* 84–109.

Lowenfeld, M. (1939). The world pictures of children: A method of recording and studying them. *British Journal of Medical Psychology, 18,* 65–101.

Masten, A. S., & Coatsworth, J. D. (1995). Competence, resilience, and psychopathology. In D. Cicchetti & D. J. Cohen (Eds.), *Developmental Psychopathology, Vol. 2: Risk, disorder, and adaptation* (pp. 715–752). New York, NY: John Wiley & Sons.

Nash, J. B. (2008). Children's social skills training: Relative effectiveness of three training models (Doctoral dissertation, Fairleigh Dickinson University, 2008). *Dissertation Abstracts International, 69(6-B),* 38–57.

Oden, S., & Asher, S. R. (1977). Coaching children in social skills for friendship making. *Child Development, 48,* 495–506.

Parker, J. G., & Asher, S. R. (1987). Peer relations and later personal adjustment: Are low-accepted children at risk? *Psychological Bulletin, 102,* 357–389.

Piaget, J. (1932). *The moral judgment of the child.* New York, NY: Harcourt.

Rennie, R., & Landreth, G. (2000). Effects of filial therapy on parent and child behaviors. *International Journal of Play Therapy, 9(2),* 19–37.

Schaefer, C. E. (1993). *The therapeutic powers of play.* Northvale, NJ: Jason Aronson.

Schaefer, C. E. (1999). Curative factors in play therapy. *The Journal for the Professional Counselor, 14(1),* 7–16.

Schaefer, C. E., & Drewes, A. A. (2009). The therapeutic powers of play and play therapy. In A. A. Drewes (Ed.), *Blending play therapy with cognitive behavioral therapy: Evidence-based and other effective treatments and techniques.* Hoboken, NJ: Wiley.

Spence, S. H., Donovan, C., & Brechman-Toussaint, M. (1999). Social skills, social outcomes, and cognitive features of childhood social phobia. *Journal of Abnormal Psychology, 108,* 211–221.

Terr, L. (1990). *Too scared to cry: Psychic trauma in childhood.* New York, NY: HarperCollins.

Webster-Stratton, C., & Hammond, M. (1997). Treating children with early-onset conduct problems: A comparison of child and parent training interventions. *Journal of Consulting and Clinical Psychology, 65,* 93–109.

Weiss, M. J., & Harris, S. L. (2001). Teaching social skills to people with autism. *Behavior Modification, 25,* 785–802.

Yalom, I. D., & Leszcz, M. (2005). *The theory and practice of group psychotherapy* (5th ed). New York, NY: Basic Books.

# Integrative Play Therapies for Internalizing Disorders of Childhood

# Cognitive-Behavioral Play Therapy for Traumatized Children

|  |
| --- |
| *7* |
| Chapter |

## Narrowing the Divide Between Ideology and Evidence

### *Janine Shelby and Karina G. Campos*

## Introduction

The benefits of directive (i.e., therapist-led) versus nondirective (i.e., child-led) play therapy have been debated by play therapists for decades. Recent discussions, however, include greater emphasis on integrating the two approaches. Several authors have proposed specific methods of integrating directive and nondirective play therapy approaches for child trauma treatment (Gil & Jalazo, 2009; Goodyear-Brown, 2009; Shelby, 2010; Shelby & Felix, 2005). Also, several authors have advocated blending play therapy with cognitive-behavioral therapy (CBT; Drewes, 2009; Knell, 1993, 2009; Schaefer, 1999; Shelby & Berk, 2009). Even outside the field of play therapy, several authors have described the importance of developmental sensitivity in CBT (Holmbeck, Greenley, & Franks, 2003; Ollendick & Vasey, 1999; Peterson & Tremblay, 1999; Shirk, 2001; Weisz & Hawley, 2002), with some proposing that play methods be increasingly integrated into cognitive-behavioral therapies (Grave & Blissett, 2004).

Despite this increased interest in integrated approaches, the directive versus nondirective play therapy debate has not yet been settled by research and continues to surface in play therapy literature. Attempts to integrate play therapy treatments—either internally among various play therapy approaches or externally with CBT—have been hindered by conceptual difficulties defining play therapy (e.g., play as a vehicle to teach CBT skills, or play as a change mechanism) and identifying what, precisely, constitutes a developmentally sensitive treatment (e.g., use of simplified language, inclusion of age-salient content, implementation of treatment via play therapy or pedagogical methods specifically designed for the age level, or selection of treatment components

107

based on the cognitive capacity or developmental level of the child). Finally, the dearth of randomized controlled trials comparing play therapy or play therapy integrated treatments to well-supported child trauma treatments (e.g., Trauma-Focused CBT [Cohen, Mannarino, & Deblinger, 2006]; Alternative Families CBT [Kolko & Swenson, 2002]) makes it difficult to draw empirical conclusions regarding the efficacy of integrated directive/nondirective or CBT/play therapy blended treatments.

Despite the challenges, we postulate that *evidence* from cognitive-behavioral treatments for young children and play therapy *ideology* are complementary in nature. In fact, considerable overlap may exist between some processes that occur in effective child-led play therapy and the hypothesized change mechanisms of CBT (Shelby, 2010). To demonstrate our point, we will describe separate treatment vignettes involving, first, CBT, and then, child-led play therapy for the same young trauma survivor. Then, we will describe a third vignette, referred to here as cognitive-behavioral play therapy for trauma (CBPTT), which involves elements of directive, and nondirective play therapy as well as CBT. Following a brief discussion contrasting the three treatments, we will highlight our view that an integrationist perspective is often advantageous for young survivors, who benefit from effective, skills-based, engaging, and developmentally sensitive treatments.

## Explanations and Disclosures

Our goal is to give readers a general impression of each treatment, rather than to delineate full treatment protocols (see Trauma-Focused CBT [Cohen, Mannarino, & Deblinger, 2006] and Alternative Families CBT [Kolko & Swenson, 2002], as well as Child-Centered Play Therapy [Landreth, 1991] and Psychodynamic Play Therapy [Axline, 1947, 1964] for more detailed descriptions of the treatments loosely described in our vignettes). Therefore, we will provide a greatly abbreviated and condensed version of selected aspects of each treatment approach. Also, we present hypothesized positive outcomes in each of the treatments we portray in an effort to present a balanced view of three potentially successful therapies. The first two treatment descriptions are fictionalized (i.e., hypothesized based on treatment experiences with other, similar children), but the third therapy description closely resembles the course of treatment the youngster actually received. As a final caveat, we recognize the existence of several research-based dyadic treatments—offering a different sort of integrated, developmentally sensitive treatment—but discussion of these therapies is beyond the scope of this chapter, which is written to compare individual psychotherapies for traumatized children.

## Case Example

Last year, 5-year-old Stephen was brought to our child trauma clinic by his devastated and guilt-ridden mother, Lauren. A month earlier, the single mother had been shuffling her three children into the family car, ensuring that lunches were packed, homework assignments were in hand, jackets were worn, and faces were, at least mostly, free of the milk moustaches acquired from breakfast. As Stephen pretended to punch his older brother in the arm, he accidentally ripped his older sister's art project, which then required Lauren to settle and calm the children. It was a particularly trying morning.

"Let's just get going," Lauren thought. She put the car in reverse gear and began backing the car out of the driveway. Suddenly, she heard her youngest child scream, and she realized that the car door on his side was open. To her horror, Lauren turned to see her son fall out of his car seat, which had somehow failed to latch. With a thud, he fell onto the pavement. Lauren immediately stepped on the brake, got out of the car, and ran to her son. However, in her panic to reach him, she failed to put the reversing car into the park gear, and she subsequently watched with disbelief as her car ran over her child. Stephen sustained extensive pelvic injuries, but remarkably, he fared quite well from a medical perspective.

A month after the accident, he appeared in the child trauma clinic in his wheelchair, endorsing numerous symptoms of posttraumatic stress disorder (PTSD). Stephen had intrusive and recurrent thoughts of the traumatic event, physiological arousal upon exposure to reminders of the event, pronounced avoidance of sitting in his car seat, and avoidance of riding in—or even discussing—cars. In fact, the family used public transportation to arrive at the session because Stephen refused car travel. In addition, he exhibited hypervigilance and excessive startle response. He experienced nightmares but endorsed this symptom only if the therapist referred to them as "morningmares," because his bad dreams always seemed to happen to him in the morning, immediately before his mother woke him up to get ready for school. He also reported other symptoms known to occur among young traumatized children (Pynoos et al., 2009), such as stomachaches and headaches, and the loss of previously acquired skills, including the ability to separate from his mother and fall asleep on his own.

## Three Possible Treatments

### Treatment Option 1: CBT
*Basic Tenets*
A basic premise of CBT is that thoughts influence behaviors and feelings, but that altering any of the three components of this cognitive triangle results in changes among the other two. Although originally attributed to the work of Beck (Beck, Rush, Shaw, & Emery, 1979) and Ellis and Gieger (1986), several specific CBTs now exist for childhood anxiety disorders. Elements common among most child trauma CBTs include the following: (a) thorough assessment and diagnostic formulation; (b) the development or enhancement of adaptive coping strategies; (c) psychoeducation; (d) hierarchical exposure to excessively or inappropriately feared stimuli; (e) the alteration of thoughts, behaviors, and feelings to alter anxiety level; (f) cognitive restructuring regarding misattributions or excessive guilt; and (g) caregiver involvement in the treatment to promote caregiver

understanding, skill-building, and reinforcement of therapy techniques used with the child (Kendall et al., 2005; Shelby & Berk, 2009). Exposure is an important constituent of the treatment. That is, as children experience—either real or imagined—anxiety-provoking situations under safe conditions, they learn to manage their distress related to the exposure.

## Research

There is little doubt as to the effectiveness of CBT for childhood and adolescent anxiety, with response rates ranging from 65% (Kendall et al., 2005) to 93% (Cohen, Mannarino, & Deblinger, 2006). Given that CBTs offer such benefit to older children, it is unfortunate that so few studies have examined the experience of children younger than 8 years of age (Grave & Blissett, 2004).

## Stephen Receives CBT

Session 1: In the first session, the therapist conducts an assessment (i.e., including use of standardized instruments, caregiver report, behavioral observations, and child interview) and assigns a diagnosis, which is then matched to a treatment known to be helpful for that particular disorder or condition. Stephen's symptoms are targeted and monitored throughout the course of therapy. After learning more about the therapy, Stephen and his mother agree to participate in future sessions.

Session 2: Stephen and his mother receive psychoeducation, via didactic instruction and reading materials that provide specific information about typical symptoms following traumatic events. The mother also learns more about CBT, the importance of practicing CBT skills at home, common response rates to treatment, and helpful caregiver behaviors.

Session 3: In this session, the therapist teaches Stephen to identify different emotions by showing him a poster with cartoon faces depicting different feelings. Stephen then learns how to recognize his experiences of calm and fear, so that he can later employ anxiety-reduction strategies to decrease his distress and recognize when these strategies are successful. Then, after the therapist conducts a functional assessment of Stephen's symptoms, the therapist targets each of his most pronounced symptoms and determines the antecedent, behavior, and consequence of each. The therapist helps mother and son create a plan to respond to trauma triggers in adaptive ways (e.g., parent alters the environment to reduce exposure to triggers; child engages in specific coping strategies in response to triggers; parent assists child in recognizing when he should use one of his coping strategies). Homework: Lauren and Stephen are to respond in designated ways when Stephen encounters trauma triggers.

Session 4: After homework review, Stephen is shown a worksheet in which a triangle with arrows and labels depicts how thoughts, behaviors, and feelings are interconnected (i.e., the cognitive triangle). Stephen hears the therapist say that there is something he can think or do that will help him feel better, which he is relieved to know. The therapist offers examples of how Stephen's thoughts or behaviors affect his anxiety level, but the therapist's discussion requires complex understanding of cause and effect relationships, metacognition, and prospective hypothetical problem-solving skills. Consequently, Stephen is focused on the only portion of the page that he comprehends—the triangle—and he draws more triangles in the margins of the diagram.

Stephen makes several unsuccessful attempts to divert the therapist's attention to activities that would be more interesting to him. Nevertheless, the therapist speaks kindly to Stephen and smiles at him often, so he is not dissatisfied with the therapy session overall. When the therapist specifically asks about Stephen's unhelpful cognitions, he reports that he thinks "I'm never going to feel better." Homework: Caregiver is instructed to verbalize helpful cognitions (e.g., "This is hard, but you can get through it," or "Things will get easier") to Stephen. The caregiver will also remind Stephen to use the helpful behaviors identified during the prior session (i.e., tell his mother when he feels scared or engage in a pleasant activity).

Session 5: After discussing the prior week's homework assignment, the therapist teaches Stephen several relaxation techniques (e.g., deep breathing and positive guided imagery), which are rehearsed during the session. The caregiver is also taught to use these skills herself. Homework: Stephen is to continue using his coping plan and incorporate relaxation practice with his mother into their daily schedules.

Session 6: From the log Lauren keeps of Stephen's anxiety reactions, coping behaviors, and outcomes, the therapist finds that Stephen has been managing trauma triggers well. Even if Stephen does not fully understand the cognitive triangle and the assumptions therein, he is benefiting from the behavioral practice that the coping plan is providing him. In session, the therapist continues to help Stephen learn to self-monitor his anxiety levels, so that he can independently engage in coping techniques (e.g., engaging in distracting behaviors, cognitive coping, or seeking social support) when necessary. During their session, the therapist and Stephen engage in a role-play activity, in which Stephen pretends to have a scary thought and then uses his newly acquired coping skills to manage the associated anxiety. The homework assignment is for Stephen to utilize these skills in response to the targeted symptoms. Lauren is also taught to remind Stephen to use these skills, whenever necessary.

Session 7: Per the mother, Stephen is successfully managing his reactions to most trauma triggers. Intrusive reexperiences show a moderate response to the interventions. Some general anxiety (e.g., high arousal) and avoidance of transportation in vehicles persist. The therapist describes how Stephen will make a trauma narrative booklet, and Stephen begins by personalizing the cover page. The therapist meets with Lauren to help her enhance her own coping skills and to explore her attributions regarding the accident. The therapist is unaware that Stephen has intrusive dreams (i.e., he denied having "nightmares" and refers to them as "morningmares"). Homework: Stephen is to monitor any remaining symptoms and use his relaxation skills to reduce anxiety.

Session 8: Stephen continues his trauma narrative by drawing a tiny stick figure being crushed by a huge tire. He then describes his drawing and retells part of the traumatic event. Stephen's distress ratings are collected using an "anxiety thermometer" at various points before, during, and after his narrative to ensure that Stephen does not become excessively anxious during the retelling. He is shown a piece of paper picturing a thermometer, with five points delineated. Level 1 indicates low anxiety and level 5 indicates high anxiety. Stephen's initial trauma narrative involves distress ratings of 4 and 5. Following this, the therapist helps Stephen participate in relaxation and cognitive coping activities to help him regulate his anxiety level. Homework: Stephen is to continue practicing coping and relaxation skills when he experiences anxiety at home or during the infrequent occasions he must ride in the car.

In the subsequent caregiver collateral session, Lauren reveals that she has not disciplined Stephen since the traumatic event because of her feelings of extreme guilt. The therapist reviews appropriate disciplinary practices and encourages the mother to engage in discipline as part of Stephen's return to normal development. Maternal Homework: Use at least one parenting technique (e.g., praise for desired behavior, contingency plans, or the time-out method) in response to two targeted misbehaviors (i.e., hitting his siblings and ripping their homework) during the week.

Session 9: After homework review and check-in, Stephen reengages in the trauma narrative, drawing an additional picture of his hospital room and describing further details of both the event and his subsequent medical care. Stephen reports distress levels of 4 and, later, another 4 during the exposure portion of the treatment; however, he quickly returns to his baseline of 2 following the exposure. Homework: Stephen is to complete additional drawings that he regards as fairly benign (e.g., his hospital discharge, physical therapy sessions, and first psychotherapy appointment) to be placed in a larger trauma narrative booklet.

In the caregiver collateral session, the therapist learns that the mother has successfully used discipline methods with Stephen to increase desired behavior and decrease misbehavior. The therapist then reviews some of Stephen's trauma narrative with Lauren individually, who expresses a great sense of guilt and cries throughout the collateral session. Lauren shares her stress as a single mother (e.g., financial burdens and insufficient child care). The therapist and mother engage in a problem-solving discussion regarding these issues and then review the cognitive triangle, applying it to Lauren's own cognitions. Maternal homework: Lauren will continue using parenting methods when necessary, implement the action plan developed in session to resolve child-care and financial issues, and substitute helpful self-statements for her own unhelpful cognitions.

Session 10: In his individual session, Stephen repeats his trauma narrative, including events that occurred prior, during, and after the car ran over him. He also adds drawings of the event to his trauma narrative booklet. Stephen reports distress levels of 3 and 4 during the narrative, but he returns to baseline immediately following the completion of his narrative. The therapist reviews the coping skills Stephen has learned and reminds Stephen to tell himself helpful words rather than words that will make him feel worse.

In the collateral session, the therapist asks Lauren about her progress with the parenting issues she raised during the last session. When the therapist reads Lauren the trauma narrative Stephen dictated to the therapist, Lauren identifies negative reactions and thoughts (e.g., "I am such a bad mother") that might impede her ability to listen in a supportive manner when Stephen eventually shares his trauma narrative directly with her. Maternal homework: Lauren will use at least three positive statements (e.g., "Most of the time, I am a very good mother" or "My children and I will get through this difficult time") when she has an unhelpful thought about her role in the accident.

Session 11: Stephen and Lauren report that Stephen had no "scary thoughts" during the past week and that most of his other symptoms have dissipated. Stephen's remaining symptoms (i.e., intense avoidance of and distress while riding in his car seat) are laddered in a hierarchy from least feared to most feared. Stephen names riding in his car to school as the most feared event. The family had resorted to taking the bus on most occasions, which added to the mother's stress level. In session, Stephen engages in a trauma narrative and reports distress levels of 3 at both points. For the first time, he is not visibly anxious during the trauma retelling. Next, Stephen's car seat is placed in the middle of the floor for an exposure task. He is asked to sit in the seat for 10 seconds, after which he earns a sticker. He successfully completes several increasingly longer trials of this task (i.e., up to 2 minutes in his car seat). With anxiety reduced, the therapist now explores Stephen's attribution as to why the event happened, and Stephen identifies that it happened because his Mommy "just watched and let it happen after I was bad." Later that day, the mother, therapist, and Stephen discuss his attributions and accurate information is provided. Lauren assures Stephen that the accident was not a punishment for misbehavior.

During the collateral session, Lauren engages in role-playing activities with the therapist, who pretends to be Stephen reciting his trauma narrative. In these activities, the mother practices responding to Stephen's narrative in supportive and genuine—but not overly distressed—ways. By the end of this collateral session, Lauren reports that she is ready to participate in the conjoint trauma narrative session. Homework: Stephen is to spend brief, but progressively longer amounts of time (i.e., 10 seconds, then 20 seconds, then 30 seconds) in his car seat outside the car each day for the next four days. Then, for the next two days, he spends 10 seconds in his car seat in the car with the engine ignited. Lauren agrees to provide verbal and tangible rewards for his participation in the exposure.

Session 12: Stephen describes his traumatic experience to his mother during a conjoint session, with low distress levels during the narrative. Lauren listens attentively to his narrative and responds in a helpful and supportive manner. Homework: Stephen will continue 10-second car-seat exposures, increasing the length of the exposure task in 10-second increments each day.

Session 13: The therapist conducts an in vivo exposure task with the family at their home, where Stephen sits in his car for 2 minutes with the engine running. He reports low fear ratings and is amused that the therapist has come to sit in his car with him. Homework: Stephen will continue his daily exposure during the week, beginning with 2 minutes of sitting in his car seat in the car with the engine on, and adding 30-second increments each day. The goal is for Stephen to reach or surpass the goal of 4 minutes in his seat by the time of the next session.

Session 14: Stephen has not only completed his homework, but he reports that the prior day he accepted his mother's invitation to take a short car ride to the ice cream store. In vivo exposure activities are the focus of the session (i.e., the therapist rides with the family in the car for 15 minutes on the hospital grounds). Homework: Stephen will continue daily exposure by riding in the car a short distance. Lauren will provide reinforcement for Stephen's progress. The subsequent session is scheduled to occur at the client's home, where the therapist will accompany Stephen on his first post-accident ride in the car to preschool—a lengthy 30-minute drive. In the collateral session, Lauren reports both her own and Stephen's successful use of helpful self-statements. She also reports that as Stephen makes progress and returns to normal functioning, she feels optimistic about his future recovery.

Session 15: Stephen practices some of his cognitive and relaxation coping skills with the therapist and then enters the car readily. Stephen's car seat is moved to the left side of the back seat, to increase the likelihood of a successful outcome with this graded exposure task. Stephen rides to school successfully, reporting fear levels of 5, 4, and 3 during the drive. The homework is to continue riding to school each day on the left-hand side of the back seat.

Session 16: Stephen has triumphantly ridden to school each day, with low distress levels by the end of the week. He even sat on the right side of the back seat once, without protest. No additional clinical issues are identified by the grateful family. The therapist rides with the family in the car to further assess Stephen's progress but agrees that Stephen's avoidance level is not clinically significant. The family agrees that Stephen has achieved his therapy goals.

Session 17: After reports that Stephen has continued to ride in the car without significant distress, a termination session is held the following week.

*Discussion of CBT*

Stephen was treated quickly and effectively. Because his symptoms were specifically targeted, he experienced symptom relief early in the course of therapy. His ability to resume car travel relatively promptly prevented additional familial distress. The skill enhancement sessions for the mother helped her cope with her own distress, which, in turn, allowed the mother to reinforce Stephen's adaptive coping efforts. As a disadvantage of the treatment, Stephen sporadically had difficulty understanding the material presented to him (e.g., cognitive triangle and discussion involving metacognition). Similarly, the cognitive triad worksheet was not interesting to him, and the verbal didactic method of instruction was not as engaging as other, more experiential methods might have been.

The therapist's focus on future events and future coping behaviors was also cognitively taxing. However, in-session and in vivo practice as well as caregiver collateral sessions were effective and probably served to offset the portions of the treatment curriculum that may have been overly taxing for Stephen's level of cognitive development. The therapist's verbal methods of assessment hindered her from identifying Stephen's "morningmares." As a final point, it is not clear how much Stephen enjoyed the treatment, methods of instruction, and activities, though it is clear that both Stephen and his mother benefited a great deal from the treatment.

## Treatment Option 2: Child-Led Play Therapy

*Basic Tenets*
The fundamental premise of child-led play therapy is that a child's self-directed play in the presence of a supportive, noncritical adult helps the child move toward greater psychological health and well-being. A core assumption of child-led play therapy is that a young child's emotionally significant experiences are best processed through play, wherein situations that are difficult to manage in reality can be symbolically expressed, manipulated, explored, and resolved (Axline, 1947; Landreth, 1991). The goals of child-led play therapy (e.g., enhancement of the child's positive self-concept, sense of control and mastery, capacity for interpersonal trust, and increased self-reliance) are more expansive than typical CBT goals. Play therapy has a long tradition, involving more than 100 years of practice. Early prominent play therapists include Freud (1909), Levy (1938), Anna Freud (1946), Klein (1955), Axline (1947, 1964), and Moustakas (1966).

*Research*
Although randomized, controlled trials of individual play therapy are scant, the field has a long tradition of publishing case studies. There are also several published research studies that include some, but not all elements of experimental design (Baggerly, 2010). Recent research projects emphasizing the use of rigorous research methods are underway, but at present, individual play therapy for childhood trauma symptoms has not been compared to well-established treatments.

*Stephen Receives Child-Led Play Therapy*
In the first session, the therapist engages in a developmental interview with the family and clarifies the presenting issue, but the focus of the treatment is on the child's play activities with the therapist. Although the play therapist might meet with the caregivers during the child's course of treatment, the specific components of caregiver collateral sessions are not well articulated in child-led play therapy literature. Therefore, interventions with caregivers are not standardized and are usually not emphasized in the therapy. Caregiver-child dyadic treatments comprise a different class of psychotherapies, and though they are sometimes used to supplement individual child psychotherapy sessions, discussion of these treatments is beyond the scope of this chapter (for descriptions of some of these treatments, see Bratton, Landreth, Kellam, & Blackard, 2006; Guerney, 1964; Herschell, Calzada, Eyberg, & McNeil, 2002; Lieberman & Van Horn, 2008; Urquiza & McNeil, 1996; and VanFleet, 2000).

Session 1: Stephen enters the room timidly. He is reticent throughout the session, but as he looks at toy animals he reveals that he received a "really cool" stuffed animal from his auntie while he was in the hospital. When told that he can talk or play in any way he likes, Stephen looks skeptical and continues to examine rather than play with objects in the room. Yet, he expresses subdued pleasure and curiosity with the toys in the playroom.

Session 2: Stephen plays with play dough and creates tall towers that he then topples to the floor. Each time, he looks quizzically at the therapist, as if to ask whether this behavior is acceptable. In a brief collateral session, Stephen's mother reports that Stephen's many symptoms concern her. The therapist normalizes Lauren's concern and then describes the "healing powers" of play therapy, through which children express, process, and resolve their problems at their own pace. The therapist responds to the mother with the same warmth and unconditional regard she offers Stephen during their sessions.

Session 3: Stephen is more interactive in this session, and he poses several questions about the therapist, the playroom, and what children are allowed to do in it. Stephen explores more of the room and plays briefly with a range of objects, without developing play themes. Stephen's PTSD symptoms remain unchanged outside of the playroom, but his exploration of the playroom expands and his communication with and sense of trust in the therapist increases.

Sessions 4 and 5: In these sessions, Stephen makes toy cars repeatedly fall off the table. After a few trials, he adds sound effects (i.e., cars "scream" as they crash). The therapist complies with Stephen's requests to return the fallen cars to the table, but she neither discourages nor suggests solutions to prevent the toy cars' peril. Rather, the therapist allows Stephen to direct his own play narrative. Stephen feels the therapist's unconditional acceptance and eagerly anticipates his weekly sessions. Yet, outside of the playroom, Stephen's trauma symptoms persist.

Session 6: Stephen now repeatedly crashes his cars into walls, other cars, and other toys. When he crashes a car into the therapist, she sets a limit regarding physical contact so Stephen understands that he can play as he wishes only if they both remain safe in the room. Later, the therapist makes an interpretation that Stephen might want her to understand that "cars can really hurt." Stephen nods without directly acknowledging his accident, but he subsequently involves the therapist in spectacular car crash scenarios (e.g., the cars land in the sand tray, topple a tower of blocks, and bang around the sides of an empty trash can). Throughout the play session, Stephen honors the physical contact boundary set by the therapist but exhibits a new sense of camaraderie with her.

Outside of the session, Stephen's mother reports that Stephen's anxiety seems to be increasing, and that his avoidance of vehicle travel has caused familial distress. Lauren reports the sense of guilt, child-care needs, and financial problems described in the prior vignette. The therapist empathizes with Lauren's experience but maintains alignment with Stephen by referring the mother to her own therapist to resolve these issues. The therapist also explains to Lauren that sometimes children's symptoms intensify as trauma themes emerge in the play, but that this process cannot be rushed and that Stephen will process his traumatic experience at his own pace.

Sessions 7–9: Stephen engages in post-traumatic play themes during this stage of therapy. Stephen plays exclusively with a large blue car, which either catches on fire, lands in the sand tray, or is eaten by a giant bug. Stephen ends his play sessions without resolution.

Sessions 10–13: Stephen's play narrative now incorporates common family scenes within a dollhouse. Sometimes, the family of figurines mimics activities that took place on the morning of Stephen's accident (e.g., eating breakfast and getting dressed for school). Sometimes, the mother figurine asks the children to hurry. Stephen plays with a father doll—though Stephen's father is not present in his own life—who sometimes drives the family to school. Occasionally, a mysterious voice tells the mother to "Calm down right now!" after she frenetically tries to rush the children through their morning routine. This play takes on a more gratifying tone for Stephen, who is experimenting with solutions to the problem he alludes to in his play narrative (e.g., a father figure prevents the accident or someone calms the mother). The therapist does not directly teach coping skills but describes and highlights Stephen's discovery or use of problem-solving and coping skills as they appear in his play. Outside of the session, some symptoms slightly decrease and others persist, but Stephen's general level of anxiety is reported to be lower. He continues to avoid his car seat and vehicle travel, however, which heightens familial tension.

Session 14: Stephen engages in a more complete trauma-related play narrative, which includes the events before and during the accident. After the pretend car rolls over the boy figurine, Stephen stops and looks quizzically at the therapist (as if to ask if this sort of play is permissible). The therapist reminds Stephen that he may play however he wants in the playroom. "He got really, really hurt," Stephen announces while pointing to a boy figurine. "And he didn't like that," the therapist reflects. "NOT AT ALL!" exclaims Stephen. Then, Stephen shares a long and meaningful gaze with his therapist. He feels not only understood but also inspired to reveal more about his experience to the therapist.

Sessions 15–19: Stephen continues to immerse himself in his post-traumatic play, which either symbolically or literally replicates his experience during the accident. He begins to add detailed content to his play narrative, including peritraumatic sensory experiences and medical intervention efforts. In the 19th session, Stephen approaches his play narrative without avoidance, and he appears less anxious while playing. His mother reports that she thinks his symptoms are improving. However, Stephen continues to refuse car travel.

Sessions 20–22: In these sessions, Stephen engages in mastery-oriented physical feats to enhance his sense of mastery and competence. For example, Stephen asks the therapist to lose as they compete in a game of basketball, and he insists on earning points even when he misses shots. The therapist continues to accept Stephen's play without criticism or instruction. Though she does not directly target Stephen's cognitions, the therapist reflects and highlights Stephen's experience of strength and success.

Sessions 23–27: Now that Stephen feels an enhanced sense of power and competence, he feels brave enough to express his anger. For instance, the mother figurine is locked in a box, punished, and told by another figurine that she is a "very bad Mommy." In the 26th session, Stephen asks the therapist to play the mother character and to say "sorry" to the children in his play scenario. The therapist is then told to give the children all the (pretend) candy and cake they want. Through the therapist's reflections and interpretations (e.g., how angry people are at the mother and how much the children want their mother to "make everything better"), Stephen has a context to begin to recognize his own desires and needs.

In the 27th session, Stephen requires the mother figurine to attend "fireman" school to learn about safety. Afterward, Stephen pretends that he is a superhero fireman. Together, the therapist and Stephen put out imaginary fires, solve crimes, and rescue toy animals. Stephen is particularly interested in his magical superhero boots, which he says give him special power. Stephen's ventilation of anger at his mother, expressed in the presence of an accepting, noncritical adult, helps Stephen process his feelings. He develops creative resolutions to the problems he presents in his play, and these solutions comfort and gratify him both in and out of the playroom. In his play, Stephen offers himself a range of solutions that are not available to him in real life (e.g., mandating that his mother attend safety school). He is comforted by his fantasies and play vignettes, and he regains faith in his mother's ability to keep him safe simply by generating play narratives that remind him of these possible outcomes.

Sessions 28–32: Stephen announces that his mother is done with fire safety school, and the therapist reflects how important it is for a mom to know about safety. Stephen then spontaneously returns to the toy car and figurines. Across three sessions, he replays a more complete version of his trauma narrative, including the roles of his siblings, mother, and hospital personnel on the day of the incident. In session 32, Stephen positions the figurines such that his mother is in the driver's seat while the boy figurine is on the ground outside the right, back seat passenger door. Suddenly, Stephen's eyes widen, and he exclaims that his mother could not have seen that he was under the car from her position in the front seat. Thus, he corrects his own misattribution (i.e., he debunks his mistaken belief that his mother saw him and intentionally ran over him). Stephen has engaged in self-directed, play-induced, cognitive restructuring regarding his perception of events that befell him that day.

Sessions 33–35: Stephen now returns to play involving his superhero boots and fantastic rescue scenarios. This play has a more normative, positive, and gratifying quality. As Stephen experiences his power via magical and fantasy play themes within the session, he becomes more capable of appropriate risk-taking outside of the session (e.g., going on a brief but unprotested car ride to get an ice cream cone). Stephen's mother reports significant improvement in his symptoms.

Sessions 36–38: In his play sessions, Stephen's play activities focus on typical childhood themes. In the 38th session, after performing magic tricks for the therapist, Stephen claims that superheroes like him are very powerful and can do anything, even ride in their car seats. Using play therapy, Stephen has resolved his post-traumatic symptoms, but he has also enhanced his sense of self-reliance, self-concept, and trust in adults.

Sessions 39–41: With reports that Stephen is riding comfortably in his car seat, the therapist discusses therapy termination, which is held in the 42nd week of treatment.

Discussion: Stephen's treatment, though lengthy, was successful in alleviating his symptoms. Though he may have had difficulty describing or using abstract reasoning to sort out his emotions, experiences, and cognitive distortions, Stephen uses play to assess and process his traumatic experience, with a level of ease that would have been difficult for him to do in any other way. As another strength of this method, Stephen's self-generated play therapy reprocessing may be qualitatively superior to reprocessing directed by adults. However, child-led play did not offer Stephen immediate or short-term relief from his symptoms, and his avoidance of his car seat resulted in significant upheaval in an already overburdened family.

Caregivers in this treatment may feel disconnected from and frustrated by the child-focused therapeutic approach. Also, Stephen may have benefited from more directive and immediate skill-building, coping strategies, and specific problem-solving skills that are not part of the child-led play therapy curricula. Furthermore, it is not clear how many children have such psychological skills and coping resources to resolve their trauma play narratives with the clarity shown here, though we believe that at least some children can. Other children, however, might continue post-traumatic repetitive play without gratification or resolution, which would reinforce avoidance and exacerbate a sense of hopelessness. Finally, the caregiver did not receive direct assistance or skill-building regarding her post-traumatic experience as a parent, which might have been helpful in reducing Stephen's symptoms.

## Treatment Option 3: Cognitive-Behavioral Play Therapy
*Basic Tenets*
This integrated treatment combines play therapy with the components of CBT identified earlier in this chapter. In this treatment approach, play is used as a vehicle to deliver CBT elements in developmentally sensitive ways. The treatment also includes elements of both directive and child-led play therapy to facilitate the play-based cognitive processing and restructuring described in the play therapy section of this chapter.

*Research*
Despite the skepticism sometimes voiced about the use of play therapy, we believe that delivering the goals and objectives of CBT via play methods constitutes an evidence-informed, developmentally sensitive approach to psychotherapy. Yet, few studies have directly examined the efficacy of such integrated treatments.

*Stephen Receives Cognitive-Behavioral Play Therapy*
Session 1: As described earlier, the CBT therapist derives a diagnosis and develops a treatment plan to target specific symptoms. However, rather than collecting assessment information or engaging in interventions using only verbal communication or worksheets, the therapist in this blended treatment also uses play-based methods of assessment. For example, index cards illustrating various trauma-related symptoms are provided to Stephen, who is then asked to place each card in one of three boxes, to indicate that he is experiencing the symptom, that he is not sure, or that he is not experiencing the symptom. The therapist discusses each of the cards with Stephen, ensuring that he understands the symptoms depicted on the cards, before Stephen places them in the appropriate boxes. Items in the unsure box are reviewed for clarity. Cards from the endorsed box are given to Stephen to either rank order or select the two or three most troublesome symptoms. Coping techniques are drawn and written on the back of all highly ranked cards, which go home with Stephen. Through the use of tangible objects, manipulative materials, and experiential activities, Stephen communicates his experiences more accurately than he would via verbal communication alone.

Similarly, subjective units of distress are collected via a 3-foot-high thermometer drawn on the wall. Stephen rates his distress level by sticking a Velcro bean bag at the accurate height to indicate low to high fear levels. Because this activity is interesting to him, Stephen is motivated to rate his fear. Moreover, the large thermometer gives Stephen the opportunity to indicate high levels of fear, without engaging in a mental conversion from something that *feels* large to him to something that *looks* small when depicted on a standard-size sheet of paper. So, many interventions used in this approach map directly onto CBT assessment techniques and therapy components (e.g., coping, cognitive processing, exposure, and cognitive restructuring) but are delivered via developmentally sensitive, play-based activities.

Sessions 2–4: The therapist conducts a functional analysis as described earlier and then uses playful activities and games to teach coping skills, psychoeducation, and symptom management techniques. For instance, a three-dimensional representation of a remote control is created for Stephen's use so that he can learn to change the channel whenever he is experiencing distressing thoughts or feelings. Using a rectangular-shaped donut box top, the therapist cuts out a rectangular area, which makes the box resemble a television screen. Then, the therapist and Stephen use the box to pretend that they are on a television show. After a few moments, the therapist demonstrates how sometimes static, the emergency broadcasting network, or a cable outage result in an undesirable noise, loss of the picture, or a blank screen. Stephen is given the cardboard remote control and asked whether he would keep watching the noisy, blank screen all day or whether he would use the remote control to do something about the problem. When Stephen responds that he would use the remote control, he and the therapist discuss all of the actions he can take with the remote control, such as changing the channel, using the fast-forward or rewind buttons, switching to a radio station or DVD, or pressing the pause button and going outside to play.

Following this discussion, Stephen then receives psychoeducation about intrusive reexperiences and how he can use his own special remote control in specific ways (i.e., personalize cognitive or behavioral coping strategies) when he experiences an intrusive recollection. Stephen decorates his remote control and takes it home with him to assist him in managing his intrusive reexperiences. In the next session, Stephen focuses on enhancing his coping skills by engaging in a game of "coping fish," in which photographs of children engaging in coping activities (i.e., both adaptive and maladaptive) have been glued to cardboard-shaped fish. The pictures are placed face down, and paper clips are affixed to their mouths to allow the magnetized fishing rod to attach to each fish when the child engages in the activity. As Stephen catches a fish, he is asked whether engaging in the activity pictured on the bottom side of each cardboard fish would make him feel better or worse.

At times, Stephen and the therapist try an activity suggested on the pretend fish (e.g., thinking of a favorite toy, using deep breathing exercises) to determine whether it would be helpful. Fish with activities that would not be helpful (e.g., telling himself that things will never get better or hitting someone) are thrown back into the pond so other, more helpful fish can be collected. Some fish are left blank for Stephen to generate his own adaptive coping fish. After several trials, Stephen collects a variety of helpful coping fish, which are discussed with the therapist and tailored to specifically address his trauma symptoms. Stephen's mother is taught to play the coping fish game and encouraged to apply useful coping techniques to manage her own anxiety.

Because the interventions are engaging, Stephen is highly motivated to continue the treatment and complete his homework assignment. As a result, his symptoms decrease rapidly. Homework: Stephen is to play the coping fish game each day as soon as he returns from preschool and use at least three of the helpful fish he catches that day in response to two targeted symptoms. In a collateral session, the mother is instructed to provide appropriate and accurate reassurance of Stephen's safety by explicitly discussing the steps she has taken to enhance Stephen's future vehicle-related safety.

Session 5: With several of his acute symptoms dissipating, Stephen experiences less distress. Rather than using a worksheet to teach the cognitive triangle, Stephen is shown how a line of standing dominoes can topple a special red domino at the end of the line. The therapist then uses dominoes to show how having an unhelpful thought can lead to undesired feelings. This concept is easy to grasp, because he sees the cause-and-effect relationship demonstrated in the physical world with the dominoes. The therapist attaches labels with pictures to the first domino (e.g., a stick figure telling himself that everything is scary or dangerous) and to the last domino (e.g., stick figure "feels scared"); then Stephen is instructed to push the first domino into the line of standing dominoes, which ultimately collapses the domino with the "scared" label. If developmentally appropriate (i.e., the child does not associate collapsing dominoes with something negative), the therapist may use another line of dominoes with a helpful cognition on the lead domino label (e.g., "say that I am okay"), which results in the last domino label ("feel happy").

This explanation of the relationship between cognition and affect is readily understandable—and even enjoyable to learn. In the second half of the session, Stephen engages in child-led play with his therapist in a different room (e.g., a traditional playroom). A toy car, family figures, and other props related to the accident are placed in Stephen's line of vision to facilitate his recollection and ability to engage in trauma-related play narratives if he chooses to do so. Because the therapist's interventions have been both enjoyable and effective, Stephen's sense of trust in the therapist is well-developed. He approaches play therapy with a positive expectation of symptom relief and change. As a result, his thematic play begins and proceeds at an accelerated pace.

In the session, Stephen repeatedly crashes a car from the table to the floor. After several trials, the therapist comments that the world is very dangerous for the car. She wonders aloud whether anything can be done to make the car safer. Stephen ponders the possibility, and then asks for a cushion to place below the falling car. This level of therapist direction enhances Stephen's perception that problems can be solved and that he is capable of directing his own problem-solving efforts. If Stephen had indicated that nothing could be done, the therapist would have asked if there was anything at all that could be done to make the car more comfortable, even if the problem could not be solved yet. If the answer were again negative, the therapist would have spoken to the car directly, saying that she and Stephen would continue to try to find a way to make the world a safer or better place for the car. In this way, the therapist instills hope, encourages problem solving, and suggests that adaptive coping is possible, while also ensuring that Stephen maintains control of the world he wishes to portray in his play narratives.

In a conjoint session, a list of car safety rules with drawings to illustrate each item on the list is decorated and posted in the car. On this list, the family commits to ensure that seat belts are fastened, doors are closed, and the mother takes a safety glance around the car before departing. Homework: Stephen is to play the helping domino game at home with his mother and use at least three helpful self-statements per day in response to trauma triggers. Maternal Homework: Mother is to perform a safety puppet show (i.e., the mother puppet conducts the daily car safety ritual, the puppet family departs in their car, and they arrive safely at an imaginary destination each child chooses) for her children several times this week.

Session 6: During a play therapy session, Stephen engages in thematic play with the therapist, who has suggestively left a first-aid kit near the car that had repeatedly crashed during the last session. Without being explicitly told to do so, Stephen uses the first-aid kit, pretending to repair the car. After Stephen announces that the car is "healed," Stephen and the therapist become superheroes with superboots that bestow upon them the power to fly. The therapist reflects Stephen's sense of power, and he smiles broadly. The therapist then recites the themes of his play session, in which he first helped something heal and then felt very powerful. The therapist asks what special power or object Stephen needs to be able to ride in his car again. After considering the question thoughtfully, he responds that he needs his superboots and the car safety list.

Homework: Stephen is to participate in play with his mother wherein they pretend that one of them is driving Stephen's favorite stuffed animals to Disneyland—his favorite destination—every day. Each time, Stephen and his mother must review the safety rules with their stuffed animal passengers before they depart for their imaginary journey. The animals may bring super-boots and safety rules if they wish, but in this parent-child play, the animals must arrive safely at the theme park. This assignment builds on the prior week's parent-child puppet play by exposing Stephen, via play, to the condition he fears most.

Sessions 7–8: After the weekly homework review, the therapist uses the first part of each session to monitor Stephen's management of trauma triggers, teach relaxation skills, or provide psychoeducational puppet shows. For example, Stephen and the therapist teach coping skills to puppets who are enacting a scenario in which they are frightened to ride on a pony. This directed play helps consolidate Stephen's coping skill set and gives him the opportunity to approach a similar situation within the safety of his play metaphors. Stephen then engages in 30-minute play therapy sessions, which proceed with trauma-related and superhero fantasy play, involving the rescue of stuffed animals from various precarious situations.

Homework: Stephen and his mother will create superhero boots from construction paper that Stephen will wear during an in vivo exposure session next week. He is also asked to decorate the car with silly faces and tape a few lollipops to the windows. In conjoint sessions, Lauren describes the concerns presented earlier (i.e., finances and child care) in the CBT portion of this chapter. Via Stephen's play-based homework assignments, the mother has already learned many CBT skills. Other collateral interventions (problem-solving skills, self-statement monitoring) take place as described in the prior treatment vignette.

Session 9: All of Stephen's symptoms have remitted except his avoidance of sitting in his car seat during car travel. In vivo exposure begins, with Stephen wearing his superhero boots, holding a shield, and sitting in his car, which is decorated in full lollipop regalia. He rides briefly but successfully in the car with moderately high (i.e., 4) and then low (2 and 2) distress ratings. Homework: Stephen will attempt three additional brief car rides, with imagined scenarios as part of the exposure (e.g., "there is a secret message from another superhero at the end of the block, and they must retrieve it by driving there," or "Stephen's superhero cape was left in the park, and they must ride three blocks to recover it").

These developmentally appropriate modifications to typical exposure-based treatments allow Stephen to tolerate his distress while engaging in his own play mastery scenarios. Using fantasy to detract from focus on the avoided situation (i.e., referred to as safety-seeking behaviors in CBT) is ultimately eliminated in most exposure treatments, but we argue that this sort of combined fantasy play and exposure might actually enhance—rather than detract from—engagement during exposure tasks, given that young children regularly use fantasy to attend to, interact with, and process information from the real world.

Session 10: After learning from the family that the mini-exposure sessions were successful, the therapist schedules an in vivo exposure car ride to school with Stephen, as described in the first vignette. In his play therapy session, Stephen plays the family morning routine (e.g., eating breakfast, getting ready for school, and then getting into the car) and the accident. After Stephen replays his traumatic experience, the therapist assesses his distress level and then asks what happened next, after the car accident. Using both words and play, he demonstrates his experiences in the ambulance and in the hospital. When asked whether any part of the experience is difficult to understand, Stephen positions the figurines to determine whether his mother saw and intentionally hurt him. When Stephen replays the trauma narrative in slow motion, analyzing what is happening during each frame of his play scene, he understands that, from his mother's visual perspective, she could not have seen him fall directly under the car. In the conjoint session, the mother is asked for further clarification and reassures her son that she did not intentionally injure him.

Session 11: During the in vivo session at Stephen's home, the therapist briefly reviews Stephen's coping skills. Then they develop a superhero play scenario involving Stephen's car travel. When Stephen is ready, he puts on his superhero boots, holds his shield, and activates his supercar to pursue his rescue (i.e., Stephen's mother is to begin their drive to school). During the in vivo exposure, Stephen's distress levels are 4 followed by 2 and another 2. The in vivo exposure is a success, though he remains reliant upon his safety behaviors (e.g., superboots, shield, and distracting play scenarios). Homework: Stephen will continue to engage in car travel exposure with safety behaviors to and from school.

Session 12: Lauren reports that all of Stephen's symptoms are alleviated and that he has successfully driven to school each day since the last session. The therapist assesses whether any remaining issues need to be targeted during the treatment. Safety-seeking behaviors would be removed in typical exposure treatments for adults, but in our view, at least some safety behaviors are normative and developmentally appropriate (e.g., sleeping with a nightlight, use of a favorite blanket from home during preschool naptime, or bringing a cuddle toy to a sleepover). So, in this session the therapist does not seek to remove all safety behaviors (i.e., his superhero boots) but only those that are impractical for long-term usage in a small, cramped car (i.e., the shield and decorations) or are dependent upon the therapist's involvement (i.e., co-constructing fantasy scenarios).

When asked about the possibility of removing the shield, decorations, and imaginary rescue scenarios, Stephen says, "Actually, I don't need any of those anymore. I can do it even without these [the boots]." The therapist accompanies the family as they ride in the car near the clinic. Stephen demonstrates and reports low levels of anxiety, and he discusses superheroes only during the initial few minutes of the drive. In the individual play portion of the session, Stephen returns to the toy car that had once crashed repeatedly to the ground. He listens to it with a toy stethoscope, taps it lightly with a toy hammer (as if to test its reflexes), and inspects it closely. "Yep, it's all better," he says matter-of-factly. After another split session wherein Stephen first rides in his car without distress during in vivo exposure and then engages in child-led play with gratifying, normative play themes, termination is scheduled for the following week.

*Discussion*
The therapist's use of well-established treatment components (e.g., coping skills, psychoeducation, caregiver support, exposure, and cognitive restructuring) combined with use of the engaging delivery methods enhanced Stephen's interest in and progress during treatment. Adding play therapy sessions allowed Stephen to more fully process the event in his own way. The therapist's sporadic suggestions, use of suggestive materials, or subtle directives optimized Stephen's ability to profit rapidly from the play therapy sessions.

# Conclusion

In this chapter, we addressed the issue of integration by depicting three methods of child trauma therapy in order to examine treatment similarities, differences, and how they may be blended. We showed how each of the three methods might have produced positive outcomes for young survivors. CBT and play therapy are often considered to be dissimilar, but we highlighted several similarities in the approaches, particularly when the young recipient of child-led play therapy has sufficient adaptive resources to engage in productive processing of the traumatic event with little therapeutic guidance. Repeatedly recounting the traumatic event (i.e., either by the child's verbalization or via play), cognitive processing, and cognitive restructuring were core components of each treatment. Perhaps, effective post-traumatic play therapy and CBT involve some of the same change mechanisms (i.e., exposure with processing and cognitive restructuring).

The three treatments also differed in several ways. We pointed out how the three treatments differed in terms of the overarching goals (e.g., to enhance self-reliance versus to learn specific skills to manage anxiety), the level of emphasis on caregiver participation in the treatment and home practice assignments, and the degree to which the child comprehended, enjoyed, or was motivated to participate in the treatment. We showed how symptom reduction occurred much more rapidly in the CBT than in the play-therapy-only treatment and how the methods used to accomplish the intervention goals were considerably different (e.g., didactic instruction with skill practice versus play-based skill-building activities versus child-led play). Now, to complete the discussion of treatment differences, we highlight the critical point that CBTs typically have high response rates, and therapists can offer these treatments with a confidence level of their efficacy that has not yet been earned for play, or play-CBT-blended therapies. Yet, many play therapists are reluctant to use CBTs, at least in part, because of concerns related to developmental sensitivity issues.

## Caveat Regarding Development Sensitivity

In this chapter, we pointed out some possible areas where developmental sensitivity might be problematic in CBT. We recognize that evaluating developmental sensitivity often involves a degree of subjectivity (i.e., presumably, all authors believe that their treatments already are sufficiently developmentally sensitive). In this chapter, we rely heavily on pedagogy literature to discuss and propose developmentally sensitive methods. In developing techniques for CBPTT, we often ask ourselves whether a highly skilled preschool or elementary school teacher would teach a concept in the way we are attempting to teach it to the child and allow the answer to shape our intervention delivery methods.

In summary, we believe that each method of treatment has the potential to be successful for some children, but we acknowledge that CBT offers the strongest research base. Even so, we seek to merge the century of play therapy tradition with CBT, and we hypothesize that CBPTT holds advantages for many young survivors. By blending play therapy and CBT, we allow children to receive the benefits of CBT (e.g., rapid symptom reduction, strong evidence base) while also providing children with the opportunity to address their traumatic experiences in ways that foster self-reliance, engagement in the treatment modules, and motivation to participate in the tasks of treatment.

A direct comparison of play therapy to an evidence-based treatment is long overdue, but until such research is completed, play therapists—particularly those who are unlikely to use CBT—may be interested in the middle ground between play therapy ideology and CBT evidence. We hope that our treatment vignettes and our commentary contribute to the play therapy literature as play therapists integrate various methods of child treatment in response to a field that is increasingly driven by research evidence. By narrowing the divide between the various forms of play therapy, as well as between CBT and play therapy, there is the potential to develop an approach to child trauma treatment that is evidence-based, pedagogically sound, developmentally sensitive, and engaging to young survivors.

## References

Axline, V. M. (1947). *Play therapy: The inner dynamics of childhood.* Boston, MA: Houghton Mifflin.

Axline, V. M. (1964). *Dibs in search of self.* New York, NY: Ballantine Books.

Baggerly, J. (2010). Evidence-based standards and tips for play therapy researchers. In J. N. Baggerly, D. E. Ray, & S. C. Bratton (Eds.), *Child-centered play therapy research* (pp. 467–479). Hoboken, NJ: Wiley.

Beck, A. T., Rush, A. J., Shaw, B. F., & Emery, G. (1979). *Cognitive therapy of depression.* New York, NY: Guilford Press.

Bratton, G., Landreth, S. C., Kellam, T., & Blackard, S. R. (2006). *Child-parent relationship therapy treatment manual.* New York, NY: Routledge.

Cohen, J. A., Mannarino, A. P., & Deblinger, E. (2006). *Treating trauma and traumatic grief in children and adolescents.* New York, NY: Guilford Press.

Drewes, A. (2009). *Blending play therapy with cognitive behavioral therapy: Evidence-based and other effective treatment and techniques.* Hoboken, NJ: Wiley.

Ellis, A., & Gieger, R. M. (Eds.). (1986). *Handbook of rational-emotive therapy* (Vol. 2). New York, NY: Springer.

Freud, A. (1946). *The psychoanalytic treatment of children.* London, England: Imago.

Freud, S. (1909). *The case of "Little Hans" and the "Rat Man."* London, England: Hogarth Press.

Gil, E., & Jalazo, N. (2009). An illustration of science and practice: Strengthening the whole through its parts. In A. Drewes (Ed.), *Blending play therapy with cognitive behavioral therapy: Evidence-based and other effective techniques* (pp. 41–70). Hoboken, NJ: Wiley.

Goodyear-Brown, P. (2009). *Play therapy with traumatized children: A prescriptive approach.* Hoboken, NJ: Wiley.

Grave, J., & Blissett, J. (2004). Is cognitive behavior therapy developmentally appropriate for young children? A critical review of the evidence. *Clinical Psychology Review, 24,* 399–420.

Guerney, B. (1964). Filial therapy: Description and rationale. *Journal of Consulting Psychology, 28,* 304–310.

Herschell, A., Calzada, E., Eyberg, S. M., & McNeil, C. B. (2002). Parent-child interaction therapy: New directions in research. *Cognitive and Behavioral Practice, 9,* 9–16.

Holmbeck, G. N., Greenley, R. N., & Franks, E. A. (2003). Developmental issues and considerations in research and practice. In A. E. Kazdin & J. R. Weisz (Eds.), *Evidence-based psychotherapies for children and adolescents* (pp. 21–41). New York, NY: Guilford Press.

Kendall, P. C., Robin, J., Hedtke, K., Suveg, C., Flannery-Schroeder, E., & Gosch, E. (2005). Considering CBT with anxious youth? Think exposures. *Cognitive and Behavioral Practice, 12,* 136–150.

Klein, M. (1955). The psychoanalytic play technique. *American Journal of Orthopsychiatry, 25,* 223–237.

Knell, S. M. (1993). *Cognitive-behavioral play therapy.* Northvale, NJ: Jason Aronson.

Knell, S. (2009). Cognitive-behavioral play therapy: Theory and applications. In A. Drewes (Ed.), *Blending play therapy with cognitive behavioral therapy: Evidence-based and other effective techniques* (pp. 117–133). Hoboken, NJ: Wiley.

Kolko, D. J., & Swenson, C. C. (2002). *Assessing and treating physically abused children and their families: A cognitive-behavioral approach.* Thousand Oaks, CA: Sage.

Landreth, G. (1991). *Play therapy: The art of the relationship.* Muncie, IN: Accelerated Development.

Levy, D. (1938). Release therapy in young children. *Psychiatry, 1,* 387–389.

Lieberman, A. F., & Van Horn, P. (2008). *Psychotherapy with infants and young children: Repairing the effects of stress and trauma on early attachment.* New York, NY: Guilford Press.

Moustakas, C. (1966). *The child's discovery of himself.* New York, NY: Ballantine Books.

Ollendick, T. H., & Vasey, M. W. (1999). Developmental theory and the practice of clinical child psychology. *Journal of Clinical Child Psychology, 28,* 457–466.

Peterson, L., & Tremblay, G. (1999). The importance of developmental theory and the practice of clinical child psychology. *Journal of Clinical Child Psychology, 28,* 458–465.

Pynoos, R. S., Steinberg, A. M., Layne, C. M., Briggs, E. C., Ostrowski, S. A., & Fairbank, J. A. (2009). DSM-V PTSD diagnostic criteria for children and adolescents: A developmental perspective and recommendations. *Journal of Traumatic Stress, 22*(5), 391–398.

Schaefer, C. S. (1999). Curative factors in play therapy. *Journal for the Professional Counselor, 14*(1), 7–16.

Shelby, J. (2010). Cognitive-behavioral therapy and play therapy for childhood trauma and loss. In N. Boyd Webb (Ed.), *Helping bereaved children: A handbook for practitioners* (3rd ed.). New York, NY: Guilford Press.

Shelby, J. S., & Berk, M. J. (2009). Play therapy, pedagogy, and CBT: An argument for interdisciplinary synthesis. In A. Drewes (Ed.), *Blending play therapy with cognitive behavioral therapy: Evidence-based and other effective techniques* (pp. 17–40). Hoboken, NJ: Wiley.

Shelby, J. S., & Felix, E. D. (2005). Posttraumatic play therapy: The need for an integrated model of directive and nondirective approaches. In L. A. Reddy, T. M. Files-Hall, and C. E. Schaefer, *Empirically based play interventions for children* (pp. 79–103). Washington DC: American Psychological Association Press.

Shirk, S. R. (2001). Development and cognitive therapy. *Journal of Cognitive Psychotherapy, 15,* 155–163.

Urquiza, A. J., & McNeil, C. B. (1996). Parent-child interaction therapy: An intensive dyadic intervention for physically abusive families. *Child Maltreatment, 1*(2), 132–141.

VanFleet, R. (2000). *A parent's handbook of filial play therapy.* Boiling Springs, PA: Play Therapy.

Weisz, J. R., & Hawley, K. M. (2002). Developmental factors in the treatment of adolescents. *Journal of Consulting and Clinical Psychology, 70,* 21–43.

# The Worry Wars: A Protocol for Treating Childhood Anxiety Disorders

## *Paris Goodyear-Brown*

## Introduction

The Worry Wars: An Anxiety Workbook for Kids and Their Helpful Adults (Goodyear-Brown, 2010b), a protocol that integrates cognitive-behavioral concepts and methods with therapeutic storytelling and play therapy, was developed by the author as a response to the rising number of children who enter treatment with overwhelming anxiety. While the specific clinical label given to the anxiety—post-traumatic stress disorder (PTSD), acute stress disorder (ASD), separation anxiety disorder (SAD), generalized anxiety disorder (GAD), selective mutism (SM), obsessive-compulsive disorder (OCD), or specific phobia—helps characterize how a specific anxiety problem manifests, the Worry Wars protocol helps families understand the core mechanisms that these disorders share and equips them to fight back against any manifestation of anxiety.

## Therapeutic Intervention Models Utilized in the Worry Wars Protocol

### Psychoeducation

Psychoeducation refers to any structured form of patient information that augments a client's understanding of a clinical problem. In order to fight your enemy, you must first know your enemy. Therefore, any effective protocol for the treatment of childhood anxiety must contain information specific to how anxiety grows and how it must be fought. The Worry Wars protocol provides psychoeducation to parents and children alike. The concepts addressed include a working definition of anxiety, information about the mechanism by which anxiety grows (i.e., avoidance), and specific examples of how avoidance reinforces the anxiety. When treating adult clients, the theoretical construct of avoidance can be taught with words and the tools for regaining one's power in relation to the anxiety producing stimuli can be delivered through talk and guided skills practice. Developmentally sensitive delivery of this psychoeducational information to children requires the integration of play, expressive arts, metaphoric storytelling, and full body involvement.

Avoidance is a deceptively charming companion, often masquerading as a friend to our child clients, perhaps even as a hero. When the anxiety gets bad, the child avoids the anxiety-producing stimuli and the child feels better, often much better and often right away. Avoidance can seem to swoop in like a savior to dispel the potent physical upset that accompanies anxiety, quickly solidifying a child's belief that avoidance is by far the best tactic for dealing with anxiety. Accurate information cloaked in playful therapeutic metaphors provides families with needed ammunition. Throughout the protocol, additional psychoeducational concepts are introduced, including the role that relaxation responses play in fighting anxiety, the need for gradual exposure, and targeted information on how cognitive restructuring techniques will augment the relaxation strategies.

## Cognitive Restructuring

A solid empirical base now exists for the effectiveness of cognitive-behavioral therapy in treating disorders that have anxiety at their core, including post-traumatic stress disorder (Beck, Emery, & Greenberg, 2005; Cohen & Mannarino, 2004; Cohen, Mannarino, & Deblinger, 2006; Friedberg & McClure, 2002; Knell, 1993, 2009). The pioneering work of Albert Ellis and Aaron Beck made clear the connections between our thoughts, actions, and feelings. Beck's cognitive triad (1995) is an elegant encapsulation of the links between our thoughts, feelings, and behaviors. Through the Worry Wars protocol, clients are taught the cognitive triad and given developmentally appropriate examples of how thoughts can influence feelings and behaviors. Children as young as 5 years old can benefit from information, playfully delivered, that helps them understand these links. The therapist can use a variety of props, including musical triangles, Magnetix, and K'nex, to anchor the therapeutic learning and provide hands-on manipulation to child clients (Goodyear-Brown, 2010a).

Furthermore, helping children identify their anxiety-ridden thoughts, practice thought stopping, and craft and rehearse replacement statements are all important components of the protocol. However, the extent to which children can identify their thought patterns will vary with developmental age, proficiency with expressive language, the extent of a child's denial of an anxiety problem, and the intensity of post-traumatic stress when trauma underlies the anxiety. Older children and teenagers can usually identify several irrational thoughts or negative thoughts that influence their anxiety. Younger children may only be able to articulate one thought or may only be able to identify the physiological feeling of anxiety experienced in certain contexts.

One way to help children through the process of identifying the anxious self-talk is to extend the use of the therapeutic metaphor that was originally chosen to represent the anxiety. Once the metaphor has been established, this "anxiety with skin on" can develop a voice. By creating a character to embody the externalized anxiety and identifying the worried thoughts repeated by the character, children are able to pinpoint their anxious thoughts. Once the repetitive anxious thoughts have been articulated, children can learn a process of thought stopping. Although adults can navigate this process internally, children are much less adept at cognitive manipulation. Because children are kinesthetic creatures, the process of thought stopping is best practiced three-dimensionally, with the therapist speaking the anxious thoughts, often through a puppet that represents the metaphoric anxiety, and children having a full-body experience of stopping the puppet from talking. This process will be demonstrated through the metaphors established in The Worry Wars protocol later in the chapter.

## Systematic Desensitization

Systematic desensitization is a treatment approach designed by Joseph Wolpe (1990), a South African psychiatrist, to help clients overcome avoidance patterns related to anxiety-laden stimuli. Based on principles of behavior modification, and classical conditioning specifically, the intervention model seeks to deconstruct the learned association between a fear-producing stimuli and the anxiety reaction by progressively pairing the fear-producing stimuli with a contradictory response involving relaxation. Systematic desensitization is a two-step process that first equips the client with relaxation strategies and then pairs the relaxation response with a series of increasingly difficult exposures to the anxiety-producing stimuli. The therapist assists the client in learning progressive muscle tension and relaxation (PMR), focused breathing techniques, or mindfulness strategies. Once the client has become proficient in producing the relaxation response, the client and therapist together design an anxiety hierarchy.

## Gradual Exposure

Once a family has become educated about the anxiety, and the child has learned relaxation responses and cognitive coping statements, then the clinician, child, and parent(s) together structure a very precise set of graduated exposures (March, 2006; March & Mulle, 1998).

The hierarchy is arranged in an intentional order, placing the easiest, or least anxiety-producing tasks at the bottom of the hierarchy. Mastery in this context means that the client can tolerate the anxiety-producing stimuli while pairing it with the relaxation response. As the client masters each task on the hierarchy, he or she moves to a more difficult task.

In other words, the hierarchy is arranged from least-feared to most-feared situations. For example, a person with a specific phobia of spiders might first look at a picture of a spider, then move to looking at a spider behind glass, and eventually attempt to be in physical proximity to an actual spider. Exposures can be done through visualization or guided imagery, but the most effective exposures are done in vivo or through new virtual reality exposure programs. The time taken with each step of the ladder is important. The exposures should not just be experienced once and borne with gritted teeth, but rather the anxiety-producing content is approached and repeatedly paired with the relaxation response until the client feels comfortable with that stimuli.

## Therapeutic Storytelling

Anxiety is a term that describes a complex set of human experiences and may involve neurochemical imbalances, physiological dysregulation, cognitive distortions, traumagenic memories, and a wide array of social processes. When adults talk to each other about anxiety, we have at least a partially shared understanding of the abstract concept and of all the other abstractions that may underlie our anxiety reactions. Children do not share this ability to grapple with abstract concepts. Many child clients are in the preoperational or operational stage of development and are concrete thinkers. They grapple more easily with things that have "skin on." The metaphors that can be drawn through therapeutic storytelling allow for the abstract concept to be given a shape, a form that can then be manipulated. In other words, the metaphor that communicates the abstraction can flesh out a concept that may be otherwise unreachable for our youngest clients.

Children love stories. Long before they are old enough to read for themselves, children sit tucked on their parents' laps and absorb both the warmth of their caregivers and bits and pieces of the human experience codified in story form. Stories are a child's first exposure to all sorts of content, and they can be used to paint new pictures or unwrap new ideas. They are a ready-made medium for painting a picture of anxiety and the mechanisms by which it grows, while giving children icons that can be manipulated. Moreover, because children often experience anxiety as an overwhelming physiological hyperarousal, it can be difficult for them to separate the anxiety from themselves. Embedding a metaphoric antagonist into a therapeutic story helps focus the child's anxiety reactions into an externalized form that can then be manipulated.

Joyce Mills and R. J. Crowley (2001), in their book, *Therapeutic Metaphors for Children and the Child Within*, talks about harnessing the power of metaphor to enlist the client's creativity in problem solving. Depicting anxiety as the antagonist in a story gives children an enemy they can see, at their least in their mind's eye. Once children have a discernable enemy, they can learn how to fight that enemy. The anxiety does not necessarily have to become an enemy. It can become the problem of a character who is younger, weaker, or less equipped than the protagonist in the story. The protagonist helps educate the hapless creature and vicariously educates clients along the way.

After children have become adept at recognizing the anxious thoughts and are effectively stopping them, replacement statements or boss back talk can be generated. Examples of both of these processes will be given later in this chapter.

## Play Therapy

Many of the therapeutic powers of play have been articulated in the play therapy literature (Landreth, 1991; Schaefer, 1993; Schaefer & Drewes, 2009). When children are truly at play, their minds and bodies are activated in ways that are completely antithetical to an anxiety reaction. The positive emotions experienced by children while playing counter the toxicity of anxiety. The natural increase in focus that accompanies the manipulation of interesting objects leaves less room for the anxiety. The kinesthetic pleasure experienced as children run their hands through the sand or knead the clay runs counter to the physiological tension that is often an outgrowth of anxiety. Toys are the words of children, and play is the language through which we can begin to communicate about children's anxiety. In cases of post-traumatic anxiety, children may choose a symbol to represent the traumatic event or the perpetrator of abuse. They may then work out a way to contain the symbol that represents the anxiety as a first step in regaining a sense of safety and security. See Goodyear-Brown (2010a) for a full explication of this process.

Children will also use the tools of the playroom as anchors, grounding themselves in the safety of familiar things. The manipulation of the toys actively mitigates the anxiety that is present as children approach their trauma content. Children begin to take risks, to face their anxiety as they play. Just as a doctor titrates doses of medications, a fully equipped playroom gives children the freedom to self-titrate their doses of exposure to anxiety-producing content. The dance they do between approaching the traumagenic material and moving away from it again arguably embodies a self-titrated process of desensitization.

## The Mechanics of the Worry Wars Protocol

The Worry Wars protocol is a comprehensive program that enhances children's adaptive coping strategies, helps children rehearse relaxation responses, externalizes the anxiety, identifies problematic self-talk, helps children create boss back talk, and leads families through a gradual exposure hierarchy while delivering all interventions in a playful, developmentally sensitive format. The protocol is divided into three sections, each of which provides a variety of modules and tools for children and clinicians to choose from.

### The Stories

The first module, The Stories, provides a series of therapeutic stories that give metaphoric form to childhood anxieties. Each story provides an externalization of the anxiety: a fire-breathing dragon, a perfectionistic princess, and a clinging octopus. Each story also has a child hero who learns effective strategies to take back control over his or her anxiety responses. The child hero learns how to recognize avoidance behavior and *do the scary thing anyway*. After each successfully navigated exposure, the child hero in the story becomes stronger and the externalized anxiety becomes weaker. Each tale ends with the child's eventual triumph over the anxiety.

Clinicians can choose the most appropriate story/metaphor to represent each child's anxiety. The story becomes the context in which the child learns about how avoidance behaviors reinforce the anxiety. The stories also provide a variety of creative solutions to battling back the anxiety and provide hope that the child can win his or her battle with anxiety.

The first story, *Daniel the Dragon Slayer*, externalizes a young boy's growing anxiety in the form of a dragon. Daniel is a typical latency-age boy who likes to play soccer and build Lego structures. One day, Daniel is playing with his Legos in the living room, while his mom is watching a news report. Embedded between other local news stories is a report about a recent earthquake in Asia. Daniel goes through his normal bedtime routine, but once he is alone in his bed, he begins to ruminate about the earthquake. As he begins to worry, a dragon egg appears under his bed. He decides to build a fort in his bed, just in case an earthquake hits and the roof caves in. Once the fort is complete, he feels better, but the dragon egg begins to crack.

The next morning, Daniel starts thinking about the earthquake again while he is walking to the bus stop. He reasons that if an earthquake happens, he shouldn't be in the bus, because the bus could crash. This possibility increases his anxiety, and he decides to walk to school, avoiding the bus altogether. He feels better, but the dragon hatches in his backpack. The story unfolds as Daniel engages in continually increasing avoidance behavior. Each time he experiences anxiety about the earthquake and does something to feel better, the dragon gets bigger. Daniel's avoidance actually feeds the dragon. The story is used to show how increased cognitive rehearsal of the anxious thoughts feeds the anxiety.

When the dragon breathes his first fiery breath, Daniel realizes that he has let the dragon get too large, and he begins to fight back. Daniel uses some boss back talk and pairs his words with a physical attack on the dragon using a sword and shield. Daniel's intentional confrontations with the dragon end as the dragon's breath is put out by a fire extinguisher. This story can be used by clinicians to represent the kind of anxiety that presents itself in post-traumatic avoidance symptoms, generalized anxiety, or specific phobias.

The second story, entitled *Polly versus Princess Perfect*, characterizes the anxiety associated with perfectionism or obsessive-compulsive tendencies as a tiny princess with a big, troubling voice. Polly is a little girl with whom many of our perfectionistic clients identify. She is good at many things. She is a terrific student, she excels at ballet, and she makes her bed without being asked. She takes pride in her appearance, but she is easily frustrated when she can't get the rows of hearts on her tights to line up. She tries to braid her hair before going to school one morning, but the princess is hiding in her hoodie so that she can't be seen but only heard. Polly listens to the voice of Princess Perfect and continues to braid and rebraid her hair. Meanwhile, her mother is becoming more and more frustrated because Polly isn't ready for school.

This scenario mirrors the conflict that often arises between parents and children when children become trapped in obsessive-compulsive patterns. It is all too easy for parents to confuse their child's anxiety symptoms with deliberate defiance. Helping parents to shift their paradigm so that they see the rigidity of their children's behavior as a way of coping with the out-of-control feeling that accompanies their anxiety equips parents to respond more effectively to their children's behaviors.

Polly goes to school and continues to hear the princess's voice telling her that her work is not good enough. While she feels sad, she also rips up her work and starts all over again, working to make it perfect. Finally, Polly realizes that she is becoming a slave to the voice, and she develops a plan to find out to whom the voice belongs. She takes the princess's wand and begins to listen differently to the words of the princess. She generates a list of truths to help her combat the voice of the princess. After she generates self-talk that combats the anxiety-driven statements made by the princess, she begins to drown out the voice of anxiety. The last image in the story has Polly using a megaphone to amplify her words as she bosses back the princess. The blast of air through the megaphone knocks Princess Perfect all the way out the window! Once again, the child takes control of the anxiety.

The third story, *Oscar versus Clyde, the Clinging Octopus*, targets the symptoms of separation anxiety. The story begins with Oscar being born to loving parents. As his parents gaze at him through the hospital nursery window, they don't even notice Clyde, the infant octopus, who is clinging to Oscar's bassinet. As Oscar grows, Clyde grows right alongside him. When Oscar wants to venture out on his tricycle, Clyde uses his tentacles to keep him driving in circles around the driveway. When it is time for Oscar to start preschool, Clyde tries to stop him. When they get to the door of the classroom, Clyde wraps his tentacles around Oscar and mom, squeezing Oscar into such a state of distress that mom takes him home again. Oscar realizes that he is going to have to stand up to Clyde. Oscar proceeds to develop several silly yet effective plans for teaching Oscar that it is safe to separate from mom, and they end the story as friends.

## The Weapons

The second phase of the protocol, called The Weapons, is devoted to equipping children to fight the anxiety both physiologically and cognitively. The anxiety is portrayed as an alarm clock. The importance of the alarm clock in ensuring our survival is conveyed through child-friendly examples. In one example, the child is getting ready to cross the street when he hears an enormous truck barreling towards him. His brain trips the alarm, and his body reacts at lightning speed. He jumps back onto the curb and is safe.

The next step is to help the client make the distinction between the alarm being tripped in perilous situations and the alarm getting stuck. A child controlled by anxiety is one whose alarm has gotten stuck. The strategies offered to these children are portrayed as ways to hit the snooze button. As the child gets better at silencing the alarm for periods of time (during exposure/response prevention exercises), the brain is retrained.

The kinds of stimuli that set off the alarm vary from client to client. Playful activities are used at this point in the protocol to help clients identify their triggers. Individual worries are characterized as wriggly worms that can be difficult to pin down. Reproducible handouts depict worry worms that can be cut out and personalized as the client and therapist play a game together. The therapist hides a variety of rubber worms around the playroom. The child looks for the worms. The therapist can give hints like "you're getting hotter" or "you're getting colder." For each rubber worm that the child finds, he articulates one worry with which he struggles. Each worry is written down on the paper worms.

The child's natural drive to play counters his equally natural avoidance of anxiety-provoking content. Each time he finds one of the hidden worms, he receives the powerful reinforcement of accomplishment. This full-body experience of momentary competence mitigates the client's approach to the anxiety and enables the child to speak frankly about the kinds of experiences that scare or worry him. Parents are often surprised at the exhaustive list of worries and fears that are generated by the end of this session. Playing Hot and Cold with the Worry Worms embeds the identification process within a comforting childhood game. Moreover, the child's continual manipulation of playful props throughout the exercise decreases the child's defensiveness toward otherwise overwhelming psychological content.

Once the list of specific fears have been identified and recorded on the paper worms, the work centers on making these fears more manageable. In an exercise called Can of Worms (Goodyear-Brown, 2010b), the client and therapist create a container for the worms. The paper worry worms are placed inside the container and sealed. The child may experience relief as the worries are contained in the playroom until the child has developed a more effective set of tools for overcoming his anxiety. After the child has increased his ability to manage the fear, individual worries can be taken from the container. The new skills can then be applied to each worry.

At this point in treatment, clients are already familiar with one or more of the therapeutic metaphors for anxiety. Child heroes from the therapeutic stories (Polly and Daniel) are used to help clients identify the physiological arousal symptoms that often accompany anxiety. Symptoms such as a pounding heart, sweating, and upset tummy are presented in child-friendly icons (Figures 8.1 and 8.2).

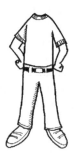

## Figure 8.1

*Source:* Goodyear-Brown, P. (2010a). *The Worry Wars: An Anxiety Workbook for Kids and Their Helpful Adults!* Nashville, TN: Author. Reprinted with permission.

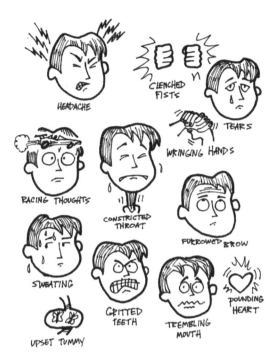

## Figure 8.2

*Source:* Goodyear-Brown, P. (2010a). *The Worry Wars: An Anxiety Workbook for Kids and Their Helpful Adults!* Nashville, TN: Author. Reprinted with permission.

The body is photocopied, and clients can choose as many physical manifestations of anxiety as they have experienced, then cut out the icons and glue them onto their bodies. Each physiological response can be targeted separately and relaxation strategies geared to the unique physical experience of each child. For example, if a client identifies clenched fists as one of his physical signals that anxiety is present, the client can be taught progressive muscle relaxation exercises (PMR), such as The Bubble Fall (Goodyear-Brown, 2002) to help the client relax his body and let go of the anxiety. Another client might identify racing thoughts as one of her signals that anxiety is present. Guided imagery, thought stopping, and thought replacement work might be most beneficial for this client. At the end of this activity, the clinician and client have a shared understanding of how the child's anxiety manifests in his or her physiology.

## Coping

The next step in the protocol is to help clients discern the differences between adaptive and maladaptive coping strategies and to enhance positive coping. It is always helpful, particularly in cases where the anxiety is traumagenic in nature, to explore the existing parameters of a client's coping repertoire before processing the anxiety-laden content (Felix, Bond, & Shelby, 2006; Kimball, Nelson, & Politano, 1993; Shelby & Berk, 2009). The Coping Tree, an intervention that

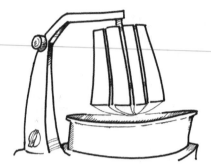

## Figure 8.3
*Source:* Goodyear-Brown, P. (2010a). *The Worry Wars: An Anxiety Workbook for Kids and Their Helpful Adults!* Nashville, TN: Author. Reprinted with permission.

helps clients identify both adaptive and maladaptive coping strategies, is one useful tool to begin this work (Shelby, Bond, Hall, & Hsu, 2004). After current coping has been assessed, clients may need psychoeducation regarding what constitutes adaptive coping.

In pursuit of this objective, clients create Copecakes over a series of sessions. During the first session, the client is introduced to four dimensions of positive coping that have been distilled from the coping literature and phrased in developmentally appropriate language. Positive coping strategies should (1) be good for you, (2) be good for others, (3) be easy to do, and (4) make you feel better. The child is given a handout that lists these four dimensions and a picture of a Copecake mixer (Figure 8.3). The client writes each of the four rules into the prongs of the mixer. This image is then used to help assess future coping choices.

Once clients have rehearsed the characteristics of positive coping strategies, they are given a picture of a Copecakes Baking Tin. Together with their parents, clients generate a list of six positive coping strategies and fill in the holes of the baking tin with these. Each of these strategies is practiced two to three times between sessions, and the parent and child are encouraged to be detectives, figuring out which coping strategies seem to work best for handling the anxiety. When the family returns, they pinpoint the top two or three coping strategies and then decorate fully baked Copecakes (Figure 8.4). These can be taken home and placed in a prominent location to serve as reminders of the child's positive coping choices.

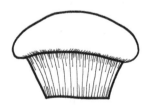

## Figure 8.4
*Source:* Goodyear-Brown, P. (2010a). *The Worry Wars: An Anxiety Workbook for Kids and Their Helpful Adults!* Nashville, TN: Author. Reprinted with permission.

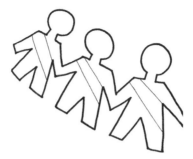

## Figure 8.5

*Source:* Goodyear-Brown, P. (2010a). *The Worry Wars: An Anxiety Workbook for Kids and Their Helpful Adults!* Nashville, TN: Author. Reprinted with permission.

Utilizing support systems is another important coping strategy. The Worry Wars protocol introduces clients to the idea of gathering a team to help fight their battles. Younger clients are given handouts with chains of paper dolls, and older clients are offered bookmarks that help identify support people (Figures 8.5 and 8.6).

Children are asked a series of questions that help them identify people who (a) build their sense of competency, (b) give them words of affirmation, (c) offer safe, nurturing physical affection, and (d) listen to them. In addition to identifying these helpful adults, it is valuable for a child to identify at least one peer relationship that is positive for that child. I will often ask, "Who is someone you like to play with?" or "Who do you like to hang out with?" Pinpointing these sources of social support can give clients a sense of being insulated from the anxiety. Moreover, once these support people have been identified, clinicians can help clients craft the specific role each support person can play in the anxiety

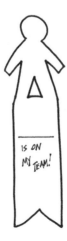

## Figure 8.6

*Source:* Goodyear-Brown, P. (2010a). *The Worry Wars: An Anxiety Workbook for Kids and Their Helpful Adults!* Nashville, TN: Author. Reprinted with permission.

management process. For example, if a client has identified his soccer coach as someone who helps him get better at something (competency building), then this soccer coach can be enlisted to help with anxiety symptoms that might manifest during practices and games. If the child is learning any specific boss back talk, the coach can be made aware of this strategy so that he can reinforce it on the soccer field.

Parents play a key role in anxiety management for their children. Clinically anxious children often require more co-regulation of affect across childhood than do their typically developing peers. The older the child, the less intuitive it will be to parents that their child's rigid or noncompliant behavior is actually an outcry for more involved soothing. An anxiety response can be an overwhelming physiological event for children. The intensity of their physical manifestations of anxiety can leave them feeling helpless, disempowered, and out of control. Many children counter this out-of-control feeling by engaging in increasingly rigid patterns of behavior. Parents who seek out help for the behavioral difficulties of anxious children are often encouraged to implement strict behavior management approaches to help curb the noncompliance without also getting the specific psychoeducation around how to effectively co-regulate their children. It is recommended that clinicians who implement the Worry Wars protocol have collateral sessions with parents to teach them the SOOTHE strategies, a series of techniques that parents can use in addition to behavior management tools to positively influence the course of anxiety in their children (Goodyear-Brown, 2010a, 2010c).

## Relaxation Strategies

Once positive coping strategies have been reinforced and a social support network gathered, clients then learn a variety of relaxation and stress inoculation strategies. One of the most important strategies is deep, diaphragmatic breathing. When children become anxious, they generally engage in more shallow breathing, which further reinforces the body's growing dysregulation. The dual processes of focusing on the simple act of breathing and taking intentionally slow, deep breaths counter the physiological arousal that often accompanies anxiety (Cyr, Culbert, & Kaiser, 2003; Gerik, 2005; Kabat-Zinn, 1990, 2005; Kabat-Zinn et al., 1992; Kajander & Peper, 1998). Several prop-based playful methods for learning and practicing deep breathing are offered in the Worry Wars protocol. Tried-and-true play tools, such as bubbles (Goodyear-Brown, Riviere, & Shelby, 2004; Paula, 2009) and personalized pinwheels (Goodyear-Brown, 2005, 2010a), become external focal points that help children practice deep breathing. A template is included in the manual that allows children to create individual pinwheels. Clients are encouraged to draw soothing pictures or write words of affirmation on the blades of their pinwheel to enhance the relaxation work.

Children are also offered an exercise called Five Count Breathing (Goodyear-Brown, 2010b). The manual includes a star template that children can trace as they are completing the breathing exercise. Each star has five points. As they trace each star, they are breathing in for a count of five, holding their breath for a count of five, and breathing out for a count of five (Figure 8.7).

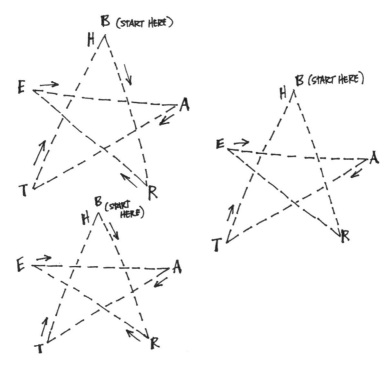

## Figure 8.7
*Source:* Goodyear-Brown, P. (2010a). *The Worry Wars: An Anxiety Workbook for Kids and Their Helpful Adults!* Nashville, TN: Author. Reprinted with permission.

Although deep breathing is a foundational skill for relaxation, other tools can be important for children in fighting their anxiety. Anxious children can benefit from the creation of safe-place imagery (Cohen et al, 2006; Goodyear-Brown, 2010a; Stueck & Gloeckner, 2005). One of the advantages of combining play therapy with more traditional exposure/response prevention programs is that children can flesh out, through the three-dimensional kinesthetic manipulation of sand, art, clay, or the play materials, a meaningful safe place. The manual offers an activity called Picture Perfect Postcards. In this activity, children are encouraged to imagine a place that they would like to go on vacation. They can draw a picture of the vacation spot on the front and then write a couple of lines about their vacation experience on the back (Figure 8.8).

Music is a natural modulator of affect and can be another powerful aid to relaxation (Goldstein, 1980; Pelletier, 2004). Another exercise, Chillin' with my iPod, encourages children to identify three pieces of music that make them feel calm and three songs that engender feelings of happiness. Their choices are written on an icon of an iPod (Figure 8.9). This intervention is particularly effective with adolescents, but the music that clients identify can be incorporated into other interventions even with younger clients. Calming songs can be used as background music for PMR exercises or guided imagery. Chosen music can also be played while the child is designing a sand tray to represent a place where she could feel happy and safe.

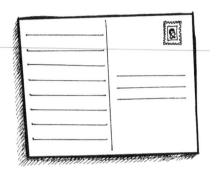

## Figure 8.8

*Source:* Goodyear-Brown, P. (2010a). *The Worry Wars: An Anxiety Workbook for Kids and Their Helpful Adults!* Nashville, TN: Author. Reprinted with permission.

Once clients have become aware of their physiological responses to anxiety-provoking stimuli, augmented their adaptive coping strategies, gathered a team to help fight their anxiety battles, and practiced inducing the relaxation response through any of these interventions, they are ready to target the anxiety-laden thoughts.

The Worry Wars protocol offers a variety of ways in which anxious thoughts can be identified and recorded. Children benefit from an externalization and playful manipulation of the anxious thoughts. When the clinician reads the child one of the therapeutic stories in the first phase of treatment, the therapist is offering a metaphoric form for a particular client's worry to take. The anxiety may take the form of a dragon, a princess, or an octopus. The client also has the option of creating his or her own worry creature after the story is read. A basic template of a worried brain can also be used (Figure 8.10). If the dragon

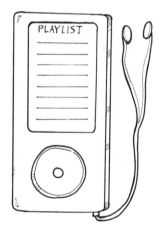

## Figure 8.9

*Source:* Goodyear-Brown, P. (2010a). *The Worry Wars: An Anxiety Workbook for Kids and Their Helpful Adults!* Nashville, TN: Author. Reprinted with permission.

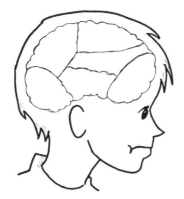

## Figure 8.10

*Source:* Goodyear-Brown, P. (2010a). *The Worry Wars: An Anxiety Workbook for Kids and Their Helpful Adults!* Nashville, TN: Author. Reprinted with permission.

metaphor is used, the handout of the dragon's fiery breath can be used to record the child's anxious thoughts (Figure 8.11).

Once the anxious thoughts have been identified, children must learn how to stop those thoughts from taking over. The protocol offers a variety of stop symbols (Figures 8.12 and 8.13).

The stop sign can be copied and personalized. The stop hand can serve as an example to clients, but clinicians are encouraged to trace and cut out each child's hand and fill it with the child's stop language that is most meaningful to that child.

Because children are kinesthetic creatures, play scenarios that allow the child to stop a physical dragon are both more fun and more therapeutically meaningful for children than the more staid methods for practicing thought stopping. Clinicians are encouraged to provide the clients with puppets that give each of the story metaphors concrete form. I keep a variety of dragons, princesses, and octopi in my office. Children can choose the puppet they find most engaging. I then play the voice of the puppet, verbalizing the anxious

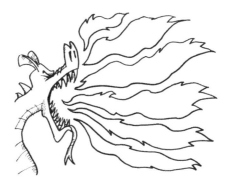

## Figure 8.11

*Source:* Goodyear-Brown, P. (2010a). *The Worry Wars: An Anxiety Workbook for Kids and Their Helpful Adults!* Nashville, TN: Author. Reprinted with permission.

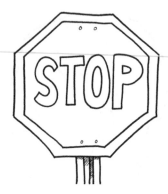

## Figure 8.12

*Source:* Goodyear-Brown, P. (2010a). *The Worry Wars: An Anxiety Workbook for Kids and Their Helpful Adults!* Nashville, TN: Author. Reprinted with permission.

thoughts while the child gets to hold up a stop sign, blow a whistle, or use a hand signal that indicates that the puppet should stop.

Once the child has practiced stopping the anxious thoughts, replacement thoughts and boss back language can be crafted. Replacement thoughts are ones that run counter to the anxious thought and can usually be crafted in direct relationship to it. For example, a child whose dragon says, "You can't handle this!" may be fought with the simple replacement statement, "I *can* do this!" Children will also use the replacement cognitions to practice positive mantras, such as "I am stronger than my fear!" Cognitive reappraisal of imagined outcomes would fall into this category of thought work as well. For example, a 7-year-old girl struggles with separation anxiety. She is plagued by the anxious thought that her mom won't come back for her. This thought leads to others, and she imagines all sorts of terrible things that could happen to mom that might keep her from coming back to pick her up at the end of the day. Reappraisal allows for the child to create a cognition that says, "She has always come back for me before. She will come back for me this time."

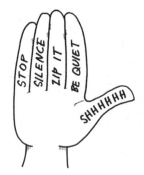

## Figure 8.13

*Source:* Goodyear-Brown, P. (2010a). *The Worry Wars: An Anxiety Workbook for Kids and Their Helpful Adults!* Nashville, TN: Author. Reprinted with permission.

The second form of cognitive warfare requires the use of boss back talk language. This set of verbalizations is aimed at increasing the child's feelings of competence and power in relation to the symbol of the anxiety. If the dragon is being used as the metaphor for the child's anxiety, the therapist will speak the anxious thoughts through the dragon puppet's mouth. The client then says things like, "I don't have to listen to you!" and "You're a liar!" to quiet the dragon. Clinicians are encouraged to help clients craft both kinds of talk. At this point in the treatment of adults, clients would be able to identify the anxious thought, stop it, and replace it—all inside of their heads. Children are best served developmentally by helping them give voice to these thoughts while combining them with kinesthetic action.

In each of the therapeutic stories, the externalized anxiety is eventually conquered through a series of weapons. Daniel uses a sword and shield to fight the dragon and finally quenches his fiery breath with a fire extinguisher. All of these icons are made available in reproducible form so that children can make their own swords, shields, and fire extinguishers. In addition to these handouts that can be individualized with a child's unique boss back language, clinicians are encouraged to keep actual shields, swords, and play fire extinguishers available in the playroom so that children can have full-body practice at bossing back their anxiety. Anxiety can be a powerful enemy for many of the children that we treat. They often experience a greater sense of personal power as they battle the externalized anxiety in three dimensions. These playful exercises also allow the client to rehearse the self-talk skills they will need as they work their exposure/response prevention hierarchies.

## The Battles

After a client has developed all of the weapons discussed in the previous section, all that remains is to structure an exposure hierarchy and work it. A pyramid icon is offered to help clients craft their hierarchies (Figure 8.14).

The least scary scenario is placed at the bottom of the pyramid, and the scariest situation is placed at the top. Tracking clients' successes as they work through exposures is a critical piece of treatment. The form that the exposure

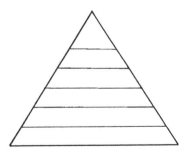

### Figure 8.14
Source: Goodyear-Brown, P. (2010a). *The Worry Wars: An Anxiety Workbook for Kids and Their Helpful Adults!* Nashville, TN: Author. Reprinted with permission.

hierarchy takes is flexible. Reproducible versions of mountains, ladders, and staircases allow for clients to track the exposures using whichever method appeals most to them. More importantly, different tracking instruments can be used at different points in the exposure process, keeping the motivation high and the exposure work more engaging.

After the hierarchy has been created, clinicians who have couched treatment within one of the therapeutic stories can continue to use this metaphor to track successful exposures. For example, if the clinician has been working with a separation-anxious client and using the octopus as the externalization of this anxiety, the client can make his own octopus out of clay and pull off pieces (to be traded for rewards) each time that he successfully completes an exposure. The client gets the three-dimensional experience of watching the octopus disappear as the anxiety is conquered. The manual also includes icons for each of the worry creatures and a reproducible set of paper bricks. One brick can be placed over the worry creature each time an exposure is completed until the creature is completely covered. I also have the child identify the subjective units of distress (SUDs) he or she is feeling before the exposure (anticipatory anxiety) and 2 to 3 minutes after completion of the exposure. Through this ongoing assessment, children learn that the physiological arousal that occurs as they anticipate the exposure quickly decreases after the exposure is complete. The SUD readings can be used to reinforce the idea that anxiety is a liar, but the truth is that children can push through the anxiety.

Fighting anxiety is difficult work for adults and children alike. For this reason, as new levels of desensitization are achieved, it is helpful for children to receive rewards. I use a two-tiered token economy system for these rewards. The child is rewarded on a daily basis for each of the small exposures and then receives a larger reward for completing a week's worth of exposures. Clinicians can help families agree on rewards using the treasure chest handout. Possible options for the daily rewards can be written in each of the four coins spilling out of the treasure chest, and larger rewards for weekly completion of exposures can be written in the two prominently depicted diamonds (Figure 8.15).

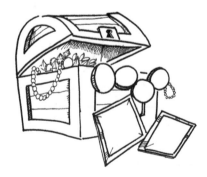

## Figure 8.15

Source: Goodyear-Brown, P. (2010a). *The Worry Wars: An Anxiety Workbook for Kids and Their Helpful Adults!* Nashville, TN: Author. Reprinted with permission.

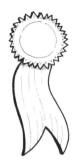
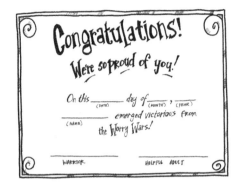
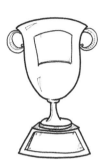

## Figure 8.16

*Source:* Goodyear-Brown, P. (2010a). *The Worry Wars: An Anxiety Workbook for Kids and Their Helpful Adults!* Nashville, TN: Author. Reprinted with permission.

The final piece of treatment is a graduation ceremony (Figure 8.16). Regaining control of one's anxiety is an accomplishment worthy of celebration. The protocol offers specific interventions that help parents and children reflect on the work done, give honor to one another, and prepare for future encounters with anxiety.

## Case Example

Sally was an 8-year-old girl referred for generalized anxiety disorder. When I met with Sally's mom, it became clear that she had been slow-to-warm-up as an infant and had bouts of fairly severe separation anxiety in her toddler and preschool years. At the time of intake, mom identified Sally as still fearful that mom might not return to pick her up from school, a fear of her teacher (but only when her teacher looked angry or stern), and fear of storms. Sally was having two to three meltdowns per day. She would scream and cry and refuse to comply with seemingly simple requests, particularly after school. According to mom this behavior often happened "for no clear reason."

When Sally and I played the Hot-and-Cold Worry Worms game, she articulated several more fears of which her mother was unaware. These included a fear of the dark, a dread of watching the news, because any scary thing mentioned on the news would "take over her brain," a fear that someone would break into her house in the middle of the night, a fear that she might fail a test at school, and a fear that she wouldn't be liked, although she had lots of friends.

Mom was given psychoeducation about the rigidity that is often engendered by anxiety, and she was taught the SOOTHE strategies at the beginning of treatment, to help Sally at home. Sally was read the story *Daniel the Dragon Slayer*, and we discussed the ways in which Daniel's anxiety grew as he gave more attention to his worried thoughts. Sally was easily able to identify the things that Daniel did to try and reduce the anxiety, and she quickly made the connection that his avoidance behaviors fed the dragon in the story. Sally was delighted by the idea of getting to fight her own worry creature, and she created a Worry Witch to be her metaphoric embodiment of anxiety.

Sally was taught deep breathing and given a bottle of bubbles and asked to practice making three big bubbles before school and three more before bed as therapeutic homework. In the next session, we created a personalized pinwheel, and she took this home to use as another prop for practicing deep breathing. She created a postcard of her safe place; she chose the beach where her family had visited the previous summer. When it was time to work on cognitive restructuring and boss back talk, we took our time. In the same way that therapists who do CBT with adults will utilize the *down arrow* technique to help clients find the thought under the thought, the strategy of *wondering with* a child can encourage her to voice other fears associated with the identified thought. In Sally's case, when she identified the thought "she might not come back" as one recurring anxious thought, I wondered out loud, "I wonder what would keep her from coming back?" She immediately listed several possibilities including, "She might have a car accident. She might get kidnapped. She might forget. She might die." Because her metaphoric creature was a Worry Witch, we drew a picture of her broom and wrote the thoughts inside the broom.

Sally chose to use a bicycle horn to practice thought stopping. I would be the voice of the witch puppet and verbalize the thoughts that Sally had identified. At any moment, she could blow the whistle on the witch. We pretended that the witch couldn't stand loud sounds and was immediately silenced by the whistle. Sally and mom worked together to identify some boss back talk to use when the Worry Witch talked to her. Sally came up with a whole host of things to say to the Worry Witch, some of which included attitude gestures like popping her hip or rolling her head. Apparently these gestures increased the client's feeling of empowerment and became fun shared actions that she and mom could do together to fight the Worry Witch.

Once Sally felt powerful in relation to the anxiety, we began to craft a set of exposures. Generalized anxiety disorder poses a challenge to hierarchy building, in that the anxiety-provoking situations are not constant. Sally could be suddenly assaulted by a new worry while consciously fighting another. In cases of selective mutism or obsessive-compulsive disorder, the hierarchy can be more straightforward. We decided to count as an exposure anything that required courage. We defined courage as *being afraid but choosing to do the scary thing anyway*. Using this definition, anytime that she felt anxious but pressed into the anxiety and resisted avoiding the situation that made her anxious, she completed a successful exposure.

Following are a couple of the tracking devices that we used to track her successes. Sally and I created a staircase (using the template in Figure 8.17) because she liked the sense that she was gaining ground with each exposure. Each time she used her courage, she wrote down the event on her staircase and was given a sticker by her mother. Each sticker translated into a daily reward. At the end of this first set of exposures, she and mom went and got joint pedicures. I wrote the numbers of the SUD scale along the bottom, and she and mom tracked

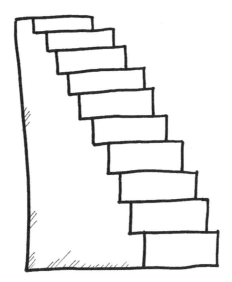

## Figure 8.17
*Source:* Goodyear-Brown, P. (2010a). *The Worry Wars: An Anxiety Workbook for Kids and Their Helpful Adults!* Nashville, TN: Author. Reprinted with permission.

her anticipatory anxiety and her anxiety 2 to 3 minutes after completing each exposure. Sally had gained confidence in her own abilities to beat back her anxiety after this first set of exposures. I invited her to draw a picture of her Worry Witch. She cut it out, and I gave her a supply of paper bricks to take home with her. Each time she finished a successful exposure, the nature of the event was written on one side of the brick and the brick was taped over a piece of the Worry Witch (See Figure 8.18 for an example of this intervention). When the Worry Witch was completely bricked in, Sally and her mother went on a little shopping spree.

## Conclusion

An integrative approach to childhood anxiety disorders is necessary in order to deliver the most efficacious treatment strategies in a form that is ingestible for children. The integration of play therapy with more traditional approaches allows for the therapeutic benefits of play to mitigate the avoidance behaviors that almost always accompany anxiety. Combining therapeutic storytelling and prop-based play therapy interventions with relaxation training, cognitive restructuring, and the establishment of an exposure hierarchy allow for systematic desensitization to occur. As the child begins to experience mastery over the anxiety, the anxiety management skills that have been learned are reinforced, equipping our child clients with tools that will last a lifetime.

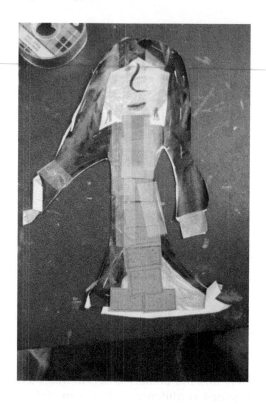

## Figure 8.18

A Worry Witch, much like the one Sally created, is being bricked in as exposures are successfully completed.

## References

Beck, J. S. (1995). *Cognitive therapy: Basics and beyond*. New York, NY: Guilford.

Beck, A. T., Emery, G., & Greenberg, R. L. (2005). *Anxiety disorders and phobias: A cognitive perspective*. New York, NY: Basic Books.

Cohen, J. & Mannarino, A. (2004). Posttraumatic Stress Disorder. In T.H. Olendick & J. March (Eds.), *Phobic and anxiety disorders in children and adolescents: A clinician's guide to effective psychosocial and pharmacological interventions*. New York, NY: Guilford Press.

Cohen, J., Mannarino, A., & Deblinger, E. (2006). *Treating trauma and traumatic grief in children and adolescents*. New York, NY: Guilford Press.

Cyr, L. R., Culbert, T., & Kaiser, P. (2003). Helping children with stress and anxiety: An integrative medicine approach. *Biofeedback, 31*(1), 12–17.

Felix, E., Bond, D., & Shelby, J. (2006). Coping with disaster: Psychosocial interventions for children in international disaster relief. In C. Schaefer & H. Kaduson (Eds.), *Contemporary play therapy: Theory, research, and practice* (pp. 307–329). New York, NY: Guilford Press.

Friedberg, R. & McClure, J. (2002). Review of Clinical Practice of Cognitive Therapy with Children and Adolescents. *Journal of Developmental and Behavioral Pediatrics, 23*(6), 457–458.

Gerik, S. (2005). Pain management in children: Developmental considerations and mind-body therapies. *Southern Medical Journal, 98*(3), 295–302.

Goldstein, A. (1980). Thrills in response to music and other stimuli. *Physiological Psychology, 8*(1), 126–129.

Goodyear-Brown, P. (2002). *Digging for buried treasure: 52 prop-based play therapy interventions for treating the problems of childhood.* Available at www.parisandme.com.

Goodyear-Brown, P. (2005). *Digging for buried treasure 2: 52 more prop-based play therapy interventions for treating the problems of childhood.* Available at www.parisandme .com.

Goodyear-Brown, P. (2010a). *Play therapy with traumatized children: A prescriptive approach.* Hoboken, NJ: Wiley.

Goodyear-Brown, P. (2010b). *The worry wars: An anxiety workbook for kids and their helpful adults.* Nashville, TN: Author.

Goodyear-Brown, P. (2010c). Play therapy with anxious preschoolers. In C. Schaefer (Ed.), *Play therapy with anxious preschoolers.* Washington, DC: American Psychological Association Press.

Goodyear-Brown, P., Riviere, S., & Shelby, J. (2004). *10 peas in a pod.* DVD. Available at www.parisandme.com.

Kabat-Zinn, J. (1990). *Full catastrophe living: Using the wisdom of your body and mind to face pain, stress and illness.* New York, NY: Delta.

Kabat-Zinn, J. (2005). *Coming to our senses: Healing ourselves and the world through mindfulness.* New York, NY: Hyperion.

Kabat-Zinn, J., Massion, A. O., Kristeller, J., Peterson, L. G., Gletcher, K. E., Pbert, L., Lenderking, W. R., & Santorelli, S. F. (1992). The effectiveness of a mediation-based stress reduction program in the treatment of anxiety disorders. *American Journal of Psychiatry, 149,* 936–943.

Kajander, R., & Peper, E. (1998). Teaching diaphragmatic breathing to children. *Biofeedback, 26*(3), 14–17.

Kimball, W., Nelson, W. M., & Politano, P. M. (1993). *The role of developmental variables in cognitive-behavioral interventions with children.* In A. J. Finch, W. M. Nelson, & E. S. Ott (Eds.), *Cognitive-behavioral procedures with children and adolescents: A practical guide* (pp. 25–66). Needham Heights, MA: Allyn & Bacon.

Knell, S. (1993). *Cognitive-behavioral play therapy.* Lanham, MD: Jason Aronson.

Knell, S. (2009). Cognitive behavioral play therapy: Theory and application. In A. Drewes (Ed.), *Blending play therapy with cognitive behavioral therapy: Evidence-based and other effective treatments and techniques,* 117–133. Hoboken, NJ: Wiley.

Landreth, G. L. (1991). *Play Therapy: The art of the relationship.* Muncie, IN: Accelerated Development.

March, J. S. (2006). *Talking Back to OCD: The Program that Helps Kids and Teens say "No Way"—and Parents Say "Way to Go."* New York, NY: Guilford Press.

March, J. S., & Mulle, K. (1998). *OCD in Children and Adolescents: A Cognitive-Behavioral Treatment Manual.* New York, NY: Guilford Press.

Mills, J. C., & Crowley, R. J. (2001). *Therapeutic metaphors for children and the child within.* New York, NY: Routledge.

Paula, S. T. (2009). Play therapy techniques for affect regulation. In A. Drewes (Ed.), *Blending play therapy with cognitive behavioral therapy: Evidence-based and other effective treatments and techniques* (pp. 353–372). Hoboken, NJ: Wiley.

Pelletier, C. L. (2004). The effect of music on decreasing arousal due to stress: a meta-analysis. *Journal of Music Therapy, 41*(3), 192–214.

Schaefer, C. E. (1993). *The therapeutic powers of play.* Northvale, NJ: Jason Aronson.

Schaefer, C. E., & Drewes, A. A. (2009). *Therapeutic powers of play and play therapy.* In A. A. Drewes (Ed.), *Blending play therapy with cognitive behavioral therapy: Evidence-based and other effective treatments and techniques* (pp. 3–15). Hoboken, NJ: Wiley.

Shelby, J. S., & Berk, M. S. (2009). Play therapy, pedagogy and CBT: An argument for interdisciplinary synthesis. In A. A. Drewes (Ed.), *Blending play therapy with cognitive behavioral therapy: Evidence-based and other effective treatments and techniques* (pp. 17–40). Hoboken, NJ: Wiley.

Shelby, J. S., Bond, D., Hall, S., & Hsu, C. (2004). *Enhancing coping among young tsunami survivors.* Los Angeles, CA: Authors.

Stueck, M., & Gloeckner, N. (2005). Yoga for children in the mirror of science: Working spectrum and practice fields of the training of relaxation with elements of yoga for children. *Early Childhood Development Care, 175,* 371–377.

Wolpe, J. (1990). *The practice of behavior therapy.* New York, NY: Pergamon Press.

# Filial Therapy for Maltreated and Neglected Children

**9**

Chapter

## Integration of Family Therapy and Play Therapy

### *Riše VanFleet and Glade Topham*

## Introduction

Children who have been maltreated, neglected, or exposed to other forms of family or interpersonal violence often present challenges to therapists because of the complex nature of their trauma and the negative impact on their attachment processes. Their trauma reactions and attachment difficulties are so entwined and their presenting problems so complicated that therapists sometimes struggle to know where to begin. At times, children's prognoses are clouded by bad experiences in the dependent care/child protection system, such as frequent placement moves, inadequate treatment, failed adoptions, and even further abuse.

Because maltreated children face numerous challenges to their healthy psychosocial development, effective treatment must address the complex needs of the children, foster families, adoptive families, or biological families with whom the children are to be reunified. Coordination of a constellation of services, including case management, residential care, foster care agencies and families, adoption workers, health-related services, and psychotherapy, is essential but often lacking. It is far too common that decisions are made about children's lives without the input of their therapists or primary caregivers.

Filial Therapy (FT) is a systemic intervention that integrates family therapy and play therapy, and offers a unique and far-reaching form of treatment for maltreated and attachment-disrupted children and their caregivers (VanFleet, 2006c; VanFleet & Sniscak, 2003). Not only does FT represent a theoretically integrative form of therapy, but it can also readily be used in conjunction with other forms of play therapy, behavior management, parent consultation, group therapy, social skills programs, or cognitive-behavioral intervention. FT is particularly useful for these children and families because it simultaneously ameliorates trauma and attachment issues in the context of a supportive family environment. Its premises and goals are consistent with the needs of maltreated and neglected children and those who care for them. Furthermore, a growing body of research spanning 45 years has demonstrated the effectiveness of FT with a wide range of problems, including those commonly reported for abused and traumatized children (see VanFleet, Ryan, & Smith, 2005).

This contribution briefly covers the difficulties commonly experienced by maltreated children and their families, the implications of the parenting style and emotion socialization literatures for their treatment, and ways in which FT can be implemented to help them. An overview of the integrative nature and methods of FT is followed by a discussion of its unique contributions to abused and neglected children and their families. Its use in combination with other modalities is also outlined, along with a transition model that bridges the gap between foster care and adoption, as well as foster care and reunification, for these children. A case illustration shows a typical application of FT within a foster-to-adopt situation.

## Rationale for the Integrative Approach

The potential negative consequences of child maltreatment are well-documented. They include (a) serious problems with self-regulation, including emotional and behavioral; (b) inability to trust and difficulties forming and maintaining healthy attachments and satisfying relationships; (c) developmental delays in language, social skills and interactions, impulse control, physical/motor development, and cognitive and sensory/perceptual functioning; (d) inability to self-soothe; (e) somatic complaints and conditions; and (f) problems with attention, focus, and memory. Furthermore, these children are at risk for a wide range of mental health problems, including post-traumatic stress disorder, depression, separation anxiety, shame, hoarding of food and other items, lack of empathy, aggression and cruelty (often directed toward animals and children), repeated victimization, sexual acting out, persistently low self-esteem and self-image, risky behaviors, isolation and peer rejection, oppositional behaviors and conduct disorders, poor boundaries, substance abuse, self-injurious behaviors, and others (Cook et al., 2005; Gilbert et al., 2009; Kim & Cicchetti, 2010; Perry, 2001; Perry & Szalavitz, 2007; van der Kolk, Roth, Pelcovitz, Sunday, & Spinazzola, 2005; Webb, 2005).

A small interview study using Adler's early recollection approach offers a glimpse into the perceptions of preadolescent and adolescent children diagnosed with Reactive Attachment Disorder (Tobin, Wardi-Zonna, & Yezzi-Shareef, 2007). The study yielded themes of children feeling alone, feeling abandoned by others, and a sense that events in their lives were unfair. The children also expressed fear and sadness accompanied by a sense of unmet emotional needs, particularly in terms of love and caring.

With so much at risk, it makes sense to intervene as early as possible with children who have histories of abuse, neglect, and attachment disruptions. Play therapy has been considered a key approach for this population for many years (e.g., Gil, 2010; James, 1994; Terr, 1990; Webb, 2005). Because their mal-treatment negatively impacts their ability to form healthy attachments, and because most long-lasting individual growth and change occurs only within the context of caring, trusting, empathic relationships, abused children can benefit substantially from involvement in FT.

## Filial Therapy

Filial Therapy was conceived and developed by Bernard and Louise Guerney starting in the late 1950s (B. G. Guerney, 1964; L. F. Guerney, 1983, 1997, 2003). They had seen the value of play therapy, and in particular, Child-Centered (nondirective) Play Therapy (CCPT), and believed that its impact would be more powerful if the play sessions were conducted by parents or other caregivers who already had formed intimate relationships with their children. Far ahead of their time, they developed and researched FT, a theoretically integrative form of family therapy in which parents/caregivers were trained to conduct special nondirective play sessions with their children under the supervision of the therapist. As the parents gained competence and confidence in conducting the special filial play sessions, they eventually transferred them to the home environment, although still monitored by the therapist. As presenting problems were resolved, the therapist helped parents generalize the skills and attitudes they had learned during the play sessions to everyday life. Initially developed as a group intervention for families, FT was easily incorporated into work with individual families (Ginsberg, 2004; VanFleet, 2005, 2006b, 2008a; VanFleet, Sywulak, & Sniscak, 2010). Filial Therapy is supported empirically by 45 years of research. Results of controlled and comparative studies have consistently shown improvements in children's presenting problems, parental acceptance and empathy, parental skills, and parental stress (VanFleet, Ryan, & Smith, 2005).

   More recently, the Guerneys and others have adapted the original model of FT for shorter-term groups (Caplin & Pernet, 2010, personal communication; Guerney & Ryan, in preparation; Landreth & Bratton, 2006; VanFleet & Sniscak, 2003, in press; Wright & Walker, 2003). Because of the complex and severe nature of child trauma stemming from maltreatment, neglect, and attachment disruption, as well as the significant family distress reported by parents and caregivers of these children, the original family systems model of FT is often most useful for this population (L. Guerney, 1997; VanFleet, 2005, 2006c; VanFleet & Sniscak, 2003, in press).

## The Theoretically Integrative Nature of Filial Therapy

The full form of FT represents a true theoretical integration, which has been described in detail elsewhere (Ginsberg, 2003, 2004; B. G. Guerney, 1964; L. F. Guerney, 2003; VanFleet, 2009a, 2009b). Included in the approach are human-istic, interpersonal, psychodynamic, behavioral, social learning, cognitive, de-velopmental, attachment, and family systems theories, integrated fully through the use of a psychoeducational model of intervention. FT is an empowerment approach that encourages parents or other caregivers to be full partners in the therapy process. A collaborative and empathic climate permeates the process for both children and parents. The method is deceptively simple, yet it embraces the entire family system and helps shift the beliefs, perceptions, and behaviors of every family member. FT strengthens parent-child relationships, and by so doing, improves co-parenting while ameliorating problems that children are experiencing. FT strengthens the family context in which change can occur.

FT helps address the needs that many researchers and clinicians have highlighted for maltreated children. These include a stable living arrangement; empathic, loving, and emotionally safe family relationships; opportunities for self-expression and healthy emotional development; developmentally appropriate methods for working through trauma reactions; assistance with trauma-reactive behaviors; improved self-appraisals; and the development of trust and attachment with trustworthy adults (e.g., Gil, 2010; Perry & Szalavitz, 2007; Terr, 1990; Webb, 2005). FT also addresses the needs of parents and caregivers who can become seriously stressed by the maladaptive behaviors of these children. Caregivers need emotional support, an understanding of the child's behavior as it relates to the trauma history, practical approaches for handling a wide range of stressful situations and behaviors, and tools for fostering healthier growth for the entire family system. FT effectively combines play therapy, which is the most developmentally appropriate form of intervention for children and adolescents, with family therapy, which strengthens family relationships, without which changes may be minimal or short-lived.

FT can be particularly beneficial to maltreating parents who are working toward or have been recently reunified with their children. These parents may lack the knowledge and skills required to foster important areas of child development. In FT, parents develop greater awareness of their children and their needs and develop a set of skills that empowers them to facilitate their children's healthy growth and development. We briefly review the research on key parenting knowledge, styles, and practices that are predictive of positive child outcomes and then link these parent competencies to FT.

## Key Parenting Characteristics, Practices, and Styles in Healthy Child Development

Several parenting factors have been shown to be key to healthy child development, including parent understanding of child development, type of parenting style, quality of parent-child attachment, level of parent respect for child autonomy, and parent socialization of child emotion. Parents' accurate understanding of the developmental level of their children and awareness of the accompanying capabilities and needs of the children are fundamental to positive parenting (Smith, Perou, & Lesesne, 2002). Absent this understanding, parenting is out of sync with children's needs and leads to increased risk for abuse or neglect. Research indicates that maltreating parents tend to have unrealistic expectations for their children (Azar & Rohrbeck, 1986), judge their children's behavior more harshly than others (Chilamkurti & Milner, 1993), and attribute more negative intent to their children's actions (Larrance & Twentyman, 1983). These problems have been shown to be interrelated in that parents' higher levels of unrealistic expectations lead to their attributing increasingly negative intent to child behavior and to more coercive and hostile parental responses (Azar, 1998; Barnes & Azar, 1990).

Research on parenting styles reveals that authoritative parenting provides the most positive outcomes for children. Children of authoritative parents have an increased sense of autonomy, self-discipline, self-efficacy, and emotional maturity (Baumrind, 1991; Baumrind, Larzelere, & Owens, 2010; Steinberg, Elmen, & Mounts, 1989). Authoritative parents are aware of and responsive to their children's needs and wishes, readily offer emotional warmth and support, and encourage their children's individuality. They set firm limits but use induction and reasoning with their children, encouraging and valuing their children's expression of their own perspectives and wishes (Baumrind et al., 2010). In contrast, neither authoritarian (high control and low warmth) nor permissive (low control and high warmth) parenting styles provide opportunities for children to develop the ability to cope successfully with challenges, and as a result, children of both types of parents are less emotionally mature and lack adequate behavioral inhibition and self-regulation (Baumrind, 1991; Baumrind et al., 2010; Steinberg et al., 1989).

The security of parent-child attachment relationships has long-lasting and profound implications for children (Ainsworth, Blehar, Waters, & Wall, 1978; Bowlby, 1969; Sroufe, 1988). Securely attached children show more enthusiasm, higher levels of positive affect, and higher levels of compliance in interaction with their caregivers; are more competent socially and are more popular with peers; are more empathic; have higher self-esteem; and have better emotional health (see Thompson, 2009, for a review). Parenting practices that have been found to be predictive of a secure parent-child attachment include acceptance, warmth, accessibility, sensitivity, and responsiveness (see Belsky & Fearon, 2009, for a review).

Another important predictor of child outcome is parent respect for child autonomy. Psychological control, which includes parental intrusiveness, guilt induction, and love withdrawal, has been shown to be particularly damaging to children's sense of identity and autonomous development (Barber, Stolz, & Olsen, 2005). Psychological control disregards emotional boundaries and child wishes in favor of manipulating a child's behavior/emotions to meet parental needs. Child outcomes of psychologically controlling parents include increased externalizing and internalizing symptoms, academic problems, low self-esteem, low self-reliance, and increased self-denigration (Barber et al., 2005; Barber & Harmon, 2002; Goldstein, Davis-Kean, & Eccles, 2005). In contrast, parents who are high on involvement but also high on autonomy foster positive academic and socioemotional outcomes in children (Grolnick, 2003).

The emotion socialization literature indicates that children whose parents discourage emotion expression or punish them for expressing negative emotions tend to be more emotionally reactive, more intense in emotional expression, less able to regulate their emotions, and more likely to use escape tactics to deal with emotional distress (Eisenberg et al., 1999; Fabes, Leondard, Kupanoff, & Martin, 2001). In contrast, children whose parents value their emotional expression, validate their experience, and provide support while they work through the emotion are more skilled at regulating their emotions, are more effective socially, and are more successful academically (Gottman, Katz, & Hooven, 1996).

In FT, parents develop awareness of their child's capabilities, struggles, feelings, and needs as they learn to attend fully to their child in filial play sessions and as they discuss their child's play in post-play discussions with the therapist. Through filial play sessions, parents learn to attune to their child's feelings and needs, to value and respect their child's autonomy, and to respond sensitively. Parents learn to calmly set and follow through on firm limits as necessary, while preserving child autonomy. Furthermore, parents learn to unconditionally accept and empathically reflect child emotion and child effort as their child works through the emotion. In developing these competencies, parents are able to provide a unique context, via the filial play sessions, for their child to heal and grow. In addition, they are able to create a relationship context in daily parent-child interaction that promotes positive child growth and development.

## The Family Therapy Perspective in Filial Therapy

Because of the emphasis in FT on fostering healthy relationships and its rejection of the medical model, which seeks to uncover and treat pathology, FT is consistent in its approach with a variety of family therapy theoretical perspectives. The family therapy perspective included in FT is shown as follows by describing the theoretical and practical alignment of FT with two popular models of family therapy.

### Consistency With Experiential Family Therapy
Experiential family therapy views problems as resulting from denial and suppression of emotional experience. The practice of emotional suppression is frequently developed at an early age as children learn that others, particularly their parents, do not accept certain emotional experiences and the expression of the emotion. Parents may view child emotion as needing to be shaped and corrected much like child behavior and so may unwittingly teach their children to look to external sources to determine what they should be feeling. The result is impaired self-awareness and self-esteem, and may also result in family relationships that are void of emotional expression and/or that are somewhat artificial (Nichols, 2009). The challenge then is to provide opportunities and experiences that will help family members develop an awareness of and acceptance of their own and other family members' emotional experience. The therapeutic solution is to foster in-session, emotional experience between family members and to help family members establish honest and sincere emotional contact with each other (Napier & Whitaker, 1978; Satir, 1972).

Similarly, a primary goal of FT is to help family members develop awareness and acceptance of their own and other family members' emotional experiences and needs. The primary experiential activity in FT is the parent-child play session. Consistent with experiential family therapy, FT play sessions provide an opportunity for children to express a range of feelings, needs, and fantasies as they engage in play. Parents learn to understand, accept, and validate their children's emotions during these sessions, and by doing so help their children to learn that their emotions are valid, accepted, and important. In turn, parents develop increased awareness of and acceptance of their own emotional experience during post-play feedback sessions as the therapist accepts and validates the parents' needs, desires, and emotions. Play sessions also introduce playful and spontaneous interaction into the parent-child relationship, which combats rigid and sterile interaction that may have previously prevailed in the relationship. Because all family members are involved in these play sessions (or "special times"), emotion acceptance and expression becomes an integrated part of family culture.

*Consistency With Structural Family Therapy*
In structural family therapy, family problems are viewed as resulting from rigid family structures that prevent the family from adapting to changing circumstances. Problematic family structures include inflexible role assignment; rigid boundaries between family members leaving them emotionally isolated; diffuse boundaries between family members undermining their autonomy; and either absent or extreme parental hierarchy, with children having either too much or too little influence in family decision making (Minuchin, 1974). In structural family therapy, family structure is observed and modified during family interaction. A primary means for accomplishing this is through the use of enactments. In an enactment, the therapist encourages specific family interaction and then works within that interaction to modify family structure, such as solidifying particular boundaries or establishing parental hierarchy. As new patterns of interaction are regularly repeated, a more functional family structure is established (Nichols, 2009).

   The enactment of FT is the parent-child play session. Similar to structural family therapy, in FT the therapist observes family interaction and works to help parents and children develop more positive patterns of interaction. The difference is that instead of shaping the interaction in the moment, as is the case in structural family therapy, the FT therapist works with the parents in post-play session discussion after each play session to modify and shape the interaction. The FT therapist works with parents to establish a healthy boundary in parent-child interaction that allows for connection, warmth, and support while also respecting and fostering child autonomy. In cases where two parents are participating, a boundary around the co-parenting relationship is reinforced as the therapist meets in executive session with the parents after parent-child play sessions. Clear and consistent limit setting combined with warmth and support help establish an appropriate parental hierarchy. Finally, FT helps parents replace rigid role assignment (e.g., disciplinarian vs. nurturer) with more flexible roles that can shift based on family need. The individual parent-child play sessions enable each parent to develop confidence and comfort in a variety of parenting roles with their children, without reflexively stepping aside for the other parent to fulfill less comfortable roles.

## Other Theories Integrated Into the FT Approach

In the ways noted previously, FT combines the theories and potential benefits of family therapy with play therapy. At its core, FT is family therapy that uses play sessions to bring about changes for the children and parents alike. Therapists also use behavioral and social learning principles to teach the play session skills to parents; they use acceptance and empathy to help parents feel safe and accepted, just as parents eventually learn to do the same with their children; and they use psychodynamic ideas to help parents understand their children's play themes and their possible relation to intra- and interpersonal dynamics. Principles and methods from cognitive therapy can help parents develop more realistic views of themselves and their children in the post-play discussions, and the play sessions typically result in cognitive shifts for children as they master their fears and trauma reactions through their play metaphors. Interpersonal theory suggests that relationships change when any party within the relationship changes. In FT, the focus of change is on the parent, and the therapist facilitates change for the child and the family *through* the parent.

In essence, FT creates an empathic, collaborative, and psychoeducational climate in which therapists guide parents on how to be better attuned to their children, how to develop and show empathy for them, how to be more supportive of children's emotions and autonomy, how to handle practical situations effectively, and how to develop and use a more authoritative parenting style. These are the very things that maltreated children need most.

## Practical Implementation

Because FT is a theoretically integrated approach, the first part of this section details how it is used for maltreated and neglected children and their families. This is followed by a brief section that shows how FT might be used in conjunction with other therapeutic modalities, including individual play therapy, group play therapy, other forms of family play therapy, parent consultation, behavior management, and animal-assisted play therapy. Finally, the unique contributions of FT for this population are outlined, and a transition model that uses FT to help children move from foster care to adoption or reunification is described.

### Parent/Caregiver Involvement

Because little true progress can be made in treating maltreated children without family involvement, it is critical for therapists to engage parents (foster parents, kinship caregivers, adoptive parents, or biological parents) fully in whatever therapeutic process they use. Parents are invited and encouraged to take part in the process as fully as possible, including participation in FT and other adjunctive interventions. In the Beech Street Program, a practice with which the first author is affiliated and which contracts with several local child protective agencies, the participation of foster parents, biological parents, or other relevant caregivers in treatment is required in order for therapists to deliver services. This enlists the agencies' help in encouraging reluctant parents to participate. Even so, the most effective method of engagement, by far, has been to offer genuine acceptance and empathy to the parents, listen carefully to their concerns, and share with them why their involvement is so important (see for example, VanFleet, 2000).

## The Sequence of Filial Therapy

Although some of the short-term individual and group FT programs follow a prescribed weekly protocol (Ginsberg, 2004; Landreth & Bratton, 2006; VanFleet & Sniscak, in press), the full form of FT described here is considered a therapeutic process, and as such, its application varies depending on the specific needs of the child and family. Even so, the chronological sequence of FT remains the same in most cases. The sequence is briefly outlined, based on a 1-hour session time frame. Greater detail can be found in VanFleet (2005, 2006b, 2006c).

- **Assessment Phase:** The assessment phase typically requires two sessions. Therapists meet with the parents alone during the first session, inviting them to share their concerns and listening carefully and empathically. The therapist suggests that parents complete any paper-and-pencil measures at home and return them on their next visit. The second session involves a family play observation, during which the therapist observes the entire family playing in the playroom and then discusses the dynamics of the play, the target child, and observations with the parents. After this, the therapist makes a more formal recommendation for FT or the suggested course of treatment. With maltreated children, this process is sometimes extended to allow parents of children with serious attachment problems to express and talk through their intense feelings and frustrations. The assessment might also require some additional interactions with the target child. Because parents can be extremely distressed by the target child, it can take some additional time to help them see the advantages of their own involvement or the need to include their other children in the treatment.

- **Training Phase:** The training phase is designed to prepare parents to conduct the filial play sessions with their children. This typically takes three to four sessions. During the first session, the therapist demonstrates a CCPT session with each of the children to be involved in the process. The parents observe, and the therapist discusses the play sessions with the parents alone afterward. Although parents frequently have questions at this time, parents and caregivers of maltreated children often express doubts about how this type of nondirective play could help with the sometimes intense behavioral and self-regulation difficulties they are experiencing.

The therapist again listens carefully and provides explanations. After the demonstrations, the therapist explains the four skills needed to conduct the play sessions and practices them with parents via role-plays. One of the most effective training tools is the mock play session, during which the therapist pretends to be a child and plays in a manner that permits parents to practice the skills. The therapist provides in-the-moment feedback as well as more detailed feedback after the short mock sessions. Emphasis is placed on the things parents have done well, with just a couple suggestions for improvement next time. While most families are ready to work with their children after two such mock play sessions, parents of maltreated children sometimes require a third mock session. The first two help them learn the skills, and the third prepares them for some of the intense play, aggression, or sexualized behaviors commonly seen in maltreated children during CCPT. The key is to set parents up for success, so thorough preparation is essential. During the training phase, the therapist also helps the family with any current crises they may be experiencing.

- **Supervised Play Session Phase:** At this point, parents begin to hold play sessions with their children, one at a time, under the direct supervision of the therapist. The therapist often observes from a corner of the room, through a one-way mirror, or from another room using a camera/computer link or wireless technology. Parents take turns holding play sessions for 20 to 30 minutes, after which the children are excused and the therapist meets with parents to discuss their skills (mostly positive feedback with suggestions for improvement as before), the child's play themes (to help parents understand the child's feelings and motivations more accurately), and the parents' reactions to the play sessions. This latter discussion often reveals parent worries, self-doubts, and concerns, and time is taken to show empathic acceptance of their feelings and to work through any immediate problems that need resolution. Typically in FT, this phase includes the therapist's direct observation of each parent four to six times before they are ready to move the play sessions to the home. In the case of maltreated children, however, it is quite common for the therapist and the parents to decide mutually to extend the number of directly supervised play sessions to 10, 12, or even more if needed to help parents understand difficult themes in their child's play and for parents to feel prepared to conduct the play sessions more independently. Even parents who were initially reluctant to participate in FT frequently request additional directly supervised play sessions, because the collaborative nature of FT helps them feel encouraged and supported.

- **Home Play Sessions Phase:** When parents have achieved competence and confidence in conducting the play sessions with their children, the therapist encourages them to shift the sessions to home. The therapist continues to monitor the play sessions through parent reports and videotapes, when available. The parents continue to meet with the therapist weekly or biweekly to report on their filial play sessions with all of their children. Often, parents observe each other's play sessions at home and provide feedback using the positive approach the therapist has modeled for them and later taught them. Each session, the therapist asks parents to review their home sessions, including what went well, what problems they encountered, the play themes the child expressed, and parents' reactions to the session. During this phase, the therapist and parents begin to discuss generalization of what the parents have learned to their daily lives and interactions. This process typically runs smoothly; however, parents of maltreated children might need extended support in this phase of treatment. The therapist helps parents develop realistic expectations of progress based on the child's abuse and attachment history and helps parents work through and maintain their hope through setbacks.

- **Generalization and Discharge Phase:** After the parents have established a pattern of regular home-play sessions, the therapist helps them generalize what they have learned. Each week, parents learn how to apply one of the play session skills to typical daily parent-child interaction. They learn to use what they have learned during the play sessions to listen empathically, structure, and set limits in a wide range of situations. The therapist also covers additional skills, such as parent messages and the use of positive reinforcement. Guerney's (1995) *Parenting: A Skills Training Manual* is a useful tool at this juncture. With families with maltreated children, this process can be more complex than usual. At times, as will be discussed later, the application of the FT skills to typical daily parent-child interaction may be taught before the start of FT. The advantage of including the generalization of skills at the end of therapy, however, is that parents have mastered the skills and are much more motivated to use them. In many parenting programs, parents report feeling overwhelmed as they try to implement unfamiliar skills within the complexities of daily life. Usually a phased-out discharge process is used, in which weekly meetings become biweekly, or biweekly meetings are shifted to once every three or four weeks. Families are discharged when presenting problems have been ameliorated or eliminated and the family feels confident to continue the play sessions and their use of the skills to tackle most problems on their own. For families of maltreated children, it is very useful to invite the family to contact the therapist for booster sessions or periodic check-ins to ensure that everything is progressing in a positive direction.

## Skills Taught to Parents

During the FT process, parents learn and master four CCPT skills that are used during their parent-child play sessions: structuring, empathic listening, child-centered imaginary play, and limit-setting. The rationale and methods of these skills are described in detail elsewhere (VanFleet, 2005; VanFleet, 2006a; VanFleet, Sywulak, & Sniscak, 2010). Parents use the *structuring skill* to start and end the play session and to set the desired tone of openness, empathy, and acceptance. The *empathic listening skill* helps parents become increasingly attuned to their child's inner world as they pay close attention to the child's verbal and nonverbal communications and in their own words briefly reflect the activities and feelings expressed in the play. The therapist helps parents develop a receptive attitude and congruent intonations and behaviors to convey under-standing and acceptance of the child's (or the toy character's) feelings.

The *child-centered imaginary play skill* is used when children invite their parents to play a pretend role. At this point, the parent's job is to enact that role as closely as possible to what the child desires. Finally, parents learn that they are ultimately in charge of the play session when the child's behavior becomes destructive or dangerous. Rarely are limits placed on the themes of children's play, but unsafe behaviors are firmly limited using a three-step *limit-setting skill* involving statement of the limit, a warning if the child tries to break the rule again, and a consequence (typically, ending the play session) if the child continues to break the rule a third time. This three-step procedure is followed separately for each play session limit.

The combination of these skills working in concert provides the safe and accepting atmosphere that is critical for the play sessions to work. Children have considerable freedom to express themselves while parents develop increased attunement and understanding. Boundaries are made reasonable and firm. Children receive warm acceptance and support and are permitted sufficient autonomy to explore and accept their *selves*. Parents learn to maintain necessary control while learning to see the world through their children's eyes. The skills contribute to the formation of healthier attachments and trusting relation-ships—the cornerstones of better child adjustment and socialization.

## Ages Relevant to Filial Therapy

Typically, FT has been used with children who are 3 to 12 years old. These are the ages during which children use their imaginations the most as they learn about the world. Slight adaptations have been applied to even younger children, and "special times" have been used with adolescents, during which parents engage in games or other enjoyable activities while remaining as child-centered as possi-ble. Because maltreated children often display significant social, emotional, and cognitive delays, it is often possible to extend the use of the usual play-session-oriented FT to adolescents as old as 15 or 16. Interactions during the assessment phase typically reveal if the adolescent is still playing imaginatively or with toys or other items.

## Integrated Use of FT With Other Therapeutic Modalities

FT is a systemic form of therapy that is designed to meet many of the funda-mental needs of traumatized and attachment-disrupted children and their families, so it is considered a core intervention for this population around which other interventions are added only as needed (VanFleet & Sniscak, 2003). Even with highly distressed children and families, the full family therapy form of FT sometimes serves as the only form of therapy needed, but there are certainly times when it must be preceded or augmented by other interventions.

Families who present for therapy in crisis have frequently exhausted their own resources trying to cope with emotional, social, and behavior problems presented by the maltreated child. These parents have lost hope, lack energy, and may be ready to give up. Sometimes, the child's behavior is so out of control that even therapists wonder if they can have an impact. In cases like these, therapists need to evaluate parents' energy reserves to determine if FT should be introduced immediately or at a later time. If parents are completely depleted, therapists can help reduce the arousal level of the family system by conducting some individual play therapy with the child while helping parents adopt more effective parenting strategies. Sniscak (2010, personal communication) recommends introducing trauma education for the parents as well as the Guerney parenting skills (1995) near the start of therapy. She helps parents understand how trauma, attachment problems, emotions, and behaviors are interlinked, helping parents shift their assumptions about the child's behavior to a more realistic view. At the same time, she offers tools for immediate use in the home.

During this period, therapists can work individually with the child, using CCPT to build rapport, learn about the child's feelings and perceptions, and give the child an opportunity to work out some of his or her dilemmas. Bibliotherapy (such as Sheppard's *Brave Bart* [1998]) is used to teach children about their trauma-reactive feelings and behaviors in a lighthearted, safe way, and other cognitive-behavioral play therapy interventions can be used to provide some immediate coping strategies, such as how to deal with triggers and rage. As soon as the parents have more energy, FT can begin.

Play therapists often see evidence of other developmental or perceptual difficulties that might need treatment. It is common to refer these children to occupational therapists to evaluate and treat sensory integration problems, or to suggest educational, psychological, or neuropsychological testing to identify deficits that need specialized intervention. Children who are taking medications may experience side effects or problematic interactions between medications, requiring therapists to establish a good relationship with a child/adolescent psychiatrist who can evaluate such situations.

During the course of treatment, the therapist and family might discuss other problems that the child is experiencing, such as poor peer relations and lack of social skills. Taking care to avoid overwhelming the family with services, the therapist might suggest that the child take part in a social skills group that employs play-based methods. For children who have been cruel to animals such as family pets, Animal-Assisted Play Therapy (AAPT) offers specific skills that help children build empathy and relationship, develop competencies, and establish trust and safety, all of which can be generalized to the home (VanFleet, 2008b). AAPT has been applied in the context of nondirective, directive, and family play therapy.

FT can be used in combination with any other therapy deemed necessary for maltreated children and their families (VanFleet, 2006c) and can be applied at any point in the treatment process. Even so, because of the potential of FT simultaneously to help children work through traumatic experiences, assist parents in developing essential skills to help their child heal and return to a healthy developmental trajectory, and to address disruptions in parent-child attachment, we see FT as a core element of the treatment of child abuse and neglect.

## The Value of FT for Maltreated Children and Families

VanFleet and Sniscak (2003) have listed the following 15 reasons why FT is applicable, often as the core treatment, for maltreated children and their families or caregivers:

1. FT creates a physically and emotionally safe environment for children. Structuring and limit-setting ensure physical safety, while parents' empathic acceptance and child-centered imaginary play demonstrate attunement and emotional safety.
2. FT offers the child acceptance of self by parents or caregivers, and this in turn can help the child learn to accept him or herself more fully.
3. FT offers children an opportunity to explore their own interests, needs, struggles, and desires, all of which can contribute to a stronger identity.
4. The nondirective play sessions that form the basis of FT facilitate the development of trust, as the child experiences empathic acceptance repeatedly from the caregivers during the play sessions.
5. Children develop better emotional and behavioral regulation during FT through the nurturance and acceptance offered by parents and the simultaneous limiting of inappropriate behaviors. This approach, nested within the context of play and relationship on an ongoing basis, offers several elements that are likely to improve self-regulation.
6. FT helps build attunement between parent and child. Parents learn to understand and attend to the child's needs better.
7. FT offers a developmentally sensitive intervention. Because play is the primary means of building attachment and working through problems, children can work through clinical, developmental, and relationship issues. In addition, the acceptance of children's feelings and play behaviors allows parents to interact with them at the social and emotional developmental levels where the children are currently functioning.
8. FT allows maltreated children to express and master their trauma-related issues.
9. FT emphasizes the reciprocity of relationships. No force is involved. The interplay of parent and child helps them understand and appreciate each other while having fun together.
10. FT gives parents the empathy, encouragement, and support that they need to try new things, tackle tough problems, and gain insight into their own and their children's feelings and reactions. The safe climate created by the

therapist offers parents a way to share their innermost concerns and fears so that they are less likely to block therapeutic progress.

11. Because the entire family is typically involved in FT, the process strengthens family identity, trust, and cohesion. It is more likely that the family will emerge stronger and with a joint sense of belongingness and appreciation.

12. FT typically involves other children in the family, including other biological, adopted, or foster children. This can alleviate problems these children experience as well as potential sibling rivalries, resentment, and competition for parent attention.

13. FT empowers families to apply what they have learned in home sessions and in daily life, reducing the amount of office-based therapy time needed.

14. Parents learn skills during FT that they can use far into the future after therapy has ended.

15. FT is transportable and can be used in many different settings and with a variety of caregivers. It offers a unique method of helping children with transitions as well.

## Filial Therapy to Help Maltreated Children Make Transitions

Maltreated children who reside within the dependent care system often face numerous transitions. Unfortunately, it is not uncommon to see children who have lived in 12, 18, or even 24 different homes before they are adopted or reunified with their biological parents. Transitions are difficult under the best of circumstances. Frequent moves can exacerbate trauma and attachment-related problems. Even when children are eager to be adopted or reunified, the transition is fraught with anxiety. Will it work? Will it last? Will the family treat the child well? Will the child's needs be met? Will the child have unexpected problems that the family is not prepared to handle?

FT has been used to stabilize foster placements and to provide an excellent transition tool to ease children's move into adoption or reunification with their biological families. This model (VanFleet, 2006c) involves the use of FT first with foster parents or kinship caregivers to help stabilize placements and provide children with an opportunity to work through some aspects of their trauma reactivity in the context of family. It encourages the development of healthy attachments and provides a template or model for children who may never have experienced this relationship. Because children quickly grow attached to their caregivers by virtue of living with them, it makes sense to help these relationships become healthy ones. It also makes sense to put the powerful tools offered by FT into the hands of caregivers, who are likely to face some significant challenges.

For foster families who eventually adopt children, the play sessions can continue through the adoption and beyond. Some foster-to-adopt families have commented that when things became rockier during the post-adoption period, the filial play sessions helped them work out the problems together while communicating to the children that the parents were "in it for the long haul."

When an adoptive family has been identified for a child, the therapist meets with them as early as possible, provides education about trauma, attachment, and trauma-reactive emotions and behaviors, and trains them in the FT play session skills. The therapist offers supervised FT sessions in conjunction with child visits with the preadoptive family. For a time, the therapist holds alternating filial play sessions with the foster and adoptive families to help the child move from one emotionally safe place to another. Over time, the filial play sessions with the foster family are diminished, and those with the adoptive family become more established.

Too often, children are uprooted from the security of foster care to the relative uncertainty of an adoptive placement. A series of visits is not enough to build emotional security. Visits combined with filial play sessions can enhance the attachment process with the adoptive family, making the transition smoother. VanFleet (2006c) has commented,

> *FT has been used successfully to help adoptive families establish meaningful relationships during the visitation process, thereby reducing transition anxieties. The adoptive child is moving from one healthy attachment relationship to another. This process provides adoptive families with specific activities to get their new relationships off on the right foot. (p. 160)*

Although no controlled research has been conducted to date on this transition model, in dozens of cases where funding has been provided, adoptions completed using FT in this way have been successful in terms of parent satisfaction reports 6 and 12 months post-adoption, as well as from reports from county protective service and adoption agency case managers and directors. With these promising clinical results, the FT transition model bears further attention and study.

The same process can be used when the plan is to reunify children with their biological parents. It is critical for the therapist to work closely with all those involved in this decision, to educate them about the child's needs, and to determine if the biological family is appropriate for FT. When uncertainty exists about the parents' commitment to the child or the therapy process, the therapist can extend the training period without involving the child in play sessions until parents have demonstrated their commitment and willingness to cooperate fully. Filial play sessions with the foster family continue. If all goes well, the therapist begins filial play sessions with the biological parents, while filial play sessions continue with the foster family. Once again, filial play sessions are conducted in an alternating fashion with the foster family and the biological family until the child is reunified. The sessions then continue with the biological family as it works to create a new and healthier environment for all its members. In this way, FT can be employed as an abuse-prevention strategy, but it should be used cautiously and only with parents who have demonstrated their commitment and motivation to make changes (with the initial assistance of the therapist during the training phase).

Too often, children are reunified with their families with relatively little intervention. This is a grave disservice to the children and to the parents, who often are parenting as they were parented. Unless something can change in the family system, there is risk for repeated victimization of the children. FT offers one method of engaging and empowering reunifying families so that they can better meet the physical, developmental, emotional, and social needs of their members. The work is challenging, but possible. A wealth of anecdotal evidence attests to the power of this approach (e.g., Children's Crisis Treatment Center, 2009, personal communication), but controlled research is needed to establish this as a viable alternative to current practices.

## Case Example

The identifying information in the case example that follows has been disguised to protect the privacy of the individuals and family. The case is a typical example of the use of FT with maltreated children and the families who care for them.

Louie first entered therapy when he was 10 years old. He had lived in foster placements from the time he was 4 years old. He had been severely physically abused by one of his mother's boyfriends and had witnessed domestic violence perpetrated by another of her boyfriends who had moved in with them. Given a choice, his mother opted to remain with the abusive boyfriend and to place Louie in foster care. At first, Louie had sporadic contact with his mother, but her increasing drug dependence made their visits nonexistent by the time he was 6 years old.

Louie had experienced one failed adoption when he was 7 years old. At first, all had gone well, but after the brief honeymoon period, he began acting out when triggered by a variety of circumstances. He quickly flew into rages, screaming and running out of the house and into the neighborhood. If one of his parents blocked his exit, he grabbed items of value and broke them. Frustrated, the adoptive parents sought help from a traditional mental health practitioner, who used talk therapy and behavior management, but relief was short-lived. They eventually gave up.

In the past 2 years, Louie had been in six different foster homes. In each case, his externalizing rampages wore out his welcome and he was moved. Foster parents had described his "don't care about anything" attitude, his "deliberately" provocative behaviors, his tantrums, and his teasing and injuring family pets as their reasons they could no longer care for him. At the time he was referred for treatment, he was living with a foster family that had indicated a willingness to adopt him. Their interest was fading, however, as his trauma-reactive behaviors surfaced once again. Staff from the foster care and adoption agencies had recently attended an in-service program on play therapy and agreed that Louie might be a candidate.

The foster parents, Ana and Rob, were frightened by Louie's rages. Initially, they tried to be understanding and loving, but when Louie destroyed one of Ana's heirlooms, she began to have second thoughts. Increasingly, they tried to control Louie's behavior by removing items from his room. It had reached a point where his room was nearly bare. Louie was sweet and well-behaved at times, but when something triggered him, he was unsafe and out of control. Ana and Rob reported that his rages seemed to come out of the blue. As they began taking away his possessions and his privileges, they noted he was becoming increasingly oppositional. They also noted that their previously satisfactory marriage was under strain. They were less patient with each other and had more arguments about how to handle Louie. They knew they needed help and asked for it.

During the assessment phase, the therapist talked and empathized with Ana and Rob. Their high hopes had been dashed. They could see Louie's kinder, gentler side, but that was insufficient to carry them through the frightening tantrums. They had read about Reactive Attachment Disorder online and wondered if Louie might be headed for delinquency. During the family play observation, Louie played vigorously with both of them. He enjoyed exploring the playroom and tried out nearly every toy. Near the end of the 20-minute observation, he began punching the bop bag and continued to do that with gusto. The therapist then discussed the observation with Ana and Rob, who were worried that his aggressive play was one more indication of his doomed future. The therapist explained how aggressive play and actual violence are two different things, and she began talking about the benefits of play therapy for emotional expression, trauma mastery, and self-regulation. She pointed out how some of Louie's play might be related to his history and also discussed FT as a valuable intervention, inquiring about Ana's and Rob's energy levels and current commitment in terms of keeping Louie. They responded that they had doubts, but they wanted to give Louie every possible chance. If the current problems could be reduced, they remained interested in having him become part of their family.

Before asking for the couple to commit to the FT process, the therapist invited them to observe a nondirective play session that she held with Louie. Louie was eager to return to the playroom and continued his aggressive play. When he tried to throw the hard plastic magic wand at the therapist (pretending it was a spear), she set the limit, "Louie, one of the things you may not do in here is throw the toys at me. You can do just about anything else." Louie glanced at her, selected another toy, and began to throw it. The therapist moved to the second stage of limit setting, "Louie, remember I said you could not throw things at me. If you try to do that again, we will have to leave the special playroom today." Louie looked surprised but turned to other play activities. Again, he explored the playroom and ended by hitting the bop bag, which Louie had identified as a villain. The therapist reflected the feelings he seemed to be expressing with the bop bag, "You're really smacking that bad guy. You're letting him know you're in charge. You feel powerful and you're not going to let him get away with anything. Pow! Whamo! You're putting him in his place." Interestingly, Louie did not attempt to break other limits.

In the discussion afterward, Ana and Rob were both distressed that he had tested the limits but impressed that he had not pushed it any farther. The therapist helped them see how the play sessions might provide a release of Louie's feelings and concerns while providing boundaries for his unsafe behaviors. They agreed to move forward.

During the first FT training session, the therapist discussed how trauma and attachment disruptions can impact children's emotions, behavior, and relationships. As she talked, Ana and Rob clearly related to the information, providing examples of the points that were being made. They admitted that they thought their loving home would be sufficient to overcome Louie's past, and the therapist empathically listened to their disappointment. Next, the therapist provided an overview of the four play session skills and practiced the empathic listening skill with Ana and Rob. For the next two sessions, the therapist held mock play sessions, first with Ana while Rob watched, and then with Rob while Ana watched. Both listened to the feedback the therapist provided. Ana quickly learned the empathic listening skill and did quite well with the imaginary play, but she had some trouble being firm with the limit setting. Rob had some difficulty with identifying feelings during the play, but his imaginary play was excellent. The therapist helped him reduce the volume of his limits to a firm, but nonpunitive tone of voice. Ana and Rob were ready to start the supervised play sessions with Louie.

Louie seemed delighted to play with them. His early play sessions with Rob were filled with battles and aggressive play. Rob had to set two limits, both of which Louie respected. Louie's play with Ana was quieter, but he tested more limits with her. After stumbling with her limits during her first play session (sounding a bit unsure of herself), Ana used the therapist's suggestions and did better in subsequent sessions. Again, Louie did not push the limits to the consequence stage, and the therapist helped Ana and Rob see this important fact.

Louie eventually engaged in more and more imaginary villain play. He battled several bad guys, beating them up, putting them in jail, and sometimes being outnumbered and being beaten down by them. He held fights with some large soft dolls. When he was down, he got back up, dusted himself off, and resumed the battle. His parents, during each of their play sessions, were able to listen empathically to his play, "You're not going to let them get away with that. You're taking care of those bad guys. You're putting them in jail where they can't do any more harm. Oh no! You're down! But now you're getting back up. They can't stop you. You're stopping them!" As their reflections got closer and closer to the underlying feelings and intentions, Louie seemed to relax. He smiled more during his play and engaged them in imaginary roles. Typically, he asked Rob to play a law enforcement officer who watched the bad guys when they were in jail. During sessions with his mother, he played a more protective role, telling her to stay home with the kids while he took care of the bad guys. Ana and Rob were amazed at his play. As their skills improved, the therapist talked more with them about play themes. They discussed the symbolic nature of Louie's battles, the way he was showing some mastery over the threats he faced, his resilience in getting back up each time he was knocked down, and his relationship-building with Ana and Rob.

Ana and Rob began to see that underlying the aggression themes were more fundamental meanings of threat, safety, and protection. They began to understand Louie's world more clearly. Even as the battles raged in the playroom, the parents noted that Louie's behavior in daily life was improving. They had tried some simple behavior management and bedtime soothing activities the therapist had suggested, but they attributed most of the change to the filial play sessions. Because Louie's history was so difficult, and because Ana and Rob wanted more help understanding and responding to Louie's intense play themes, they continued with the supervised play sessions for nearly three months. The therapist observed a total of 16 play sessions, eight with each parent. At that point, the play sessions were shifted to home.

At home, Louie played out some of the familiar themes, but near the end of each session, he typically engaged in attachment-themed play. In one session, he handcuffed himself to Ana, saying that they would be safe if they stuck together. Ana was touched by this. Louie also engaged in some regressive play, where he pretended he was a toddler crawling on the floor and Ana was his mother taking care of him, offering the baby bottle and singing (his instructions to her). He continued to ask Rob to help him with the bad guys and ended the sessions by pretending he and Rob were dragons who protected their land together. The parents were able to see how Louie was gradually trusting them more and allowing them to take the caretaking roles in the play.

The therapist followed the case and helped Ana and Rob use their skills in daily life. They continued weekly play sessions because they saw profound changes in Louie. He still had some meltdowns, but they were much less frequent. Ana and Rob also reported that they were in much better agreement about how to handle Louie's misbehavior. They also reported that the stress in their relationship had been largely replaced by more empathic attitudes toward each other. As problems diminished and Ana and Rob gained confidence in their play session and parenting skills, they began seeing the therapist once every three weeks. The therapist monitored their progress at least monthly until several months after Louie was adopted. Although some reactive behaviors and testing returned after the adoption was finalized, it was short-lived because Ana and Rob continued holding play sessions, during which the issues played themselves out. A follow-up at six months post-adoption indicated that the family was still enjoying play sessions and feeling good about their lives together.

## Conclusion

Child neglect, maltreatment, and other forms of interpersonal violence leave serious developmental and psychosocial damage. Without effective treatment, these children and their families or caregivers are likely to suffer in significant ways. The children need to work through their traumatic experiences and reactions in the context of a safe, warm, and supportive family environment. Because attachment processes are often impacted negatively by complex trauma, it is important to help these children build trust and to create healthy relationships. Parents and caregivers can be frustrated and exhausted by the trauma-reactive behaviors and poor self-regulation often exhibited by these children.

Filial Therapy, an empirically supported therapeutic intervention that blends family therapy and play therapy, offers considerable assistance to maltreated children and their families. It provides the context of a warm, supporting environment in which children can form healthier attachments with caregivers and master their trauma-based difficulties. Through therapist-supervised nondirective parent-child play sessions, FT provides parents with the tools and confidence to parent these children in a positive and effective way. FT helps all family members heal while forming healthier attachments and more satisfying relationships with each other. Its integrative nature harnesses the power of play therapy and family therapy to help strengthen families coping with some of the most difficult circumstances and offers real hope for their futures.

# References

Ainsworth, M. S., Blehar, M. S., Waters, E., & Wall, S. (1978). *Patterns of attachment: A psychological study of the strange situation.* Oxford, England: Lawrence Erlbaum.

Azar, S. T. (1998). A cognitive behavioral approach to understanding and treating parents who physically abuse their children. In D. Wolfe and R. McMahon (Eds.), *Child abuse: New directions in prevention and treatment across the life span* (pp. 78–100). New York, NY: Sage.

Azar, S. T., & Rohrbeck, C. A. (1986). Child abuse and unrealistic expectations: Further validation of the Parent Opinion Questionnaire. *Journal of Consulting and Clinical Psychology, 54,* 867–868.

Barber, B. K., & Harmon, E. L. (2002). Violating the self: Parental psychological control of children and adolescents. In B. K. Barber (Ed.), *Intrusive parenting: How psychological control affects children and adolescents* (pp. 15–52). Washington, DC: American Psychological Association Press. doi:10.1037/10422-002.

Barber, B. K., Stolz, H. E., & Olsen, J. A. (2005). Parental support, psychological control, and behavioral control: Assessing relevance across time, culture, and method: I. Introduction. *Monographs of the Society for Research in Child Development, 70*(4), 1–13.

Barnes, K. T., & Azar, S. T. (1990, August). *Maternal expectations and attributions in discipline situations: A test of a cognitive model of parenting.* Paper presented at the annual meeting of the American Psychological Association, Boston, Massachusetts.

Baumrind, D. (1991). The influence of parenting style on adolescent competence and substance use. *Journal of Early Adolescence, 11,* 56–95.

Baumrind, D., Larzelere, R. E., & Owens, E. B. (2010). Effects of preschool parents' power assertive patterns and practices on adolescent development. *Parenting Science and Practice, 10,* 157–201.

Belsky, J., & Fearon, R. M. P. (2009). Precursors of attachment theory. In J. Cassidy & P. Shaver (Eds.), *Handbook of attachment: Theory, research, and clinical applications* (2nd ed., pp. 295–316). New York, NY: Guilford Press.

Bowlby, J. (1969). Disruption of affectional bonds and its effects on behavior. *Canada's Mental Health Supplement, 59,* 12.

Chilamkurti, C., & Milner, J. S. (1993). Perceptions and evaluations of child transgressions and disciplinary techniques in high- and low-risk mothers and their children. *Child Development, 64,* 1801–1814. doi: 10.2307/1131470.

Cook, A., Spinazzola, J., Ford, J., Lanktree, C., Blaustein, M., Cloitre, M., . . . & van der Kolk, B. (2005). Complex trauma in children and adolescents. *Psychiatric Annals, 35* (5), 390–398.

Eisenberg, N., Fabes, R. A., Shepard, S. A., Guthrie, I. K., Murphy, B. C., & Rieser, M. (1999). Parental reactions to children's negative emotions: Longitudinal relations to quality to children's social functioning. *Child Development, 70,* 513–534.

Fabes, R. A., Leonard, S. A., Kupanoff, K., & Martin, S. L. (2001). Parental coping with children's negative emotions: Relations with children's emotional and social responding. *Child Development, 72,* 907–920.

Gil, E. (Ed.). (2010). *Working with children to heal interpersonal trauma: The power of play*. New York, NY: Guilford Press.

Gilbert, R., Widom, C. S., Browne, K., Ferguson, D., Webb, E., & Janson, S. (2009). Burden and consequences of child maltreatment in high-income countries. *Lancet, 373,* 68–81.

Ginsberg, B. G. (2003). *An integrated, holistic model of child-centered family therapy*. In R. VanFleet & L. F. Guerney (Eds.), *Casebook of filial therapy* (pp. 21–47). Boiling Springs, PA: Play Therapy Press.

Ginsberg, B. G. (2004). *Relationship enhancement family therapy* (2nd ed.). Doylestown, PA: Relationship Enhancement Press.

Goldstein, S. E., Davis-Kean, P. E., & Eccles, J. S. (2005). Parents, peers, and problem behavior: A longitudinal investigation of the impact of relationship perceptions and characteristics on the development of adolescent problem behavior. *Developmental Psychology, 41,* 401–413. doi:10.1037/0012-1649. 41.2.401.

Gottman, J. M., Katz, L. F., & Hooven, C. (1996). Parental meta-emotion philosophy and the emotional life of families: Theoretical models and preliminary data. *Journal of Family Psychology, 10,* 243–268. doi:10.1037/0893-3200.10.3.243.

Grolnick, W. S. (2003). *The psychology of parental control: How well-meant parenting backfires.* Mahwah, NJ: Lawrence Erlbaum.

Guerney, B. G., Jr. (1964). Filial therapy: Description and rationale. *Journal of Consulting Psychology, 28*(4), 303–310.

Guerney, L. F. (1983). *Introduction to filial therapy: Training parents as therapists.* In P. A. Keller & L. G. Ritt (Eds.), *Innovations in clinical practice: A source book* (Vol. 2, pp. 26–39). Sarasota, FL: Professional Resource Exchange.

Guerney, L. F. (1995). *Parenting: A skills training manual* (5th ed.). North Bethesda, MD: Institute for the Development of Emotional and Life Skills.

Guerney, L. (1997). *Filial therapy.* In K. J. O'Connor & L. M. Braverman (Eds.), *Play therapy theory and practice: A comparative presentation* (pp. 131–159). Somerset, NJ: John Wiley & Sons.

Guerney, L. (2003). The history, principles, and empirical basis of filial therapy. In R. VanFleet & L. Guerney (Eds.), *Casebook of filial therapy* (pp. 1–20). Boiling Springs, PA: Play Therapy Press.

Guerney, L. F., & Ryan, V. M. (in preparation). Manual of group filial therapy.

James, B. (1994). *Handbook for treatment of attachment-trauma problems in children.* New York, NY: Free Press.

Kim, J., & Cicchetti, D. (2010). Longitudinal pathways linking child maltreatment, emotion regulation, peer relations, and psychopathology. *Journal of Child Psychology and Psychiatry, 51*(6), 706–716.

Landreth, G. L., & Bratton, S. C. (2006). *Child parent relationship therapy (CPRT): A 10-session filial therapy model.* New York, NY: Taylor & Francis.

Larrance, D. T., & Twentyman, C. T. (1983). Maternal attributions and child abuse. *Journal of Abnormal Psychology, 92,* 449–457. doi:10.1037/0021-843X.92.4.449.

Minuchin, S. (1974). *Families and family therapy.* Cambridge, MA: Harvard University Press.

Napier, A., & Whitaker, C. (1978). *The family crucible: The intense experience of family therapy.* New York, NY: Harper & Row.

Nichols, M. P. (2009). *Family therapy: Concepts and methods* (9th ed.). Boston: MA: Pearson.

Perry, B. D. (2001). *Bonding and attachment in maltreated children: Consequences of emotional neglect in childhood.* www.childtrauma.org/images/stories/Articles/attcar4_03_v2_r.pdf (August 28, 2010).

Perry, B. D., & Szalavitz, M. (2007). *The boy who was raised as a dog.* New York, NY: Basic Books.

Satir, V. M. (1972). *Peoplemaking.* Palo Alto, CA: Science and Behavior Books.

Sheppard, C. H. (1998). *Brave Bart: A story for traumatized and grieving children.* Grosse Pointe Woods, MI: Institute for Trauma and Loss in Children.

Smith, C., Perou, R., & Lesesne, C. (2002). Parent education. In *Handbook of parenting, Vol. 4: Social conditions and applied parenting* (2nd ed., pp. 389–410). Mahwah, NJ: Lawrence Erlbaum.

Sroufe, L. A. (1988). The role of infant-caregiver attachment in development. *Clinical implications of attachment* (pp. 18–38). Hillsdale, NJ: Lawrence Erlbaum.

Steinberg, L., Elmen, J. D., & Mounts, N. S. (1989). Authoritative parenting, psychosocial maturity, and academic success among adolescents. *Child Development, 60,* 1424–1436.

Terr, L. (1990). *Too scared to cry: How trauma affects children . . . and ultimately us all.* New York, NY: Basic Books.

Thompson, R. A. (2009). Early attachment and later development: Familiar questions, new answers. In J. Cassidy & P. Shaver (Eds.), *Handbook of attachment: Theory, research, and clinical applications* (2nd ed., pp. 348–365). New York, NY: Guilford Press.

Tobin, D., Wardi-Zonna, K., & Yezzi-Shareef, A. M. (2007). Early recollections of children and adolescents diagnosed with reactive attachment disorder. *The Journal of Individual Psychology, 63*(1), 86–95.

van der Kolk, B. A., Roth, S., Pelcovitz, D., Sunday, S., & Spinazzola, J. (2005). Disorders of extreme stress: The empirical foundation of a complex adaptation to trauma. *Journal of Traumatic Stress, 18*(5), 389–399.

VanFleet, R. (2000). *A parent's handbook of filial play therapy*. Boiling Springs, PA: Play Therapy Press.

VanFleet, R. (2005). *Filial therapy: Strengthening parent-child relationships through play* (2nd ed.). Sarasota, FL: Professional Resource Press.

VanFleet, R. (2006a). *Child-centered play therapy [DVD]*. Boiling Springs, PA: Play Therapy Press.

VanFleet, R. (2006b). *Introduction to filial therapy [DVD]*. Boiling Springs, PA: Play Therapy Press.

VanFleet, R. (2006c). Short-term play therapy for adoptive families: Facilitating adjustment and attachment with filial therapy. In H. G. Kaduson and C. E. Schaefer (Eds.), *Short-term play therapy for children* (2nd ed., pp. 145–168). New York, NY: Guilford Press.

VanFleet, R. (2008a). *Filial play therapy*. (Part of Jon Carlson's DVD series on children and adolescents.) Washington, DC: American Psychological Association.

VanFleet, R. (2008b). *Play therapy with kids & canines: Benefits for children's developmental and psychosocial health*. Sarasota, FL: Professional Resource Press.

VanFleet, R. (2009a). Filial therapy. In K. J. O'Connor & L. D. Braverman (Eds.), *Play therapy theory and practice: Comparing theories and techniques* (2nd ed., pp. 163–201). Hoboken, NJ: Wiley.

VanFleet, R. (2009b). Filial therapy: Theoretical integration, empirical validation, and practical application. In A. A. Drewes (Ed.), *Blending play therapy with cognitive behavioral therapy* (pp. 257–279). Hoboken, NJ: Wiley.

VanFleet, R., Ryan, S., & Smith, S. (2005). Filial therapy: A critical review. In L. Reddy, T. Files-Hall, & C. Schaefer (Eds.), *Empirically-based play interventions for children* (pp. 241–264). Washington, DC: American Psychological Association Press.

VanFleet, R., & Sniscak, C.C. (2003). Filial therapy for attachment-disrupted and disordered children. In R. VanFleet & L. Guerney (Eds.), *Casebook of filial therapy* (pp. 279–308). Boiling Springs, PA: Play Therapy Press.

VanFleet, R., & Sniscak, C. C. (in press) *Filial therapy for child trauma and attachment problems: Leader's manual for family groups*. Boiling Springs, PA: Play Therapy Press.

VanFleet, R., Sywulak, A. E., & Sniscak, C. C. (2010). *Child-centered play therapy*. New York, NY: Guilford Press.

Webb, N. B. (Ed.). (2005). *Working with traumatized youth in child welfare*. New York, NY: Guilford Press.

Wright, C., & Walker, J. (2003). Using filial therapy with Head Start families. In R. VanFleet & L. Guerney (Eds.), *Casebook of filial therapy* (pp. 309–330). Boiling Springs, PA: Play Therapy Press.

# Integrating Art Into Play Therapy for Children With Mood Disorders

## 10

### Chapter

## *Sarah Hamil*

## Introduction

Integrating art modalities and materials into play therapy provides a rich and personal depiction of how mood disorders are experienced in childhood. The unique imagery in the child's art can be used to assess the child's strengths and needs as well as a guide in treatment planning. As the imagery is created, observed, expanded, or altered, the child and therapist have the opportunity to evaluate treatment progress. The client art becomes a visual and tangible personal depiction of how the mood disorder is experienced and expressed by the child (Pifalo, 2009). Furthermore, the child, family, and therapist have the opportunity to observe and discuss the mood disorder in the imagery (Gil, 2003). This type of dialogue (verbal and nonverbal) validates the child and provides safety and containment for the symptoms of the mood disorder.

As the child portrays the mood disorder, the impact the symptoms have on the child's behavior and the impact on relationships is further understood. This allows coping strategies to be introduced within the art (Findler, 2009; Malchiodi, 1998), thus beginning the change process within the art and play, allowing for adjustments that are uniquely attuned to the child's particular needs. Furthermore, the therapist and family observe and participate in the alterations within the imagery, introducing a picture of what changes or modifications are potentially needed from all those involved with the child, including siblings, parents, teachers, and so on.

Integrating the art throughout the play therapy process allows for transitions that have the potential to add depth to the therapeutic process. For example, the child with major depressive disorder experiencing sadness, tearfulness, and isolation will often demonstrate restrictive and lethargic play, selecting few miniatures and props with limited expressiveness (Briesmeister, 1997; Newman, 2006). The play therapist bears witness to the child's painful symptoms and supports the child's self-expression. Inviting the child to create an image using art materials engages an expanded selection process and provides a multidimensional understanding of the child's strengths and needs. The nuances of the mood disorder, such as the degree of sadness, can be expressed and rated for intensity or severity, providing a baseline for treatment objectives. For example, the therapist asks the child to draw a person or self-portrait and to select colors that represent feelings such as sadness, happiness, loneliness, or excitement. The child uses the colors and the image to express the degree of each feeling state in regard to the intensity and frequency of the symptoms (Hamil, 2008).

Another tool that may be adapted to assess the impact of mood disorder symptoms is O'Connor's (1983) color-your-life technique, in which the child is invited to use a circle in a similar manner. The child assigns an emotion to a color and fills in the circle with the amount of color or emotion that is experienced. In this way, the art assists in treatment planning specific to the presenting problem and the current presentation of symptoms. The symptom presentation in color can be rated by the child and family in describing symptoms and features of the mood disorder. An additional benefit is recognized in the dialogue regarding the association of color to symptomology, which provides the opportunity to educate the child and family about the characteristics and features of the mood disorder. This is of particular importance with mood disorders, because the symptoms include problems in multiple biopsychosocial domains, including concentration, energy, appetite, sleep, self-worth, and interest in activities such as play. A salient feature of mood disorders is that these symptoms emerge and are experienced on a fluctuating continuum. Accurate assessment of the symptoms and how they are experienced by the child leads to effective treatment planning and improved coping, enhancing the quality of life for the child and the family.

## Understanding Mood Disorders in Childhood

Health professionals and the general public are very familiar with the term *depression*. It is understood that depression, the vernacular for a myriad of symptoms associated with mood disorders, can have a devastating effect on the functioning of the individual. The Diagnostic Statistical Manual-IV-TR (DSM-IV) provides specific diagnostic criteria for Mood Disorders, including Major Depressive Disorders, Dysthymic Disorder, and Bipolar Disorders. Each of the mood disorders has features that impact and impair the individual's ability to function adequately in numerous biopsychosocial domains, including psychomotor activity, concentration, sleep, appetite, self-care, self-worth, self-esteem, socialization, interpersonal relating, and mood problems such as irritability, sadness, or hopelessness (American Psychiatric Association, 2000). The mood disorders are differentiated depending on the combination, frequency, degree, and duration of the features.

The National Institute of Mental Health (NIMH) provides specific guidelines for understanding how mood disorders are recognized in children and teens. For example, children experiencing major depressive disorder or dysthymic disorder will express the symptoms differently than will an adolescent, and certainly very differently than an adult. A child with bipolar disorder may exhibit extreme behavior changes and demonstrate significant impulsivity, exaggerated excitement, and/or silliness when experiencing mania. Alternately, the symptoms of a depressive episode may be expressed by the child as heightened fearfulness, pretending to be sick, refusing to attend school, disinterest in play and socialization, as well as significant negativity in appraisal of self and others (NIMH, 2010).

Understanding mood disorders in childhood requires considering how the criteria for each disorder are expressed cognitively, behaviorally, emotionally, and physically by the child relevant to the individual's developmental stage (Gilbert, 2004). This imposes a requirement of specific knowledge of developmental characteristics and recognition of the disruption the mood disorder has on the child's development (Newman, 2006). The play therapist is in a unique position of suspending negative evaluations of the child's behavior by providing "the opportunity to be viewed by the therapist as a positive and growing self in an atmosphere of permissiveness and acceptance" (Sweeney & Landreth, 2003). In this respect the child may explore and distinguish the self apart from the mood disorder. The mood disorder is then understood as an influence on the child rather than the child's identity. Furthermore, the influences of the mood disorder are expressed spontaneously in the child's art and play, facilitating a fluid and dynamic treatment process.

## Risk and Protective Factors for Mood Disorders in Childhood

The symptom expressions of mood disorders are overwhelming and at times paralyzing for the child and family. These problematic features must be considered with respect to both the risk and resiliency factors that exist, and when treating childhood depression, it is important to assess for these factors upon first contact with the child and family. Risk factors in childhood have been defined as "any influences that increase the chances for harm or, more specifically, influences that increase the probability of onset, digression to a more serious state, or maintenance of a problem condition" (Fraser, Kirby, and Smokowski, 2004). From this perspective, the very experience of mood disorders in childhood serves as a significant risk factor for the child and family. Furthermore, the symptoms of mood disorders certainly contribute to and influence any existing risk factors that are present. The risk factors should be identified and recognized with particular regard also given to the resiliency or protective factors that exist. Protective factors are defined by Fraser, Kirby, and Smokowski, (2004) as "both internal and external resources that modify risk." Regard or acknowledgment of the protective factors provides a starting point for effective treatment, matching client strengths directly to resolution of client needs.

Certainly careful attention must be given to any indications of recurrent thoughts of death or suicidal ideation that may emerge in the language, play, or art of the child experiencing a mood disorder. The child's play and art should be carefully observed for any indicators of suicidal ideation. Thoughts of suicide or frequent thoughts of death demonstrated in play behavior or depicted in art or drawings must be acted upon immediately. A plan of action should be made with the family, child, and any related parties to ensure the child's safety.

Treatment of mood disorders in childhood requires a multidimensional approach to support optimum coping and to provide the opportunity to develop adaptive and functional life skills (Gilbert, 2004; NIMH, 2010; Shelby & Berk, 2009). This includes psychoeducation for the client regarding the symptoms and features of mood disorders, providing the child and family with a factual understanding of the mood disorder. Features such as cognitive distortions or negative self-talk can be described to the child and family as:

- Thoughts you have over and over that make you feel very sad or afraid
- Thoughts you have about hurting yourself
- Thoughts that nobody likes you or loves you
- Thoughts that race in your mind and confuse you

Even the very young child can identify fears, emotional pain, and erratic thoughts when the play therapist employs puppetry, songs, and imagery as metaphors that speak about the influence the symptoms are having on the child and family.

At times, ideas of hopelessness and worthlessness are clearly evident in the art. For instance, a foster parent brought a 12-year-old female for a clinical evaluation. The chief complaint related to the therapist by the foster parent was "The child has a bad attitude about everything." The parent reported negative communication patterns, including daily arguments that frequently elevated to shouting matches, and disrespectful language. The child's grades had significantly dropped, and she was rejecting her friends and having numerous peer conflicts. The mother further reported that the child became emotional often "for no reason." The client stated she was "fine," but she also said she "wished everyone would just leave me alone." When asked to create a House Tree Person Drawing (Hammer, 1997, 1980), the client quickly sketched the requested drawing. The therapist noticed that the figure portion of the drawing was drawn as an outline lying flat on the ground. The person had a phrase bubble above stating "Help Me." When the child was asked to tell the therapist more about the person, and what kind of help was needed, she quickly crossed out the person with a large X, and created another phrase bubble stating "Never mind."

Further assessment revealed that this young person was at significant risk for self-harm. When her expressions of hopelessness and worthlessness were validated by the therapist, the client reported having thoughts of death and ideas about harming herself for weeks. Immediate action was taken to ensure the child's safety, and a treatment plan was made by the child, family, and therapist to utilize art and play to correct cognitive distortions, to improve her functional expression of thoughts and feelings, and to identify and cope with shifts in mood and affect. This was achieved by recognizing the child's protective or resiliency factors in the same drawing that indicated her risk. The child's resiliency factors were also evident in her art. She was able to clearly express herself and her needs in drawing, and this skill was expanded in the treatment process. The client was interested in creating a journal in which she could include drawings, pictures, letters, and poems. The journal became a valuable tool for the child to share her thoughts, self-worth, identity, and her ideas about her relationships. In this venue, the art and play mediated the risk and resiliency. The journal contained the child's experience in a way that provided a reparative and coherent narrative related to the challenges she was facing in coping with a mood disorder.

## Addressing Mood Disorders in Childhood Utilizing Play and Art

When a mood disorder emerges in childhood, it is important to differentiate the clinical indicators of the mood disorder with consideration of the symptom manifestation related to the child's developmental stage (Briesmeister, 1997). Developmental considerations should include a comprehensive assessment of the child's biological, psychological, and social functioning (Newman, 2006; NIMH, 2010). These developmental considerations are seen in the child's art and play in a variety of ways. As the child depicts biological needs such as appetite, sleep, stimulation, and so forth in play behavior, the therapist may evaluate the child's level of need, with consideration given to the child's developmental stage assessing for congruence or incongruence as valuable treatment information. Furthermore, the child has the opportunity to demonstrate or develop effective coping within the play therapy process. Integrating art through the use of drawings expands the play therapy process and "children's drawing provide a unique frame of reference for thinking about and evaluating the children's overall development in many areas and for this reason they offer the therapist a unique way of understanding children from a variety of developmental perspectives" (Malchiodi, 1998).

Additionally, an environmental assessment is needed to evaluate the reciprocal influences of the mood disorder, which often manifest in academic problems, family conflicts, and problems in socialization (Fraser, Kirby, & Smokowski, 2004). Risk and protective factors for the child and family may be understood or "classified as broad environmental conditions; family, school, and neighborhood conditions; and individual biopsychosocial conditions" (Gilbert, 2004). Using art in play therapy assists in understanding each of these domains in a unique manner, and when incorporating these modalities into the assessment of the child and family, "sources of information and opportunity multiply quickly" (Gil, 2003). The child's developmental nuances emerge in drawings and may be utilized to understand the child biopsychosocial needs.

For instance, a 10-year-old girl with major depressive disorder was referred for treatment because of social withdrawal, frequent episodes of crying, school refusal, and failing grades. The aforementioned problems were also contributing to significant conflicts within the child's family. The client was compliant yet very hesitant in engaging with the miniatures, sand tray, or other play materials. She made no eye contact and offered no spontaneous comments. Her responses to questions about school concerns were "I don't know," and when asked about her functioning in general, she responded "Okay, I guess." She was offered a variety of art materials, including various papers, pencils, and markers. She was invited to create an image of "anything you would like to draw, or what's on your mind right now." The client took her time and created a detailed drawing using only white paper and a lead pencil. The drawing depicted a school building, including her image with an obvious frown. Her image was framed in a window, and she was throwing her books out the window. She also drew a teacher with a witch's hat glaring with hostility in her direction. As the client slid the picture to the therapist, tears were welling in her eyes. This drawing provided the valuable information needed to understand the emotional pain and turmoil being experienced by the child, as well as clear communication of the client's main concern at the time.

From this vantage point, the drawing is certainly a tool for self-expression and an opportunity for the therapist to provide empathy while validating the child. Moreover, the art imagery functions as a stable container grounding the content for cognitive processing or restructuring (Hamil, 2009). The client and therapist engage in a verbal and nonverbal dialogue in which the art is observed and processed. The child is invited to consider her options, and a decision can be made by the client to accept, expand, or alter the art in a way that assists the child's ability to manage or understand the mood disorder. This option allows the child to take an active role in the change process that is thoughtful, purposeful, and meaningful.

## Purposeful Treatment Strategies for Mood Disorders in Childhood

After careful assessment indicating the type of mood disorder, and a medical evaluation to determine if medication is needed, a treatment plan is created to establish specific strategies utilizing art and play to assist in making lifestyle changes that support healthy functioning at home, at school, and in relationships. Whether medication is prescribed or not, it is essential to integrate adaptive cognitive and behavioral skills through play and art to ensure adjustments for lifelong coping with the symptoms of a mood disorder. This approach responds to and capitalizes on the child and family protective factors for successful resolution of mood disorder problems.

Utilizing a child-centered approach allows the child to be "self-directed and naturally curious" (Landreth, 2002) in selecting art or play materials needed for expressing and coping with mood disorder symptoms. In this venue, the therapist serves as a witness to the child's experience, and both child and therapist rely on the safety and freedom of the therapeutic relationship and therapeutic space to facilitate the resolution of biopsychosocial needs. For mood disorders in childhood, the child-centered approach may be augmented by utilizing a prescriptive approach, allowing the therapist an opportunity to prompt or cue the child to use play and art in a way that guides the child and family to recognize and repair cognitive distortions, negative self-talk, and problematic mood shifts. In this form the play therapy becomes a tool for implementing the evidence-based protocol of Cognitive-Behavioral Therapy (CBT), a "well-established and empirically validated treatment for depression" (Newman, 2006), which is "active, problem-focused, and collaborative" (Reinecke & Ginsburg, 2008).

The therapist allows the client to portray the unique features of the mood disorder in the play and art imagery. This provides an opportunity for the therapist to recognize the impact of the mood disorder by observing the child's cognitive and behavioral expressions. The therapist continually observes and responds (verbally and/or nonverbally) to what is presented by the child, and through fluid assessment may identify needs that function as the *target of intervention* in the therapeutic session. Opportunities are offered in art and play strategies, allowing the child to adapt coping options that are most effective for the presenting concerns.

## Targets of Intervention for Mood Disorders in Childhood

As previously stated, a clinical assessment regarding the specific mood disorder the child experiences is an essential component of appropriate treatment. The child should be referred for a medical and psychiatric evaluation to determine if medications are needed and to rule out any comorbid medical conditions. An integral part of the assessment phase is the identification of any suicidal thoughts or thoughts of death the child may be experiencing, so that these risk factors may be intervened upon immediately.

Regardless of the type of mood disorder the child experiences, there is an impact on the child's capacity to relate to self, others, and the environment. This injury to interpersonal and intrapersonal relatedness is the hallmark feature of mood disorders (NIMH, 2010; Weller, Weller, & Danielyan, 2004) and is directly linked to the child's "vitality affects" or "external expressions revealing the primary or the differentiated nature of emotional states, respectively" (Siegel, 1999). The child's impaired vitality effects may have any number of origins, including the continual impact of the mood disorder over time (Siegel, 1999), parental depression (Gilbert, 2004), and negative outcomes from impaired social reciprocity (Avenevoli, Knight, Kessler, & Merikangas, 2008). Furthermore, the problems in relatedness are perpetuated by a schema based in fear and confusion from experiencing the biopsychosocial fluctuations associated with the mood disorder. This results in cognitive distortions, negative and self-depreciating self-talk, as well as overwhelming feelings and emotions. The primary biopsychosocial domains influenced by mood disorders in childhood are exquisitely tied to relatedness to the self and others. The mood disorder may significantly impair the child's understanding of self in relation to identity, relating to others, and the function of self in the environment. A mood disorder disrupts the child's ability to cope adequately in each of these domains. Play therapy provides an opportunity for the child to express the impact of the mood disorder and, most importantly, the arena to establish coping and resolution. The aforementioned domains become Targets of Intervention for the play therapist, providing options in the play and art that assist the child in developing adaptive skills for coping with the complex symptomology of the mood disorder.

## Integrating Art Into Play Therapy for Targets of Interventions

The child's spontaneous expressions and improvisations in play therapy provide unique insight into the child's experience. As the child's strengths and needs emerge in the play themes and art imagery, adaptations can be made to facilitate optimum coping for mood disorder symptoms. The art and play provide options for the child to meet and cope with challenges of mood swings, emotional dysregulation, and impulse control. Specific strengths and needs may be identified by the client and therapist as the focus of treatment. In this regard the focus of treatment is what this writer terms the Target of Intervention. Establishing a target or treatment focus structures the therapeutic process in a manner that is meaningful and attainable for the child and family. Furthermore, this structured format provides treatment goals or Therapeutic Objectives that are observable and measurable for the child, therapist, and family, contributing valuable information for the evaluation of treatment progress.

Targets of Intervention selected for review in this chapter include the following:

1. Psychoeducation
2. Self-Care
3. Communication
4. Cognitive Restructuring
5. Mood Recognition and Affect Regulation
6. Problem Solving Skills
7. Functional Relatedness

## Integrating Art Into Play Therapy for Children With Mood Disorders

### Targets of Intervention and Therapeutic Objectives

Child therapists are encouraged to utilize the selected Targets of Intervention when relevant to the child's presenting needs, and to use them as a guideline in structuring unique treatment objectives to meet the therapeutic goals. Targets of Intervention may be incorporated into group, individual, or family models of therapy.

*Target: Psychoeducation*
*Therapeutic Objectives*: (1) Learn specific features of mood disorders in childhood; (2) Identify and communicate how the symptoms of mood disorders are experienced; (3) Role-play or create a drawing to demonstrate coping with symptoms.

The initial focus of treatment for mood disorders in childhood is based in effectively communicating to the child and parents the characteristics, features, and symptomology of the specific mood disorder the child is experiencing. In play therapy this is achieved by connecting terms, universal concepts, and images to the symptoms. Clinical terms such as *depression, mania, lethargy,* and *impulsivity* are described to the child and family in universal concepts such as weather conditions (e.g., highs, lows, stormy, foggy, cloudy, frozen, and raging like a fire), animal behavior (e.g., buzzing, flying, screeching, howling, soaring, and hibernating), and in other relevant characterizations (e.g., race car, volcano, turtle, bumblebee). For instance, the fluctuating symptoms of bipolar disorder can be understood in terms such as a race car that speeds around at certain times and then unexpectedly has four flat tires, causing it to not be able to drive at all. The play therapist invites the child to identify the characterization and assists the child and family in exploring the symptom frequency, intensity, and duration from the characteristics and descriptions provided.

A meaningful way to educate children and families about mood disorders is the use of children's books, stories, poems, and personal narratives. The quote at the beginning of this chapter is from *Harold and the Purple Crayon* by Crockett Johnson (1955). This story beautifully illustrates the use of creativity and improvisation (both inherent to art and play) as a means of navigating the unknown, solving problems, forming relationships, gaining sustenance, and establishing safety. Stories such as this establish characters and themes of narratives as metaphors for the problematic symptoms of the mood disorder, allowing for identification and discussion of problems in a way that does not shame the children or families. Assisting children in creating a personal narrative provides a structured container for an otherwise chaotic and overwhelming life experience. The children may be encouraged to identify an animal or character they would like to represent themselves, and then children are invited to engage in storytelling, role-play, or drawing to portray "The Story of the Brave Warrior" (example). The children may begin the story or myth with the phrase "Once upon a time" to further prompt creativity and improvisation. This type of prompt allows the children to expose ideas, thoughts, core beliefs, and values in a way that is nonthreatening. Art may be integrated at any juncture of the psychoeducational process, affording the play therapist opportunities to respond therapeutically to children's presenting strengths and needs.

*Target: Self-Care*
*Therapeutic Objectives*: (1) Establish routine and consistent skills in self-nurturance and self-soothing; (2) Demonstrate the knowledge of caring for self and others through play and art; (3) Schedule and engage in fulfilling and pleasant activities.

As a result of erratic mood changes, such as the fatigue and lethargy with depression, or erratic mood shifts associated with bipolar disorder, a child may demonstrate problems with self-care. Self-care includes the practice of important but ordinary tasks such as hygiene, exercise, taking meals, and interpersonal socialization. When a child is experiencing the symptoms of a mood disorder, basic tasks such as washing and combing hair, brushing teeth, bathing, and getting dressed in clean clothes require extraordinary effort and concentration. Also, the child's effort to play or engage with others is interrupted by symptoms such as hyperactivity, impulsivity, and irritability. The child may withdraw from play or may have been removed from play because of impulse control problems or problems in socialization. In play therapy, the child is allowed to utilize dolls, miniatures, costumes, puppets, and props, such as baby bottles, bandages, blankets, and pillows to model self-care, personal likes and dislikes, preferences in socialization, and nurturing needs. The objective is for the child to gain a sense of knowing what makes him or her feel clean, nurtured, and satisfied. This basic function provides the child with balance and a starting point to build additional skills.

Art tasks that bridge this form of play in therapy include allowing the child to make or create a doll from paper, fabric, wire, or clay. The skills used in creating a self-object such as a doll or a pet can be generalized into a daily routine of self-care. This fosters a sincere care of the self, which occurs when the child demonstrates care for the object created. As children build self-care skills, they become aware of their own needs and establish the ability to identify and express what helps them cope with the symptoms and problems of a mood disorder. Furthermore, the child and family are prompted to schedule times for pleasant activities so the coping may be demonstrated and reinforced. A dry-erase board serves as a wonderful tool for scheduling pleasant activities and for drawing images that portray positive interactions and motivating symbols. The dry-erase board or a poster board is also useful for portraying lists or images of accomplishments to affirm the child's success.

*Target: Communication*
*Therapeutic Objectives*: (1) Increase functional communication of needs, concerns, and interests; (2) Practice expressing thoughts and beliefs; (3) Identify communication style and utilize personal style to communicate thoughts and feelings effectively.

One of the most devastating aspects of a mood disorder in childhood is children's inability to adequately express to family, teachers, or friends the overwhelming feelings and thoughts that occur with the disorder. A mood disorder stifles children's desire to play and create, thereby cutting them off from their intrinsic forms of communication. It is imperative that therapists, teachers, and parents stimulate children's innate capacity to communicate through play, movement, and art. Careful and nonjudgmental observation of children's behavior and expressions will instruct adults in the needs and concerns of these children. The greatest benefit to children with mood disorders is to establish an age-appropriate way to identify and express the complex and painful experience of a mood disorder. In child-centered play therapy, children are provided the opportunity to "lead the way" (Landreth, 2002) and to utilize or play with the materials available in any way they deem beneficial (of course without harming the self or others). This freedom to improvise prompts children to communicate the impact of mood fluctuations, current physical needs, and behavioral and cognitive styles.

In this arena, the child exposes her schema and the influence the mood disorder has had on her concept of self and her experience of the environment or her worldview. This is an excellent opportunity to integrate art into the play therapy process. The child is provided with an assortment of art materials, such as oil pastels, crayons, colored pencils, or paint, to depict any number of schematic representations. Suggested directives would include (a) create a picture using these materials, (b) draw what you are thinking right now, (c) paint or color your feelings, (d) draw your world, and (e) draw you and your family doing something together (Hamil, 2008; Malchiodi, 2007). It is important that the play therapist allow the child to identify what the drawing means to her. The child's response or lack of response is the opportunity for the child to express verbally or nonverbally what she is experiencing. It is not necessary for the play therapist to interpret the drawing unless there are overt expressions of self-harm or intent to harm others. This type of communication in the art is managed exactly the same as a verbal or a behavioral gesture of suicidal or homicidal ideation. Any time an individual communicates intent to harm self or others, immediate action must be taken to ensure safety. This includes a medical evaluation and possible hospitalization.

*Target: Cognitive Restructuring*
*Therapeutic Objectives*: (1) Recognize and communicate core beliefs about self, others, and the environment; (2) Identify and correct cognitive distortions; (3) Establish a coherent sense of self and a functional identity.

The negative self-image perpetuated by experiencing a mood disorder facilitates a sense of shame and self-loathing related to self-expression (Riley, 2003). The child observes the apparent carefree behaviors of other children and yearns for similar experiences. The child perceives the observed experiences of others as out of reach because of cognitive distortions created by the experience of a mood disorder. These experiences support an internal sense of self that is chaotic and unpredictable resulting from erratic shifts in mood. Cognitive distortions need to be expressed in art and play to allow positive and functional thoughts to be internalized by the child. A child with a mood disorder can learn healthy self-expression to communicate the personal experience of a mood disorder. As self-expression improves, the child gains insight into his or her personal needs and how to get those needs met appropriately.

The experience of a mood disorder contributes to the impression in the child and in others that the child *is* a problem rather than that the child *has* a problem (Newman, 2006). The mood disorder leads a child to feel disoriented and overwhelmed, and in turn the child begins to distrust herself and misreads interpersonal gestures as threatening and harmful. These problems interfere with family and peer relationships. In play therapy, children experience acceptance and freedom to express themselves (Landreth, 2002), learning to see themselves as special in regard to family and group dynamics, thus building a coherent sense of self. For example, the child learns to distinguish a sense of self apart from the mood disorder by role-playing symptoms such as irritability or impulsivity and tagging the symptom to the disorder rather than the self. A delightful way to assist the child in this process is to play a game I call Pin the Tail on the Problem. The problem may be depicted in several ways, such as a large circle with the word Bipolar. Symptoms or "tails" are identified on strips of paper, which are "pinned" (taped, glued, stapled, etc.) to the problem. Furthermore, the child is encouraged to clearly identify the symptom in association with the mood disorder and empathically state, "It's not me!"

This process is expanded with miniatures, puppets, and art materials to depict the child's understanding of both the self and the disorder. A distinction can be made supporting a coherent sense of self, which is understood as influenced by the mood disorder symptoms rather than consumed by it. Utilizing art materials in this process with the child is an essential part of developing a unique sense of self through creativity. The child is invited to engage in creating images of "the problem" (depression, feeling lonely, racing thoughts, etc.) by making a "moody mask" or creating a drawing of "what depression looks like in your mind." Other associations that separate the mood disorder from the child can be made by identifying a metaphor to represent the problem, such as a race car, a black bear, or a turtle. The metaphor is explored in drawings, sculpture, or collage. This exploration begins the task of nurturing a coherent sense of self in relation to the mood disorder. The child gains a sense of mastery and begins to think "I can" cope with this problem.

### Target: Mood Recognition and Affect Regulation

*Therapeutic Objectives*: (1) Establish a functional appraisal of mood states and expressed emotions; (2) Identify and cope with shifts in mood and affect; (3) Develop skills to direct behavior based on an informed understanding and recognition of feeling states.

The experience of a mood disorder in childhood is complex and includes overwhelming mood and affect shifts. This makes it difficult for children to find an adequate way to express their feelings and to make an objective appraisal of their emotions. In play therapy, children learn the terms for mood states and practice behaviors and gestures to convey specific feelings. This is accomplished by recognizing how mood and affect are actually experienced in the body. Mood disorders in childhood are associated with numerous somatic complaints (Gilbert, 2004; Weller, Weller, & Danielyan, 2004). For example, children may complain of stomachaches and headaches in an effort to address the overwhelming affect shifts. In play therapy, children practice differentiating physical pain and emotional pain as the therapist helps them find the words and expressions that reflect what is being experienced. The children may use puppets to show how the character behaves with a physical pain and then demonstrate how the puppet character behaves in a feeling state. This play strategy can also be utilized to differentiate emotional and cognitive responses. Art can then be integrated into the play therapy and bridge the process, facilitating a personal understanding of how the behaviors, thoughts, and emotions are differentiated by the child when influenced by the symptoms of the mood disorder. The play therapist establishes an image collection, including a variety of facial expressions from magazines, pictures, or drawings, and engages the child in playing with emotional appraisal. It is important to acquire a diverse image portfolio, including as many different cultures and ages as possible.

The children and families can be involved in the search for images representing moods and feelings as homework between sessions, encouraging active participation in the learning process. The first task is to assist children in establishing a rich vocabulary of terms to describe various mood and feeling states. The therapist allows the children to select images of interest and then asks the children to identify the mood and feeling states they perceive. The children and family may also enjoy using pictures of animals, providing an opportunity for associations with animal expressions. The children may even identify with the roar of a tiger and learn to describe what triggers the roar or what quiets the roar.

If a child identifies strongly with an animal or character, further exploration into the other characteristics of the animal or character is beneficial in helping the child understand the connection between mood states and behavior. As children explore the character's moods and emotions, they learn to recognize the embedded relationship of these feeling states. Art and symbols enhance this process when the moods and feeling states are paired with selected metaphors such as weather conditions. Children can easily draw symbols, such as the "burning" sun, the "lonely" moon, a "furious" storm, and so on. As children create these symbols, the feeling state is processed and managed in the art. Beneficial adaptations for expressing fluctuations in mood and affect are begun by creating and altering the art imagery, and are then generalized to alterations in the children's behavior.

### Target: Problem-Solving Skills
*Therapeutic Objectives*: (1) Establish competent age-appropriate problem solving; (2) Practice collaborative problem solving; (3) Demonstrate conflict-resolution skills.

Mood disorders have a significant impact on concentration and cognitive functioning, which may result in the child having difficulty in making small daily decisions. At times a parent or teacher may be inclined to make all the decisions for the child, interrupting the child's ability to practice problem solving and conflict resolution. Children need the opportunity to demonstrate age-appropriate competency in problem solving and in making personal decisions regarding daily functioning and interactions. Problem solving is an intrinsic feature of drawing, sculpting, painting, and collage (Hamil, 2008, 2009; Malchiodi, 2007; Pifalo, 2009). The child contemplates a multitude of options in content, use of materials, and color selection, as well as how to utilize the time and space available. Each of these components poses a problem for the child to resolve. At times the depressed or hesitant child will avoid art making. A dry-erase board is an effective tool for these children, because errors may be easily corrected, minimizing their influence as obstacles in starting or completing tasks.

Creating a map is a valuable problem-solving strategy that integrates art into the play therapy process (Hamil, 2009; Pifalo, 2009). The child and family identify a goal or destination and work together to create a map to reach the destination. Mapping involves the child and family in a wide range of problem-solving steps, such as identifying a starting point, considering options, selecting a direction, and visualizing the results. The child becomes competent by facing structured challenges and experiencing different levels of success through trial and error, or considering alternate routes. Furthermore, the child and family engage in accepting each person's creative efforts, which supports collaborative problem solving. The child can practice frustration tolerance while considering expectations of self and others. Cumulative success facilitates skill acquisition, and the child establishes a pattern of creative thinking for solving problems.

*Target: Functional Relatedness*
*Therapeutic Objectives*: (1) Improve social skills; (2) Establish relational boundaries; (3) Practice limit setting and self-control.

The symptoms of mood disorders manifest in various boundary challenges. For example, a child experiencing the symptoms of mania with bipolar disorder will demonstrate impulsivity, inattention, and hyperactivity in the environment. This can result in many boundary problems with others and may even present a safety concern. The child will benefit from role-play with the therapist using puppets and miniatures to identify boundary issues regarding personal space, interpersonal interactions, and behavioral modifications. The child practices identifying personal preferences related to boundaries and respecting the boundaries of others in the art and play. Some children like for others to get close to them, whereas others are frightened by proximity.

The child establishes improved appraisal of interpersonal gestures and appropriate behaviors for social settings by using art and play directives, such as creating a comic strip. This format depicts the child's perception of interactions with family, peers, and even pets. This provides unique insight into the child's preferences and understanding of sequences in socialization. Problematic or uncomfortable boundary issues can be framed in a comic manner to provide the distance needed to reflect on each person's part in the interactions. For example, if the child relates well to the comic strip *Garfield*, the therapist and child would collect comic strips that demonstrate how Garfield the cat sets limits with others or does not respect limits others request of him. This directive may be expanded in several ways, and certainly the child could create a cast of characters to represent different scenarios of socialization that are influenced by one's mood state.

## Case Example

This case shows how the Target Interventions can be used to meet Therapeutic Objectives for cognitive restructuring and regulation of mood and affect. A 5-year-old male was experiencing significant problems with irritability, sadness and crying, aggression toward his peers and family, as well as sleep and appetite problems. The child was also refusing to engage in activities he previously found pleasant. He was easily frustrated when playing and became enraged when he was dissatisfied with general play activities. These symptoms had been ongoing for three months and emerged after numerous biopsychosocial changes occurred for the family (i.e., moving, illness, new sibling, and school changes).

The reported symptoms were demonstrated in the first session of play therapy, as the child moved quickly from one activity to the other. Eventually, he expressed his frustration and sadness by standing rigidly in the center of the room with his hands balled into fists, and he yelled, "I'm not okay! I'll never be okay! I'm not okay! I'll never be okay!" This is a salient example of a child clearly communicating his thoughts, feelings, and fears during the play therapy session. I asked the child what was needed for him to be okay. I also invited him to identify anything that was "okay" in the playroom. The child went directly to the sand tray and selected what he identified as a "brave warrior." The child was prompted to use the costumes, shields, helmets, belts, and swords in the playroom to become a brave warrior. As he became the brave warrior, the child's mood and emotions stabilized, and he fully engaged in the characterization. He moved around the playroom with confidence and expressed the things he liked about brave warriors. The terms he used were *strong, brave, smart, mean,* and *friendly.*

When the session was over, the child asked to take the brave warrior accessories with him, but he was reminded that these items must stay in the playroom. After thinking about these requirements, the child stated, "But I don't have the tools I need to be a brave warrior." Again the play assisted the child in expressing his main concern of not having the skills to be "okay" in managing the mood shifts and emotional turmoil of the mood disorder. A picture was taken of the child in character, and he was prompted to continue to imagine and act as if he were the brave warrior he wanted to be. The brave warrior character was used to assist the child in developing the skills and tools he needed to cope effectively. The family was engaged in supporting the brave warrior in his battles with mood and affect regulation by joining him in creating a narrative of The Brave Warrior. The child created drawings and selected pictures of scenes he found empowering, and these were incorporated into his story as he and his family identified the tools and coping skills needed for him to be "okay."

## Conclusion

Appropriate treatment of mood disorders in childhood has a profound effect on the quality of life for the child and family. Improving relationships and strengthening a cohesive sense of self in the child are beginning steps in fostering a sense of hope and purpose. Play therapy provides the child with a sense of being in charge of the mood disorder and the forum for open self-expression. The child and family learn in play therapy how to build on their progress and enjoy other benefits, such as pleasing performance in school, satisfying peer relations, and the ability to face stressful situations with confidence. The child and family are restored by an empowering sense of balance as they are equipped with the tools and adaptive skills for lifelong coping.

## References

American Psychiatric Association. (2000). *Diagnostic and statistical manual of mental disorders* (4th ed., text revision; DSM-IV-TR). Washington, DC: American Psychiatric Association.

Avenevoli, S., Knight, E., Kessler, R. C., & Merikangas, K.R. (2008). Epidemiology of depression in children and adolescents. In R. Z. Abela & B. L. Hankin (Eds.), *Handbook of depression in children and adolescents*. New York, NY: Guilford Press.

Briesmeister, J. M. (1997). Play therapy with depressed children. In H. G. Kaduson, D. Cangelosi, & C. E. Schaefer (Eds.), *The playing cure: Individualized play therapy for specific childhood problems* (pp. 3–28). New York, NY: Rowman & Littlefield.

Findler, E. (2009). Playful strategies to manage frustration: The turtle technique and beyond. In A. A. Drewes (Ed.), *Blending play therapy with cognitive behavioral therapy: Evidence-based and other effective treatment and techniques.* (pp. 401–422). Hoboken, NJ: Wiley.

Fraser, M. W., Kirby, L. D., & Smokowski, P. R. (2004). In M. W. Fraser (Ed.), *Risk and resilience in childhood: An ecological perspective* (2nd ed., pp. 13–66). Washington, DC: National Association of Social Workers Press.

Gil, E. (2003). Family play therapy: The bear with the short nails. In C. E. Schaefer (Ed.), *Foundations of play therapy*. Hoboken, NJ: Wiley.

Gilbert, C. (2004). Childhood depression: A risk factor perspective. In M. W. Fraser (Ed.) *Risk and resilience in childhood: An ecological perspective* (2nd ed., pp. 315–346). Washington, DC: National Association of Social Workers Press.

Hamil, S. (2008). *My feeling better workbook: Help for kids who are sad and depressed*. Oakland, CA: Instant Help Books.

Hamil, S. (2009). *Latest considerations in integrating art into child therapy*. Association for Play Therapy Mining Report (November, 2009 ed.). Retrieved from www.a4pt.org/download.cfm?ID=28409

Hammer, E. F. (1980). *The clinical application of projective drawings* (6th ed.). Springfield, IL: Charles C. Thomas.

Hammer, E. F. (1997). *Advances in projective drawing interpretation*. Springfield, IL: Charles C. Thomas.

Johnson, C. (1955). *Harold and the purple crayon*. New York, NY: Harper Collins.

Landreth, G. L. (2002). *Play therapy: The art of the relationship*. New York, NY: Brunner-Rutledge.

Malchiodi, C. (1998). *Understanding children's drawings*. New York, NY: Guilford Press.

Malchiodi, C. (Ed.) (2003). *Handbook of art therapy*. New York, NY: Guilford Press.

Malchiodi, C. (2007). *The art therapy sourcebook* (2nd ed.). New York, NY: McGraw-Hill.

National Institute of Mental Health. (2010). *Bipolar disorder in children and teens: A parent's guide*. U.S. Department of Health and Human Services. National Institutes of Health. NIH Publication No. 08-6380. Retrieved from http://www.nimh.nih.gov

Newman, E. (2006). Short-term play therapy for children with mood disorders. In H. G. Kaduson & C. E. Schaefer (Eds.), *Short-term play therapy* (2nd ed., pp. 71–100). New York, NY: Guilford Press.

O'Connor, K. J. (1983). The color-your-life technique. In C. E. Schaefer & K. J. O'Connor (Eds.), *Handbook of play therapy* (pp. 251–258). New York, NY: John Wiley & Sons.

Pifalo, T. A. (2009). Mapping the maze: An art therapy intervention following disclosure of sexual abuse. *Art Therapy: Journal of American Art Therapy Association, 26*(1), 12–18.

Riley, S. (2003). Using art therapy to address adolescent depression. In C. Malchiodi (Ed.), *Handbook of art therapy*. New York, NY: Guilford Press.

Reinecke, M. A., & Ginsburg, G. S. (2008). Cognitive-behavioral treatment of depression during childhood and adolescence. In R. Z. Abela & B. L. Hankin (Eds.), *Handbook of depression in children and adolescents*. New York, NY: Guilford Press.

Shelby, J. S., & Berk, M. S. (2009). Play therapy, pedagogy, and CBT: An argument for interdisciplinary synthesis. In A. A. Drewes (Ed.), *Blending play therapy with cognitive behavioral therapy: Evidence-based and other effective treatment and techniques* (pp. 17–40). Hoboken, NJ: Wiley.

Siegel, D. J. (1999). *The developing mind: How relationships and the brain interact to shape who we are.* New York, NY: Guilford Press.

Sweeney, D. S., & Landreth, G. L. (2003). Child-centered play therapy. In C. E. Schaefer (Ed.), *Foundations of play therapy* (pp. 76–98). Hoboken, NJ: Wiley.

Weller, E. B., Weller, R. A, & Danielyan, A. K. (2004). Mood disorders in prepubertal children. In J. M. Weiner & M. K. Dulcan (Eds.), *Textbook of child and adolescent psychiatry* (3rd ed.). Washington, DC: American Psychiatric Association Press.

# Integrating Play Therapy and EMDR With Children

## A Post-Trauma Intervention

### *Victoria A. McGuinness*

## Introduction

Play therapy and EMDR are two powerful methods of therapy for children independent of each other and have proven to be helpful in assisting children who have experienced traumatic events in their lives. A working definition of trauma needs to address both single incident trauma VS. repeated traumas and be measured, *by the child* by intensity, frequency and duration. A thorough parent or legal guardian report/intake is necessary too but no one can measure the effect of other people's trauma, not even parents, so the child's responses provide the ultimate key to the process.

Simply put, there is single-incident or devastating trauma and/or repeated, even ritualized trauma that occurs for days, weeks, or even years—that weave themselves into a child's sense of identity so deeply that utilizing all methods of helping the child process traumatic events need to be available to the clinician. Although the structure may remain essentially the same, each child's process is entirely unique.

The interplay of child-directed play therapy and therapist-guided EMDR is like an infinity symbol that involves balancing the interplay of opposites; specifically, the two hemispheres of the brain. Combining the two dynamic methods of play therapy and EMDR offers children ways to process both experientially and cognitively according to their developmental ability. The therapeutic relationship provides a container for holding the child's intense

---

Note: Formal training in both play therapy and EMDR are necessary to provide these therapies; this chapter is not intended as an actual training but simply as an overview of the two methods combined.

feelings. This relationship becomes the safe, creative, and effective bond that allows the processing of feelings and confronting cognitive beliefs that cause misery and anxiety to the traumatized child.

There are many similarities and differences if one compares and contrasts the dynamics of play therapy with EMDR. EMDR is a more cognitive approach while play therapy tends to be more experiential in nature although both appear to positively and directly affect a child's negative cognitions, beliefs and themes. Themes are important in both experiential play therapy and directive play therapy and appear often as targets within the EMDR process. Children's themes reflect back to the adult world what their experience in life is like, what issues they struggle with, and essentially reveal the effects of trauma on their minds, hearts and souls. Children can be absolutely poetic, absolutely raw in their response to trauma.

## Play Therapy and EMDR With Traumatized Children

The first step in child therapy is to meet with the child's parents or caretakers. Because traumatic events can be a source of shame as well as anxiety and maladaptive behaviors, it is important to meet with the child's parents or caretakers before meeting with the child. This initial meeting provides a wealth of information about the child for the therapist and helps parents to understand and anticipate the possible effects of experiencing both play therapy and EMDR.

Exploring the traumatic event from the parents' perspective relating to any symptoms they experience their child as having are vital beginning elements in child's therapy. Asking parents to imagine and relate the fears or negative cognitions their child might be suffering from and then exploring the positive beliefs and cognitions they would like their child to have or regain contributes positively to the therapy process. It is also important to be aware that not all parents or caretakers will be able to provide all the information that a clinician would like to obtain in the first meeting or at all. It is critical to remember that the child's *experience of being honored on the journey* helps the child to heal.

During the parent or guardian intake, the traumatic event is usually known and is the primary reason for bringing the child for therapy. At times, the child's behavior causes the parent or guardian to bring the child to therapy, and the traumatic event is basically guessed at or unknown. Regardless, the therapist must recognize the differences between healthy, normal play themes and traumatic play themes. Themes or targets tend to be dualistic in nature: good vs. evil, powerlessness vs. empowerment, power/control, vulnerability and protection/defenses, male/female, destructive vs. constructive, violence vs. creativity, and so on. Targets, the pictures a child will focus on during EMDR processing, can be accessed through pictures, drawings, sand trays, verbalizations, and/or provided through parent observation.

Targets in EMDR and themes generated through the play therapy illustrate the specific emotional experience of each child and can be especially helpful for even the youngest child. Both therapy methods have the power to positively alter a child's feelings about him or herself and the traumatic event(s). Combining these two methods has the power to change the direction of a child's life! Both methods can teach children that they can be the boss of their thoughts and behavior—a powerful lesson, indeed.

Regardless of how a clinician and a child weave together the fabric of the child's journey in the playroom or office, it is essential that the child have true choice in the process. Giving children a choice is essential to seal this container of safety to hold children's often overwhelming feelings by respecting the pace of their personal processing. Teaching all children ages six and over that behaviors and actions, thoughts and feelings are all connected helps empower them with knowledge. Find experiential ways to validate this theory for children by exploring how trauma affects behaviors and actions by causing disturbing or frightening thoughts and bad feelings in order to facilitate understanding by providing some concepts for children to ponder in their own way.

Both EMDR and play therapy offer a path to raising self-esteem, lowering fears and anxieties, and offering healing from even the most traumatic events. Both methods open the door to unconscious material and reveal beliefs that cause emotional pain. Children can play about, draw pictures about, and create sand trays about their inner world without having to verbalize. In fact, their communication is enhanced precisely because they don't *have to* verbalize. EMDR requires more verbal feedback from children, but even this feedback can be modified by experiential means to limit the need to verbalize when a child is not yet comfortable doing so.

The second session generally invites both the child and the child's parents into the playroom; older children might prefer to come into their session alone. Again, giving the child this choice is the first step toward empowering the child. The parents are usually included in the second session for younger children or highly anxious children. Children, especially those younger than 7 who have experienced trauma often benefit from playing first, discharging energy through play. Allowing children to tell their story through play first takes pressure off of them prior to introducing EMDR, while showing them that the therapist is willing to enter their world. I once saw a 5-year-old child whose father literally chased tornados and she was terrified and dreamt repeatedly that he would be swept away in one. During the second session, I mentioned a game that could help her with her bad dreams, not ever mentioning this again. In her eighth session, *she asked* to play the game and within 3 minutes she experienced relief from her nightmares in the months to follow.

When following a basic structure for play therapy, mentioning other forms of treatment to the child within the first three sessions seems to work best. Letting children know that you have a way, a game, that can help them with their negative thoughts and feelings, nightmares or memories early on also gives them a chance to choose and time to think about what you said to them. Usually within minutes, unless they are immobilized by anxiety, traumatized children will pick a self object and start to tell their story through play, or the child will explore the playroom and more slowly decide how to play.

Sadie was 6½ years old when I met her. Her story as told in the Case Example later in this chapter illustrates the power of play therapy and EMDR combined to alleviate the negative effects of trauma.

In her first session, Sadie chose a tiny red wagon and a tiny, tiny shovel from the miniature collection. Playing in the sandbox, she carefully placed one tiny shovelful of sand at a time into the miniature red wagon. It was like Sadie was saying, "This is how much feeling I can allow myself to feel and not become overwhelmed by the process." Sadie needed a strong feeling of being in control.

When children are ready for EMDR processing, the first thing to teach them is the use of the word "STOP!" as well as the attendant hand gesture. Children of all ages need to be able to stop the EMDR processing at will, again returning the power to the child and reinforcing feelings of safety and control. Whenever a child chooses to play the "game that can help them"—or engage in EMDR processing—*always* start with helping the child create a "safe place" or "peaceful or happy place." One way to explain the safe or peaceful place is by saying: "This is a place that can be real, imaginary, or both where you are in total control and you feel *totally* safe and comfortable; this is a place where *nothing* bad can happen." Then, collect as much sensory data as possible to include odors, sights, tastes, textures, scenery, people or animals who the child might imagine to be there with them, whether they are alone, and so on. Many traumatized children choose the playroom as their safe or peaceful place.

Using hand-taps, puppets, toys or the Thera-Tapper (see Reference Section) is generally the easiest way to install a safe place in children. Make sure all children are armed with the ability to say "STOP!" and halt the EMDR processing as well.

Pretending to hold an imaginary remote control to fast-forward, skip, pause, delete and so on, memories or scenes that are too upsetting for them is a great tool too. (Children do not ever seem to say "Stop!" during the safe or peaceful place installation.)

Installing a safe place and seeing the depth of response in the positive will be your measuring tool for assessing the child's depth of response when processing traumatic events. A lot of joy equals the potential for a lot of pain. This is not hard science, but it tends to be accurate. Practicing "STOP!" and using the imaginary commands on the remote control before eye movements also lowers a child's anxiety by giving them more control. (Using actual eye movements with children can feel invasive, so other ways of achieving bi-lateral brain stimulation are preferred.)

If there is nowhere in the child's mind that can serve as a container for safety, be *very* cautious about using EMDR until the child has engaged in reenactment play, has experienced some relief from the trauma and has developed more trust in the relationship with the therapist. Even when no other EMDR processing takes place, installing a safe or peaceful place is a powerful addition to therapy and is highly recommended. This provides the structure of the container used to hold a child's intense feelings and functions as a grounding exercise after a difficult session or to just help lower a child's anxiety. Including the child's favorite color and using that color in a guided meditation to fill the whole body is an amazing way of calming down a child.

There is increasing evidence that the brain is flexible and literally rewires itself based on the *experiences* a person has. The more trauma a person experiences, the more poorly brain functioning develops, and the healthy pathways are blocked or become nonfunctioning or misfiring, causing socio-emotional delays for children of trauma. But it is also true that this marvelous elasticity of brain development allows the intensity of emotional trauma to be significantly reduced, sometimes even eliminated entirely, by providing positive experiences, thoughts and feelings to replace the traumatic ones. These traumatic experiences are translated into themes and targets for processing.

Target selection and measuring Subjective Units of Distress (SUDS) and Validity of Cognition (VoC) is a process that varies, often widely, from the adult protocol for EMDR processing. The EMDR process with children is often more imagery-based while children may need more help than adults to make the associative connections. There is less focus on the articulation of cognition, feelings and sensations. Children may draw these images or even keep those thoughts private, if requested. Use hand-taps, knee-taps, toys, puppets (one in each hand) or the Thera-Tapper to help facilitate EMDR processing with children.

Children who suffer from post-traumatic stress disorder or other disorders caused by trauma may find the actual eye movements to be invasive or even too difficult to engage in. Using a two-handed or two-puppet approach helps children younger than 8, who cannot cross the midline between brain hemispheres. Certainly, shorter sets of eye movements are generally sufficient for children; they often process more quickly because they have shorter channels (of association.) Traumatized children are more likely to experience abreaction so safeguards need to be built into the process. Going slowly and observing the child's response to intensive therapy are critical to a successful outcome.

The adult protocol for using EMDR does not work very well with children. Letting go of measuring SUDS with numbers is a good idea, too. Simple hand gestures, rulers, drawing thermometers, and so on are better alternatives when measuring SUDS with children. With severe trauma or prolonged or repeated trauma, less resolution may be possible in the immediate time-frame. Allowing non-directed play or, in some cases, more directive play therapy to be woven into the therapy process literally takes the reporting pressure off of traumatized children by solidifying the therapeutic relationship first.

Other ways to measure SUDS and VoCs include drawing events or feelings before processing and then after EMDR processing. For very young children and many older children as well, just using the distance between their hands to show a small, medium, and large distance is sufficient for measuring SUDS.

Again, in general, introducing the concept of EMDR to children within the first three play therapy sessions is the ideal. Using Norton's experiential model as a structure for therapy (Norton & Norton, 1997), the idea of EMDR is introduced to the child during the Exploratory Stage and/or the Testing for Protection Stage thus building EMDR into this structure. For example, by way of introduction the therapist might say, "I have a game that helps with nightmares or with the bad pictures in your mind or scary feelings in your body. This game helps to make these pictures and feelings change and make them better." This is also a time to look for *any* positive beliefs a child holds about him or herself or a situation as well as considering any themes and targets.

Another way to create a feeling of safety and empowerment for a child is to say: "Today we are going to work to help make your power stronger. Pick a toy to help you out, and show me where you want to be in this room." The advantage of having parents in the room at this point is so you can offer even more safety by suggesting: "You can sit in Mommy or Daddy's lap while we make your power stronger."

One way to introduce EMDR with children of about 6 or 7 years of age is drawing on a whiteboard. Draw a circle, dividing it in half to represent the two sides of the brain and explain the basic functioning of each hemisphere to the child. Then, draw dots on the right side to show children that that's where the trauma/upsetting event(s) "got stuck," which is something they can relate to. Next draw lines going from the left to the right hemispheres and talk about how this mysterious process will help them to think and feel differently about what they experienced. This makes sense to children and is often intriguing to them. This method has captured the attention of many children and encouraged them to choose EMDR for processing.

Telling children that by holding the controls for the Thera-Tapper, for example, the bad stuff can get unstuck encourages them to try the process. Letting them know that this game might dissolve the bad stuff and turn it into something much better also encourages children to attempt EMDR processing. Children intuit that they have the power to alter their perceptions for the better and this awareness can help them throughout their lives, especially for children who experience trauma.

Some important considerations are involved when working with traumatized children. The first is the child's age or developmental stage when the trauma first took place. The second identifying consideration is to discover if any healing has already taken place or if the child just lives in almost constant fear. Traumatized children live in a state of hyper-arousal. Moving from one polarized behavior to another, traumatized children may withdraw totally inside themselves or strike out and decide that attacking others (verbally or behaviorally) is the way they have learned to protect themselves.

Single-event trauma, such as being the lone survivor of an automobile accident in which your entire nuclear family dies, is an incomprehensible loss for anyone. Major influences affecting the outcome of the healing process can result from, for example, being taken in quickly by family members following a major loss as opposed to going into foster care. The circumstances immediately following the trauma influence the child's readiness to face his or her painful life situation.

In addition to the quality of support a child has, the child's temperament is always a consideration. The level of support, temperament, and resiliency will impact a traumatized child's ability to heal. Other single-event traumas such as having a house burn down but the child and family remaining intact can be resolved more quickly through play therapy and EMDR than can the loss of a loved one. The death of a pet and death in general is in some important ways more chronic than acute but the initial grieving process sets the tone for dealing with a major loss throughout life.

During the hard work stage of therapy, the "working stage" according to Norton's experiential model (Norton & Norton, 1997), the therapist has the opportunity to work with negative cognitions/beliefs by developing themes and targets for processing. The working stage can be intense in the playroom and at home or elsewhere.

Parents, guardians, teachers and so on need to be informed ahead of processing with either play therapy or EMDR that most children regress or get worse before they get better. This is particularly true of the traumatized child who one way or another has to face the trauma again and work through it to a more adaptive resolution. Re-entering or facing the trauma stirs up the actual terror that occurred for the child *during* the traumatic event or events. This is just like having to go through it again. (Reminding children that the event is over and that they survived the actual trauma can help some children.) Children and their parents need a lot of support and validation during this stage.

In the working stages, using directive play therapy with children who experience intense anger regarding life's events provides information that children need. This is when teaching the very direct connections between thinking–feeling–behavior to educate children about how we, as human beings, function gives them a framework for understanding themselves. Using a myriad of child-level worksheets that explore both cognitive and sensory data for describing how their anger *feels* in their bodies, where it is located in their bodies, and what color it is gives the clinician valuable information for helping. Gently addressing maladaptive behaviors and mis-thoughts and connecting these thoughts and behaviors to the trauma provides even more safety and resources for the child's healing process.

After imagining a safe or peaceful place, and when the therapeutic relationship is more solid, during the working stage a therapist can say: "Your power is so strong now; you can still feel safe when you remember the bad man, scary night, your mother going away, etc.; just tell me what you see. Tell me when it feels better or say "STOP!" if it feels too scary.

Try to discover the child's body sensations. Using colors for feelings in the body seems to work for almost every child. Asking children to associate feelings with colors and then using markers or crayons to identify feelings in their bodies works well and they enjoy this process. Having a drawing of a body and a list of colors/feelings on the same page facilitates this exercise. An example might be purple for happy with that color going in the heart or head area. Often red is the chosen color used to represent anger but black, sickly green and so on tend to be chosen as well. Hands, hearts, head and feet are often colored in red or black or the "angry" color. After the child has identified about seven to eight feelings, including jealousy, guilt, worry, sadness, then ask the child's favorite color. When a child feels comfortable with this process, the favorite color is used to push out the other colors and is anchored to the safe or peaceful place at the same time. This experience is intensely relaxing for the child who is open to this process. It's almost like a guided meditation, enhanced by bi-lateral stimulation and is essentially child created.

Because children re-experience the original pain during both play therapy and EMDR processing, acting out behaviors often ensue—the getting worse before getting better part of the working stages of play therapy. It is of vital importance that children are not punished for acting out during this difficult stage of therapy. Alerting parents to this distinct and almost predictable event, as well as teaching a simple and effective but nurturing system of discipline to the adults in the child's life before starting therapy, is essential to ensure the safety of the whole process.

So much processing also takes place between sessions. Many parents and caretakers feel so sorry or so guilty for the child that they neglect to include the safety and love that correct, nurturing discipline provides. Encouraging parents to use a simple, effective form of discipline not only helps organize the household but provides an ever larger container for the entire process. There are many effective discipline models for parents to choose from. *All* children are entitled to all feelings but all behaviors are not okay and this is the time to teach that difference. When the time comes and therapeutic growth is happening and the child feels safer, calmer, and the initial storm resulting from processing trauma begins to recede, EMDR is used to install the positive growth experience as well as positive beliefs about the self. This is what all the work has been for—a more empowered child restored to facing the more typical developmental challenges of growing up.

The final stage of experiential play therapy, the Termination Stage, is also vitally important to the process. Choosing the number of remaining sessions enables children to disengage from the supportive environment of therapy slowly. However the number of good-bye sessions is determined, it is important that children be informed of how many more times they will be coming to see you. This enables them to let go of the process, finish up unfinished business, and still feel protected. When EMDR is woven into the therapy, this is the time to use eye movements and bi-lateral stimulation for processing "friends saying good-bye." It is so important, this cannot be emphasized enough. In a perfect world, all children would have the time to safely say good-bye. Because the world is not perfect, it is generally wise to let children know verbally that you won't always be together after a period of growth. This gives children a time to prepare for an ending as well as allowing an update to their safe or peaceful place which may have changed by the last stage of therapy.

The following is a condensed version of a post-traumatized child's journey in therapy using both play and EMDR processing.

## Case Example

Sadie was 6½ years old when I met her. Sadie's father had hanged himself while in prison for drug trafficking. When Sadie's mother received a phone call with this news she cried out loud: "Oh my God! Denis hung himself!" and basically freaked-out. Both Sadie and her brother overheard her mother and witnessed their mother's hysterical reaction to this tragic news. There was no going back to protect the children from the harsh reality of this situation and tell them of their father's death more gently. Essentially a single-incident trauma, there was naturally *some* previous trauma or upset from living in a home involved with drug trafficking and all the chaos that lifestyle brings with it.

Sadie presented as an extremely intelligent, self-controlled (mostly), and resilient child. Silent and withdrawn when feeling angry, Sadie appeared to experience confusion and mild dissociation after feeling powerful emotions. Sadie's reaction to hearing the news of her father's sudden death by his own hand was one of denial and emotional numbing. She entered a terrifying labyrinth of emotional turmoil to traverse and find her way out of darkness. It was very helpful that Sadie's mother recognized her daughter's need for therapy right away and did not wait months or even years to start her process.

In Sadie's case, as determined in the initial parent intake session, there was no disclosure of pre-trauma events in the chaotic household. Her mother was unaware of Sadie's "scary dad" memories, which came up later during therapy, but she understood the actual trauma of the death of her father, further complicated by suicide, and had some understanding of the natural grieving process that would follow. Sadie's mom knew enough to accept that it would be difficult, if not impossible, for Sadie to process all of these feelings on her own. Of course, her mother and her older brother were in the throes of their own grieving process. Her mother did not feel equipped to help Sadie without support. Sadie experienced some unusual symptoms including forgetting the alphabet which she had completely mastered, sleep-walking, refusing to speak when angry and experiencing difficulty with the rules at school and possibly, hallucinations and dissociative episodes.

Sadie needed a strong feeling of acceptance, safety, and security to be established before any other form of treatment might be utilized, so the first three sessions consisted of non-directed play therapy. Sadie's response to the playroom was so positive that it made working with her easier, and her feelings of safety with women emerged.

In her first session, after using the miniature shovel and red wagon to let me know that her feelings were closed off or held in tight control, she started to recite her ABCs. After reciting the first three or four letters of the alphabet, she would start over. Most of her first session consisted mainly of this repetitive behavior of re-reciting the alphabet. Sadie also spent her time trying to arrange magnetic letters of the alphabet on a board in order.

When Sadie came to her second session, it was as if she didn't remember being there the first time in the beginning. I just let her be, and little by little she re-oriented herself and appeared present. Sadie repeated her alphabet recital and arranging letters in her second session in an almost compulsive fashion. Then in her third session, Sadie reported that "a man with no head" came into her bedroom at night and stood at the side of her bed, scaring her terribly. She started to report that a "fake, invisible man" was in the playroom with us; in her play she used the word *pretend* often. It was important to Sadie that I agreed that her play themes were "fake." Sadie was simply not ready to accept the loss of her father.

One of her coping methods was to play that she was a 2-year-old again when her father was still alive. In this role-play, Sadie took the role of "Mommy" and I was assigned the role of "kid." As the Mommy she would prepare dinner for aunts, brother, father, grandmother and grandfather, say grace, and we would eat. At the end of the third session, she froze and declared that the "invisible man" was looking at her. The "fake, invisible man" seemed to be literally haunting this child both inside the playroom and at home at night.

At this point, when there were 15 minutes left in Sadie's third play session, I asked her if she wanted to make a safe and peaceful place for her to feel better in. Sadie hesitated so I asked if she wanted her mother to come into the room. (Sadie had chosen to come in alone each time.) Her mother came in, and I had Sadie sit in her mother's lap. I explained that her safe and peaceful place could be real or pretend or both and that the main thing was that *nothing* scary or bad could happen to her in her safe and peaceful place. I told her that she could be alone or pretend other people were there, and we detailed the sensory data, including as much of the sights, smells, sounds, and so on she could come up with.

Sadie chose her mother's bed, snuggled under the covers with her mother, older brother, and their purring cat. After gathering as much detail as she could provide and learning that her favorite color was pink, we tried hand-taps (upturned palms), which Sadie felt comfortable with. As I tapped her hands, I recited back to her the details of her safe and peaceful place while sending a sparkling pink light through her entire body and filling her with a feeling of calm. After just a minute or two of this processing, Sadie visibly relaxed into her mother's arms. Sadie's positive response to installing her safe and peaceful place was the measure of the strength of the EMDR processing for her.

At home, her mother would take out the family albums about once a week and sit with the children and talk about memories. Per her mother's report, Sadie would sit in silent withdrawal. Her mother was afraid that Sadie would hurt herself sleepwalking and moved her into her mother's own bed.

In Sadie's fourth session, it took less time for her to get through reciting the alphabet, and in the middle of the role-play she stopped and asked, "Can we play that other game?" After a minute of installing her safe and peaceful place, I asked her what happy memory she had of her father. Her memory was eating dinner at the table with her family, including her grandparents, brother and aunts so I tapped her hands for less than a minute and she smiled. Instinctively, as if lead by a mysterious force, Sadie crawled over to a small feeling faces chart and brought it over. Sadie pointed to the happy face and said, "I feel happy, but sometimes I feel like this." She pointed to the mad face, then the sad face, and finally the scared face. I asked her what face she wanted to think about today. (Sadie just taught me a new way to select targets!) Sadie pointed to the scared face.

Seeing that Sadie was frightened we called her mother into the room again and had Sadie sit on her lap. I asked her if she could think of the scared face and tell her mother the scary parts. After a few seconds, Sadie yelled, "Stop!" We stopped and she buried her head in her mother's chest. I suggested we go back to the happy place. Sadie snuggled for a few minutes and then we just hand-tapped her happy/safe place. These sets of hand-taps were short, less than minute.

It didn't appear that much was happening with Sadie's therapy but her mother reported a reduction in her angry silences and, in fact, Sadie started to act out her anger. This broke the frozen rage inside of her and released a lot of pent-up energy. Sadie felt like she couldn't do anything "right." This came out in her play as well as other issues with authority. Over the next several sessions, Sadie did not want to play the game. She continued to practice the alphabet, then her numbers, and she continued in the role-play where the toddler had an alive father who now was "out in the yard."

In her tenth session, Sadie took out the feeling faces chart again. She pointed to the mad face and held out her hands. I tapped her hands for about 10 seconds and she said, "I'm mad about my Dad." This was the first verbalization Sadie had ever made about her father. Then she pointed to the sad face and said, "He makes me sad too." I reminded her that she could say "Stop!" at any time, and she agreed to the hand-taps. Before 15 seconds had passed, the first tears streamed down Sadie's face. She fell into a heap on the floor and cried as I just sat next to her patting her back and told her very quietly how brave she was and how important it was for her to let her mad and sad feelings out. Later, her mother told me she slept all the way home and slept until the next morning, undisturbed by sleep walking or the "invisible, fake headless man."

Sadie attended five more sessions. In those sessions, her play took on similar themes of coming to terms with the loss of her father and being 6½ and no longer a toddler. Sadie stopped reciting the alphabet but did write it out on a white board in her 14th session in perfect order backwards Z and all. Sadie said about her father, "He is my guardian angel now." Sadie was able to verbalize that she missed him. After that breakthrough tenth session, EMDR was used only to fill her body with pink, sparkling light or to revisit her safe and peaceful place.

After checking in with her mother recently to see how Sadie was progressing in her life, her mother reported that she was now able to look at the family albums and be okay, ask questions, and share some of her feelings. The "headless, invisible man" no longer appeared in her room, and Sadie was able to sleep in her own bed again. Sadie's mother also mentioned that the safe and peaceful place was the way that Sadie learned to go back to sleep when she woke up or had trouble falling asleep.

Sadie's story, one of so many stories of trauma, demonstrates the power and speed with which young children can recover and begin to heal from a tragic and sudden traumatic event. Although her grief will be life-long, Sadie became able to ground herself back in reality and move on with her development more naturally and easily and stop being haunted by the memories of her father.

## Bibliography

Gil, E. (1991). *The healing power of play: Working with abused children*. New York, NY: Guilford Press.

Kotulak, R. (1996). *Inside the brain: Revolutionary discoveries of how the mind works*. Kansas City, KS: Andrews McMeel.

Norton C. C. & Norton, B.E., (1997) *Reaching children through play therapy: An experiential approach*. Denver, CO: The Publishing Cooperative.

Shapiro, F. (1995). *Eye movement desensitization and reprocessing: Basic Principles Protocols and Procedures*. New York, NY: Guilford Press.

Shapiro, F. & Forrest, M. S. (1997). *EMDR: The breakthrough therapy for overcoming anxiety, stress and trauma*. New York, NY: Basic Books.

The *Ever-Changing Brain* (training workshop presented by John Preston, Psy.D., ABPP, Alliant International University, Sacramento, CA. Sponsored by The Institute for Brain Potential, March 2010.

The Thera-Tapper, DMS Institute, LLC, 6421 Mondean Street, San Antonio, TX 78240; www.theratapper.com. A simple instrument used for tactile stimulation and bilateral processing for EMDR and other therapies; used to facilitate the process for children and to provide another alternative to actual processing with eye-movements.

# Utilizing Bibliotherapy Within Play Therapy for Children With Anxieties and Fears

<table>
<tr><td>12</td></tr>
<tr><td>Chapter</td></tr>
</table>

## *Dale-Elizabeth Pehrsson*

## Introduction

Libby stepped lightly and slowly as she skirted the parameter of the playroom. Tentatively her fingers traced the base of the shelves, her fingertips barely touching a toy here and there. She said nothing, but when she completed her circle of the room, her eyes locked onto the bookshelf in the corner. She stood frozen. "Looks like you are wondering if those books are for using," Dr. Nellie calmly stated. Libby's eyes grew wide as she focused on one book, titled *No, David!* (Shannon, 1998). Dr. Nellie continued, "In this room you can play with many things in a lot of different ways." Libby reached out for the book but dropped her hand slowly. "In here, touching books is okay; that is something you can decide to do." Libby no longer hesitated. She grabbed the book. She plopped down on the beanbag in the corner and turned open the first page. She exclaimed, "No, David! No, Jasmine! No, Libby!" Libby's story had begun, and Dr. Nellie listened with her whole essence.

This chapter is an introduction for play therapists who wish to include book work in their practices. This chapter offers general guidelines for competent use of bibliotherapy within play therapy. Particular applications for work with children with fears, worries, and anxieties are offered.

Every child at play tells a story; children are born storytellers. Telling stories is what they do. Play therapists listen; we are lucky participants. We get to witness children's stories as they unfold hour by hour, week after week. Each session overflows with mini-tales evolving into a larger story that tells of events, experiences, and feelings in a child's life. Children sometimes express their stories verbally, but more often they do so by their interactions with objects and most specifically with their chosen toys. Children use their stories in play as metaphors that represent their knowledge, ideas, concerns, fears, and an array of mixed feelings. A wise and well-prepared play therapist reads such stories, recognizes their messages, and works to fulfill the needs told by each tale. The simple telling of a story has therapeutic value. Working through and moving the storyline forward provides therapeutic growth.

Libby knew immediately that the book *No, David!* (Shannon, 1998) told a story very much like her own and added clarity to her life situation. It represented her anxieties and her struggles. Libby was an anxious child, and she was much afraid to take risks. This book also helped her generate solutions and offered opportunities for change. Stories often provide such opportunities. Some are only somewhat related to a child's situation. However, Libby found a direct connection in this story, *No, David!* Among all the objects in the room, Libby chose this book. Children, even the very youngest ones, seem to know exactly what tool, toy, or book will fit their needs. Sometimes, a play therapist makes the choice by deliberately inserting a story into the process of therapy. In such cases the therapist provides more direction and structure. However, the selection of a story, the right story, requires very careful judgment. The play therapist attempts to match the story with the child's situation. This involves knowing both.

Hynes and Hynes-Berry define *bibliotherapy* as the use of "literature to bring about a therapeutic interaction between a participant and facilitator" (Hynes & Hynes-Berry, 1994, p. 10). For most of us, *bibliotherapy* means to engage with clients using books to bring about psychological healing. Although *bibliotherapy* is the most recognizable term for using books in this way, several other names are also used. A partial list includes biblio guidance, reading therapy, literatherapy, bibliocounseling, bibliopsychology, bookmatching, and library therapeutics (Pehrsson & McMillen, 2005).

Many of us play therapists employ the use of stories and books as part of our practices (Gardner, 1992; Pardeck & Pardeck, 1993; Pehrsson & McMillen, 2010). It serves us well, especially those who practice brief or solution-focused, cognitive-behavioral, and Adlerian therapies (Ackerson, Scogin, McKendree-Smith, & Lyman, 1998; Barrett, Duffy, Dadds, & Rapee, 2001). Several strategies are utilized by play therapists, but generally interventions include reading to or with a child. However, occasionally the child reads or relates a story using a book. Interventions tend to fall into three major categories: (1) counselor-initiated (those techniques chosen and facilitated by the therapist), (2) interactive (those processes that are used conjointly by therapist and child), and (3) client-initiated (processes that use books but are child driven) (Pehrsson, 2007; Pehrsson & McMillen, 2006).

## Bibliotherapy and Children With Anxiety Concerns

Children with anxieties and worries are often brought into therapy by over-anxious caretakers who fear for their children's well-being. The symptoms can be perplexing and frightening. These may include fear, nightmares or terrors, obsessive thoughts and behaviors, high-risk or self-harming behaviors, withdrawal from social situations, insomnia, or hypersomnia to name a few. These can develop if untreated into severe symptoms that over time can be debilitating. For all of us, we experience anxiety every day; it is a normal warning sign that something is not quite right. But normal levels of anxiety can become pathological. When this occurs, physical symptoms like headaches, nausea, and palpitations can develop. For children, these symptoms are terrifying and, coupled with other emotions such as guilt, can become overwhelming.

Anxiety affects our thinking patterns and problem-solving ability. It skews our interactions with others and our daily world, and it is exhausting. This can lead to more physical problems, such as gastrointestinal pain and respiratory distress. Some of the disorders children suffer from include generalized anxiety disorders, panic disorders, obsessive-compulsive disorders, post-traumatic stress disorders, acute stress disorders, social phobias, specific phobias (such as school or animals), adjustment disorders with anxiety, and anxiety disorders caused by a general medical condition (like a child dealing with diabetes). Anxiety and stress play no favorites; they are equal-opportunity disorders, impacting all across the life span (Rapoport & Ismond, 1996). Children are not immune. Short-term interventions that include a cognitive or structured intervention seem to have positive effects on children (Barrett et al., 2001), and that is where bibliotherapy can be of great assistance.

## Bibliotherapy Origins and Theoretical Premises

Bibliotherapy is not new. The application of literature and books for therapeutic value has a rich history that can be traced to the ancient Greeks. Aristotle proposed the notion of emotional catharsis through literature (Pehrsson & McMillen, 2005). Throughout the ages, elders and parents have employed literature to guide their children's decision making and to strengthen their character development and moral reasoning. Samuel Crothers, in an early issue of *Atlantic Monthly*, suggested using books in hospitals to help patients with insight, self-understanding, and to help solve problems. He coined the term *bibliotherapy* (Crothers, 1916, p. 291).

In her hallmark dissertation, Carolyn Shrodes (1950) developed the seminal theoretical model from which numerous bibliotherapy models and applications have emerged. Shrodes postulated that the effectiveness of bibliotherapy lies with our clients' abilities to identify with storylines or with protagonists and other characters. Through this identification, clients realize that others have similar problems; they align with the characters, their plight, and their solutions. Thus, the sense of aloneness or isolation decreases. Along with a character, the client is emotionally engaged in the struggle and works through a problem. Ultimately, clients achieve insight about their own situations (Shrodes, 1955, p. 24). For children, who naturally learn about life and consequences, not only through action (play) but also through stories, this process provides learning and empowerment (Pehrsson & Pehrsson, 2007). According to Shrodes (1950), bibliotherapy includes the three-step process of identification, catharsis, and insight.

Play therapists assist children in identifying and relating to characters and storylines as they pertain to their situations. The play therapist facilitates the clients' growth by assisting in verbally expressing emotions, cognitions, and concerns. This process is made possible within the safety of the play therapy relationship and within the playroom setting. The articulation (whether verbal, through play, or both) of emotions, cognitions, and concerns enables the play therapist to guide the client toward insight. A story can be a valuable tool that leads to a beneficial dialogue regarding thoughts, feelings, and emotions. The therapist and client can discuss the issues and characters in the story. For example, focusing on a character's problems can be a safe initiation into a discussion about the client's concerns that may otherwise be difficult for the client to express. A story is a helpful way to begin a discussion about the client's current concerns and issues (Gardner, 1992; Hynes & Hynes-Berry, 1994).

## Bibliotherapy and Play Therapy

While Dr. Bertocchi awaited her next client, she busily wrote her case notes. Although her computer was directly in front of her, she penned in a journal, a book of notes that would not be easily changed. She clicked her pen shut, backed away from her desk, sipped some herbal tea, and sighed in quiet silence. The quiet moment abruptly ceased. *Thump! Thump! Thump!* The thumping on her door grew louder. Dr. Bertocchi smiled, rose from her chair, and opened the door. There stood a breathless Cassie, who exclaimed her usual greeting, "Dr. B., I'm ready for action!" This was followed by her smiling face proclaiming, "I brought you my favorite book, *Go Away, Big Green Monster!* (Emberley, 1993) and I am going to read it to you right now!" Cassie marched into the playroom, claimed the beanbag as her throne, and opened the book to the first page. She held the book above her head and grinned. Cassie had taken charge. Dr. Bertocchi had rules, or at least a routine, for how play sessions started. However, Cassie's excitement could not be ignored. Her way of starting this session was to be honored. Dr. Bertocchi's usual comments would not apply at the beginning of this session. Dr. Bertocchi's own words emerged in her mind, "Cassie, you know just what to do." Instead, she said, "Hello, Cassie, it looks like you've decided we need to begin our session with a story."

When I set up my first playroom, I considered adding books, but I was initially trained in play therapy using Virginia Axline's (1947) model and, therefore, books were excluded. It was not until little Cassie burst into the playroom so enthusiastically with her book in tow that I began to ponder if this form of book therapy could fit within play therapy.

Kottman (2002) applied individual psychology to clinical work with children and supported the use of books within Adlerian play therapy. This form of therapy focuses on the four stages: (1) establishing a therapeutic relationship, (2) exploring client and family lifestyle, (3) promoting insight, and (4) re-educating and re-orientating (Jackson, 2001). Book use works well within all four of these stages of Adlerian play therapy. Counselors who draw from brief and solution-focused theories, as well as cognitive-behavioral models, in their practices also rely on books regularly (Pehrsson & McMillen, 2010).

Currently, bibliotherapy experts divide this form of therapy into two primary practice categories: developmental (educational) and clinical (therapeutic) (Rubin, 1978). Developmental bibliotherapy deals with normal life transitions and stages and is usually practiced by educators and non–mental health individuals. Clinical bibliotherapy involves a treatment plan, a deliberate and planned intervention, employing literature or books within a psychiatric or mental health paradigm with specific outcomes and goals in mind (Hynes & Hynes-Berry, 1994). Most mental health therapists who use bibliotherapy draw from both categories.

Some play therapists might suggest that the use of books is not congruent with the principles and practices of play therapy (e.g., client-centered play therapy; Landreth, 2002). For those who practice Axlinian play therapy, this might be true. However, for those who utilize other theoretical constructs, bibliotherapy enhances the treatment process (Kottman, 2002). In addition to the benefits suggested by Shrodes, bibliotherapy has a host of advantages (Pehrsson & McMillen, 2005), and in some interventions it is appropriate when combined with play therapy. Therapeutic use of books can enhance a child's self-awareness, promote clarification of values, and assist in the development of empathic understanding. Books promote self-discovery and self-awareness and therefore can help children learn about themselves. For children, both imaginative and nonfiction stories increases understanding of other cultures, people, places, and times and encourages flexibility and tolerance of difference. The child's own ethnic and cultural identity can be appreciated at a deeper level (Pardeck & Pardeck, 1998a; Tway, 1989).

Children learn to cope with painful and challenging situations and therefore build up their own coping skills with realistic and constructive responses to challenges. Communication skills, emotional maturity, and self-efficacy can be strengthened. Children who tend to be more isolated, perhaps even withdrawn, can learn to connect more readily with others as they realize that others share similar feelings and have experienced similar events. A child can learn about the values of friendships and social skills can develop; for a lonely child, relationships become possible. Youngsters become motivated to behave in innovative and healthier ways. By reading to a child, a trustful and warm bond is established that helps even the most resistant child feel comforted. Bibliotherapy offers a respite, because it can provide a temporary escape from life's worries. Literature puts forward advice and recommendations for problem solving and decision making. Books provide a safety net that helps children communicate a bit more openly. Books provide a buffer for emotional intensity, a buffer that children often require (Pehrsson & Pehrsson, 2007).

Research indicates that bibliotherapy as an intervention has been utilized by many professional groups (Marrs, 1995). These include but are not limited to school counselors (Gladding & Gladding, 1991), nurses (Farkas & Yorker, 1993), social workers (Pardeck & Pardeck, 1998a), psychologists, physicians, psychiatrists, mental health counselors, marriage and family therapists, addictions specialists, educators (Kramer & Smith, 1998), and librarians (Bernstein & Rudman, 1989; Pehrsson & McMillen, 2007).

## Bibliotherapy Applications

Bibliotherapy has applications across the life span and can address many concerns. It has been used for many specific disorders and mental health problems that present within the context of therapy with children, some of which include aggressiveness (Shechtman, 1999, 2000), adoption/foster care (Pardeck, 1993; Sharkey, 1998), diversity awareness, cultural valuation and ethnic identity (Holman, 1996; Pardeck & Pardeck, 1998a; Tway, 1989), death and dying (Meyer, 1994; Todahl, Smith, Barnes, & Pereira, 1998), chemical dependency (Pardeck, 1991), divorce and family dissolution (Early, 1993; Kramer & Smith, 1998; Meyer, 1991; Pehrsson, Allen, Folger, McMillen, & Lowe, 2007), obsessive-compulsive disorders (Fritzler, Hecker, & Losee, 1997), giftedness (Hebert, 1995), conflict resolution (Hodges, 1995), child abuse and parental neglect (Jasmine-DeVias, 1995; Pardeck, 1990), night fears and night-mares (Barclay & Whittington, 1992), depression (Ackerson et al., 1998), separation & loss (Bernstein & Rudman, 1989), family violence (Butterworth & Fulmer, 1991), homelessness (Farkas & Yorker, 1993), and self-destructive behavior (Evans et al., 1999). It has particular utility with children who deal with worries, anxieties, and fears (Pehrsson, 2007).

### General Guidelines

Competent therapists follow general guidelines and cautions when including books in their play therapy work with children. They always consider client growth. They ask this simple question before they use a book: "What will this book do for the therapeutic movement of my client?" Therapists must know their clients and postulate what particular books might do for them. Assessment is critical. Shrodes argues that clients react differently, and no one size fits all in the clinical world. She states, "[for] no two persons can there be an absolute equivalence of symbols, for no two people have identical psychological fields" (1950, p. 85). Zaccaria and Moses (1968) argued that bibliotherapy is not a cure-all and that it may not work for all individuals. Bibliotherapy might not be helpful with children who have attention difficulties, learning disabilities, or visual impairment, and for those who have experienced academic trauma or acquired reading phobias. Although bibliotherapy may not work for everyone, for various reasons, nevertheless books are often very appropriate interventions for many children.

As a matter of practice, play therapists should be well acquainted with the content of materials they intend to recommend or use with children, just as good play therapists know they must play with their new toys before they put toys in the playroom. Likewise with books, play therapists need to read books first for content and to assess reactions; this prevents surprises from surfacing during the session. Play therapists know their clients, and thus they anticipate client readiness for specific materials.

## Book Selection

Good books for therapy are a lot like good books in general. They engage, they excite, and we relate to them and to their characters. Play therapists look for several components as they examine books for therapeutic work, especially with children. This matters because such developmental variation exists in our client populations. Younger children have needs that differ from those who are past the concrete operational stage. Tweens (9- to 12-year-olds) are a whole specialty themselves. But there are some guidelines that therapists must consider.

First, the cultural, ethnic, and religious messages in material must be inclusive, accurate, and respectful. The early 1990s exploded with diversity-laden titles and materials, but some books were actually inaccurate and stereotypical. When searching for materials, check the author's bio and see if material was written by someone with expertise and cultural awareness of a given topic or population. When in doubt, ask a librarian. Librarians are a major resource for play therapists and are very underutilized by clinicians.

Second, factual material needs to be correct and current, as when dealing with a topic that pertains to health or history. For example, a child who is learning about living with diabetes should read material that is current, medically relevant, and not frightening. Stories dealing with addictions, grief, and death and so forth should be clearly presented and have timely information and suggested resources. Stories about history should be told in a manner that is true yet engaging, with compelling characters with whom children can relate.

In bibliotherapy, characters matter because children identify so closely with them. Therefore, therapists choose stories with characters and situations similar enough to facilitate some level of identification. Some stories can increase empathic understanding for those from different backgrounds and yet provide needed distance from painful emotions. Stories should include characters who provide constructive solutions and instill hope. Otherwise, they are antithetical to bibliotherapy mandates.

## Bibliotherapy Cautions

Bibliotherapy is not about reading or teaching reading. It is about the use of literature to create therapeutic growth. Therapists must not confuse this. If reading the story becomes like a school lesson, then the process is altered, and for many youngsters intended benefits can be lost. Some children have experienced much trauma within educational settings, and this could prompt responses that get in the way of building a therapeutic alliance and impede growth (Pehrsson & Pehrsson, 2007). Not all children like to read or be read to, thus making bibliotherapy an inappropriate intervention for these children. Play therapists need to be skilled in evaluation, including clinical and developmental readiness of children. They will need to assess if this intervention is the right fit for their child client.

Furthermore, within the context of private practice, it may be necessary to share materials with parents or primary caregivers. This may require that they understand the purpose for using books and even give their permission for specific books. This ordinarily can be included in the informed consent process. For those counselors who work within agencies, obtaining administrative support and authorization is a must. Finally, for those who work within school contexts, the surest way to gain approval is to use materials that have already been approved for use in the school library. This may not avoid all political problems but does provide a strategy for choice that may be the least controversial (Pehrsson & Pehrsson, 2007).

## Bibliotherapy Interventions

Bibliotherapy offers many creative choices and is limited only by the therapist's imagination and skill (Hynes & Hynes-Berry, 1994). The suggestions discussed next have been useful in play therapy practice with children ages 3 through 13, but especially for children dealing with issues of anxiety or fear (Pardeck & Pardeck, 1993, 1998b). Bibliotherapy can provide a structure that is either prescribed and formal or flexible. The framework provided by a story is useful, in that it generally has a beginning, a middle, and an end. Such stories offer predictability that is often comforting. The traditional structure of a story can help mollify children's feelings of uncertainty and fear. Poems offer creativity, catharsis, and playfulness but nevertheless provide order (Robbins & Pehrsson, 2009). Informational books and historical biographies offer data and real-world knowledge that can help youngsters deal with specific issues (like a chronic illness or a hero's challenges). Creating stories offers direct character development and empowerment. Children can test out strategies and become brave, which is a major benefit for fearful children (Pehrsson & Pehrsson, 2006). Whether reading literature or creating stories, there are benefits that overlap, and the advantages are multifaceted (Pehrsson, 2007).

Among the many interventions available within the clinical play therapy session, play therapists often select a book and read to children or read with them during a session. But it is the processing of the information and the facilitation of discussion of the material, the story, or the characters that helps clients learn more about themselves and their life circumstances. Processing material can occur through discussion, but for children it is usually discussion accompanied by playing, drama, sandwork, or art that is the most beneficial and that creates therapeutic movement and healing. When therapists work with teens (13- to 18-year-olds) and tweens (9- to 12-year-olds), recommending a book for client reading can prove beneficial. However, for younger clients (3- to 8-year-olds), reading to them or with them during the session, in my experience, yields the most gain (Pehrsson et al., 2007).

Therapist-initiated bibliotherapy techniques are therapist driven; they are developed and facilitated by the therapist. If we know our books and we know our clients, then our judgment about what might provide client connection and therapeutic growth should not be ignored. A therapist can select materials that fit the child's stage of therapy. The activity can be introduced in several ways. The following story illustrates this technique.

Dr. Stevie looked at Joshua, and softly said, "Josh, we have been working together a long time now. I think you are ready for a story about death and losing someone you love. I think this story is a lot like your own story. I'd like to read it to you today. We can stop any time you say so." Josh's eyes grew wide, he swallowed hard, and he sighed and said, "Okay." He paused and asked, "Can I pick my reading spot today?" "Yes," replied Dr. Stevie. "That is something you get to decide." Josh went over to the red beanbags and said, "We'll read it over here!" Dr. Stevie walked over to the bookshelf, reached for the book, *Goodbye, Rune*, and gently settled onto the chair next to Joshua. She read the title and opened the first page.

Joshua was referred to counseling because of nightmares and severe symptoms of anxiety that developed six months after his brother's death from drowning. The book, *Goodbye Rune* (Kaldhol, 1987), provided the mechanism to introduce a more direct discussion about his own feelings. This was at a stage when deep trust between Joshua and the therapist had developed. After reading the story to Josh, the therapist asked Josh if he wanted to talk about the story or draw a picture. Josh chose to draw, and then the therapist discussed the picture and related it to the story and to Josh's life; the picture provided an additional container, a safe one for discussing Josh's concerns. The goals of assisting the client in gaining insight were met through this process.

Use of therapist-initiated activity requires that the play therapist be knowledgeable about a wide variety of materials, books, and literature, and it also requires an understanding of the client's ability to grow therapeutically from their use. Reading a story to children clients also gives the play therapist many chances to model the courage to be imperfect. When I read, I make lots of miscues.

Interactive bibliotherapeutic techniques engage children and produce the energy and positive results. These processes are used conjointly by therapist and child during the session as the two interact. Often the therapist chooses the material but invites the child to participate in the reading or the storytelling. In the case illustrated as follows, the child was engaged completely, the resulting catharsis intense and the insight most meaningful.

Gigi pushed the small green action figure deep into the sand and poured a handful of sand on top of it. The sand sifted off, leaving the figure still visible. Gigi grabbed another handful and poured more sand on top. Three more handfuls of sand failed to completely bury the action figure. Gigi sighed deeply, sat back on her heels, and shook her head. Then she glanced at the bookshelf. Her eyes locked, and without hesitation she reached for the book. Gigi stated, "I want you to read this, Dr. Jonna." Dr. Jonna looked at the cover; a big green monster stared back at her. Dr. Jonna said, "Okay, sounds like you made a decision about what you want." Dr. Jonna sat down on the beanbag next to Gigi and read the title, *Go Away, Big Green Monster!* She slowly turned to the first page.

It was a cooperative effort. Dr. Jonna read, and Gigi eagerly turned each page. When they got to the end, Gigi exclaimed "Again!" "You've decided we need to read this book one more time. Sounds like a plan." Dr. Jonna started to read. This time Gigi echoed all the words as they read together. Gigi read in a low voice except for one repetitious phrase. "Go away, big green monster!" she yelled in her loud voice, which seemed to surprise her. Each time these words appeared, Gigi's voice grew stronger, as if she were demonstrating her power. At the end of the second reading, Gigi exclaimed, "This time I get to read!" Dr. Jonna handed the book to Gigi, who prompted, "Now you have to follow me!" Dr. Jonna smiled and replied, "You are in charge and you want me to follow your lead. You can let me know what to do." Gigi exclaimed, "That's right! I am in charge."

This time Gigi stood, held the book open, and read with the serious purpose of exhibiting her newfound sense of power. Her voice grew stronger each time she demanded the monster to go away. When Gigi opened to the last page, she shouted her last command, "And don't come back until I say so!" Gigi smiled broadly, placed the book back on the shelf, and marched directly to the sandbox. She reached up to the toy shelf and grabbed a puppet that she had previously named "the scary guy." She took the small action figure out of the sand and placed him on the floor. Then she threw "the scary guy" into the sandbox. Next Gigi reached for the lid and covered the sandbox. She placed two heavy blocks on the lid and then turned and sat on top of it. Gigi took a deep breath and said, "Now we are finally safe."

Gigi had been referred to Dr. Jonna's practice by the county court system. Because of accusations of alleged sexual abuse, the court had mandated that visitations with her father were to be supervised. Although her physical safety was an issue, Gigi's severe anxiety, night terrors, and hypervigilant behaviors were of primary concern to Dr. Jonna. Each week that followed, Gigi would start her session by reading this book. It became a touchstone of their sessions. However, each week Gigi read fewer and fewer pages as her confidence grew. It was soon time to terminate their sessions. At the end of their last session, Gigi asked, "Dr. Jonna, do you know what my favorite toy in the playroom is?" "Sounds like you'd like to tell me," answered Dr. Jonna. Gigi smiled and exclaimed, "Why it's the monster book, Dr. Jonna. You know that!"

Some bibliotherapeutic interventions are completely client initiated; these are book selections and processes that start with the client. When children bring in books or choose books during the session, these books matter, and wise play therapists pay attention. A child might say, "I want to read this book to you." Let them. As they read, do not correct reading miscues. This is not a time to correct language or mistakes; this is a time to listen to the child's interpretation of what is meaningful to them. I have been read to when the story being read had absolutely nothing to do with the written text, but the story gave me much information into the child's worldview. The therapeutic benefits were measurable in the change and growth that occurred. By providing freedom for children to read, to interpret, and to give the story their own meaning, we offer children choice, power, and control. These are critical components for children with anxieties and fears. Let me illustrate in the following case synopsis.

Zoë arrived to her appointment as per usual, right after school on Tuesday. She entered the office with her school backpack packed with her important stuff. She plopped onto the rocking chair and dropped her backpack onto the floor. "I brought a book for you to read. It is important that you read it by next week, because this is a really great story. It is my favorite. You can borrow my copy, but you can't keep it." Dr. Johns smiled as Zoë searched her backpack, digging and looking through its content. "Here it is!" Zoë tenderly placed in Dr. Johns's hands a dirty, torn, ripped, and curled-paged well-loved copy of *Summer of the Monkeys* (Rawls, 1998).

Zoë had been referred for counseling for a severe anxiety disorder and for somatization of her anxiety-related symptoms. After extensive medical testing, it was determined that her gastrointestinal symptoms were stress induced. Within her family of origin, she was the oldest child and was primarily responsible for caring for her younger sibling, Tara, who had some ambulatory impairment resulting from multiple surgeries and interventions to deal with spina bifida. The family suffered from severe financial challenges because of ongoing medical bills. Zoë related to a key character in the book and through that connection was able to talk about how she cared for Tara and the stress that comes from being responsible while also worrying about money, siblings, schoolwork, and family matters. Zoë was able to come to terms with her own stress and anxieties and find acceptable alternatives to managing her worries. She developed a plan to destress and allow herself some alone time. Even though the family would continue to experience stress, Zoë was able to manage her own and plan for some time to replenish herself. This may seem like a lot for a 12-year-old to manage and learn. It was the story that helped her articulate her own issues and allowed her a chance to develop workable solutions. As a therapist, Dr. Johns was also able to assist the family in developing some coping strategies. Had Dr. Johns not invested in the homework reading assignment that Zoë gave, an opportunity would have been lost, and perhaps Zoe would never have gained insight and experienced re-education.

Play therapists can employ many strategies within the playroom; the choices are limited only by their imaginations and willingness to take creative risks. I recommend that play therapists pursue interventions that fit well with their theoretical underpinnings and their personal clinical style. That way, their work with child clients will be comfortable for them, thus the process and therapeutic gain will more likely be enhanced.

## Book Selection

When selecting books, several categories should be considered before putting a book on your bookshelf. Assess books for their general format and structure, subject matter, reading level and developmental suitability, book density and length, text and pictures, diversity factors, therapeutic use, context/situation, and overall impression. These categories are discussed as follows.

When considering the book's format and structure, the therapist looks at the reading material in a general manner. Books such as a narrative, historical fiction and biography employ different formats, and their language structures differ. However, these are generally structured in a story format. Content or expository books provide information, and some even offer helpful suggestions about solving problems. Books that relate a positive message are usually more effective than those that could be depressing. Attractiveness is important, especially for children and teens. Works of fiction should be assessed for factors such as plot cohesiveness, character development, universality of the story line, and general quality of the writing. Attempt to assess the general feel or the Gestalt of the book.

Examining the subject matter requires play therapists to identify major subjects and themes covered within the book. Books offer themes, and whether the book is fiction or nonfiction, there is usually a topic (or multiple topics) addressed within the material. Consider factors such as relevance of material, interest level, and writing style to determine general client–subject fit. The guiding question here should be "Is this book a good match for my client?" Knowing the client and what the client needs is critical to this process.

Play therapists do not have to be reading specialists to address appropriateness of reading level and suitability for their clients. Yet, it is important to evaluate material regarding reading level. If a child is to read the material, the play therapist would want to avoid creating frustration by asking the child to read material that is too difficult. Some materials identify reading or age level, but some do not. So it is often up to the helper to make a best guess as to the appropriateness. Play therapists are advised to consult with a teacher or librarian. However, therapists should consider how the material will be applied. If the clinician is reading to the client, the reading level matters less, but the vocabulary and other language structures, such as sentence lengths, should be considered.

With an approach called echo reading, the child reads along as the therapist takes the lead, which can be less intimidating to the child. Sometimes even the words may be ignored when turning the pages of a book. A discussion about the pictures may be very useful for both assessments and interventions.

The length of the book is related to the time of a session. Clinicians look at book format and length and decide how the text will be utilized. For older children, a book that may take more time may be read in portions such as chapters. Clinicians may plan to assign clients some reading at home, or they may assign parental or family reading. Sometimes a book is used in therapy as a one-time read with an activity to follow, so brevity matters. Individual client characteristics influence how long it will take to use a book and in what manner.

The text and pictures can influence the message and the mood of the book, and therefore the therapeutic process, so it is incumbent for play therapists to evaluate the print (text) and graphic illustrations. Therapists should check the congruence and mood created by the combination of print and pictures. Furthermore, examine if the artwork is age appropriate. For example, although abstract art may be visually attractive to the adult reader, the picture may not be of interest to the younger child. For children, the art within the book must make emotional sense and match the context and story of the book. Children rely heavily on visual cues. The art must be accurate, culturally representative, and ethnically respectful. Illustrations should be engaging and tell a story along with the written narrative. Printed text must be readable and not too crammed or crowded on the page. If a play therapist is facilitating group bibliotherapy, a picture with each turn of the page creates anticipation, and likewise each written page needs to be short enough not to lose children who have shorter attention spans. Examine the pictures for quantity and quality. Once an intervention strategy is identified, then assess whether the text will create a positive therapeutic effect for this particular client.

Play therapists need to consider the developmental level of their clients. Play therapists know firsthand the huge variations and range in child clients. Three-year-olds have particular needs and skills that differ from tweens and teens. Clinicians should consider clients from a holistic perspective, taking into account culture and ethnicity, language, age, diagnosis, presenting concerns, family dynamics, school difficulties, and academic standing. Therapeutic readiness and the stage of counseling are considered when analyzing types of books that will work best. Wise clinicians evaluate fit and match of the text, the characters, and the subject matter addressed to their child clients. They also assess the appropriateness of a text for populations who may be at multiple developmental levels.

Play therapists must be culturally responsive to be effective and ethical practitioners; therefore, they evaluate material from the vantage point of diversity, community, religion, race, ethnicity, and culture. They ensure that materials are presented in a respectful manner. That is to say that books are culturally appropriate, expand the worldview of children, and match the needs of clients. They check materials (especially dated books) to ensure that stereotyping does not exist. They examine books for relevancy and determine that it is current. One strategy is to check for the authenticity of authors and illustrators. This can be done with a fast search on the Internet to determine if the authors or illustrators have cultural knowledge of the group for which they are writing or drawing.

Always determine if using a particular book in a particular setting might have administrative or political impact. A general rule in the school setting is that if the school library has it, it is okay to have in the playroom. In a clinical or agency setting, parental or caretaker permission might be needed, especially when using a book that deals with sexual abuse or one that contains anatomical illustrations of human body parts.

The context, environment, and situation where books are used within play therapy matters. Play therapists assess the environment or clinical situation in which the material will be used. If a clinician does home visits, obviously book selection will be limited. In this case, the book choice is usually therapist initiated, and therefore selecting appropriate material is important. The setting in which play therapists practice often determines the book selection. Those who practice within health-care contexts may use more materials related to diseases and health diagnoses (such as cancer and diabetes). Mental health settings often deal with acute and long-term diagnoses such as bipolar disorder, anxiety, depression, and post-traumatic stress disorders, requiring a different range of books topics.

For those who practice within school settings, books may be included that help with academic success, problem solving, friendship and social skill development, and anxiety and phobias. School counselors and social workers who conduct play therapy have complex roles with the added pressure of time limits, typically 20- to 30-minute sessions. Private practitioners plan their playroom books based on their specialty and the client population that they serve. For example, a play therapist who deals with children of divorce would have books that focus on divorce and related topics, such as anxiety, anger, change, and hope (Pehrsson et al., 2007; McMillen & Pehrsson, 2010).

How the book will be put to therapeutic use is another consideration in bibliotherapy. Play therapists must plan for the way in which a text will be used during their play session. A book that is read to a child during a session that takes the whole session to read allows for nothing else but the reading. That is fine if the therapist is planning for that, but if the therapist wants to allow for reading, reaction, play, and art time, then it might be better to choose a book that takes 10 to 12 minutes to read. If the therapist is considering a treatment intervention such as choral reading (children reading in unison and reacting to the main reader, the therapist) for a group, then the book should allow time for preparation and presentation. Short poems and rhyming materials, such as Shel Silverstein's (1974) work, may be appropriate for group reading. Picture books with repetitious phrases also allow for choral or echo reading. One such book that was mentioned earlier is *Go Away, Big Green Monster!* (Emberley, 1993). Short and plucky responses to the scary monster can bolster a child's confidence and minimize anxiety related to those scary monsters that many children fear. Some books are best read alone, others by the therapist. However, the therapist should plan for the time needed to facilitate the best outcome. When planning to use books with games, art, play, puppets, or whatever, therapists should always have this question in the forefront of their minds: "What will this do for the therapeutic movement of my client?"

After prereading a book and assessing the clinical applications to a client, the play therapist will have a definite sense of its overall value. Give the book a ranking on a scale of 1 to 10, 10 being the best clinical value. Is this book worth the cost, and will it be used for multiple clients? Other practical questions might arise: Is this book such a perfect fit for little Sookie and for many other children that buying it is worth the cost? If it seems a perfect fit for Sookie but not necessarily for other children, it would be wise to consider borrowing it from the library.

## Bibliotherapy Playroom Construction

Building a good playroom first starts with the play therapist's theoretical framework. Because my primary approach draws from both Axlinian and Adlerian premises, that is how I constructed my playroom. All standard tools (toys) that promote catharsis, role-play, creativity, mastery and problem solving are placed for easy access and use within the therapy room. Additionally, tools that assist with re-education and re-orientation are carefully selected as well. Adlerian tools include books. How books are placed within the playroom matters. It is a mistake to place books on a shelf as one might at home or in a library. The books should be easily seen, and they should invite the child to touch, to take, and to open. I recommend that books be placed on narrow shelves with easy access to the child. Picture books are deliberately placed at lower levels. The pictures must be facing the child. The pictures, not the words in the title, are what the child will connect with at first, so it is critical that the pictures face out from the shelves. A therapist should select and display about 20 to 25 books based on the population and treatment issues. More than 25 books can overwhelm children. Create a reading or story corner within the playroom. Beanbag chairs create a comfortable place for children to snuggle up with a good book.

## Conclusion

Countless advantages for integrating bibliotherapy and play therapy exist. This chapter has touched on the most obvious and those supported by research (Pehrsson & McMillen, 2010). Play therapists will discover their own strategies over time and with practice. I see play and bibliotherapy as a perfect companion set. The emphasis in bibliotherapy is on reception, while the emphasis in play therapy is on expression, but certainly there are elements of both in the two modalities. Bibliotherapy is largely a receptive avenue for learning about problems and solutions, and identifying with the feelings of others. In play therapy, children can express their feelings in symbols, analogies, and metaphors and through actions work to solve their own problems. I have now observed many children telling their own stories and also retelling a story read to them. How best do children learn from and tell their stories? Through play—and sometimes books can help!

## References

Ackerson, J., Scogin, F., McKendree-Smith, N., & Lyman, R. D. (1998). Cognitive bibliotherapy for mild and moderate adolescent depressive symptomatology. *Journal of Consulting & Clinical Psychology*, 66(4), 685–690.

Axline, V. M. (1947). *Play therapy*. New York, NY: Ballantine Books.

Barclay, K. H., & Whittington, P. (1992). Night scares: A literature-based approach for helping young children. *Childhood-Education*, 68(3), 149–154.

Barrett, P. M., Duffy, A. L., Dadds, M. R., & Rapee, R. M. (2001). Cognitive-behavioral treatment of anxiety disorders in children: Long term (6-year) follow up. *Journal of Consulting and Clinical Psychology, 69*(1), 135–141.

Bernstein, J. E., & Rudman, M. K. (1989). *Books to help children cope with separation and loss: An annotated bibliography, Volume 3.* New York, NY: R. R. Bowker.

Butterworth, M. D., & Fulmer, K. A. (1991). The effect of family violence on children: Intervention strategies including bibliotherapy. *Australian Journal of Marriage & Family, 12* (3), 170–182.

Crothers, S. M. (1916). A literary clinic. *Atlantic Monthly, 118,* 291–301.

Early, B. P. (1993). The healing magic of myth: Allegorical tales and the treatment of children of divorce. *Child & Adolescent Social Work Journal, 10*(2), 97–106.

Emberley, E. (1993). *Go away, big green monster!* New York, NY: LB Kids.

Evans, K., Tyrer, P., Catalan, J., Schmidt, U., Davidson, K., Dent, J., . . . & Thompson, S. (1999). Manual-assisted cognitive-behaviour therapy (MACT): A randomized controlled trial of a brief intervention with bibliotherapy in the treatment of recurrent deliberate self-harm. *Psychological Medicine, 29*(1), 19–25.

Farkas, G. S., & Yorker, B. (1993). Case studies of bibliotherapy with homeless children. *Issues in Mental Health Nursing, 14*(4), 337–347.

Fritzler, B. K., Hecker, J. E., & Losee, M. C. (1997). Self-directed treatment with minimal therapist contact: Preliminary findings for obsessive-compulsive disorder. *Behaviour Research & Therapy, 35*(7), 627–631.

Gardner, R. A. (1992). *The psychotherapeutic techniques of Richard A. Gardner.* Cresskill, NJ: Creative Therapeutics.

Gladding, S. T., & Gladding, C. (1991). The ABCs of bibliotherapy for school counselors. *The School Counselor, 39*(Summer), 7–13.

Hebert, T. P. (1995). Using biography to counsel gifted young men. *Journal of Secondary Gifted Education, 6*(3), 208–219.

Hodges, J. (1995). *Conflict resolution for the young child.* (ERIC Document Reproduction Service ED 394624)

Holman, W. D. (1996). The power of poetry: Validating ethnic identity through a bibliotherapeutic intervention with a Puerto Rican adolescent. *Child & Adolescent Social Work Journal, 13*(5), 371–383.

Hynes, A. M., & Hynes-Berry, M. (1994). *Biblio/poetry therapy, the interactive process: A handbook.* St. Cloud, MN: North Star Press.

Jackson, S. A. (2001). Using bibliotherapy with clients. *The Journal of Individual Psychotherapy, 57*(4), 289–297.

Jasmine-DeVias, A. (1995). Bibliotherapy: Books that can play a role in helping children work through some of the effects of abuse and neglect. *New England Reading Association Journal, 31*(3), 2–17.

Kaldhol, M. (1987). *Goodbye Rune.* La Jolla, CA: Kane/Miller.

Kottman, T. (2002). *Partners in play: An Adlerian approach to play therapy* (2nd ed.). Alexandria, VA: American Counseling Association.

Kramer, P. A., & Smith, G. G. (1998). Easing the pain of divorce through children's literature. *Early Childhood Education Journal, 26*(2), 89–94.

Landreth, G. L. (2002). *Play therapy: The art of the relationship.* New York, NY: Brunner-Routledge.

Marrs, R. W. (1995). A meta-analysis of bibliotherapy studies. *American Journal of Community Psychology, 23*(6), 843–870.

McMillen, P., & Pehrsson, D.-E. (in press). Contemporary children's literature recommendations for working with preadolescent children of divorce. *Journal of Children's Literature.*

Meyer, M. J. (1991). Split decision: A bibliotherapy guide for children who are experiencing divorce. *Lutheran Education, 126,* 252–266.

Meyer, M. J. (1994). Mortal thoughts: A bibliotherapeutic guide to books for children about death and dying. *Lutheran Education, 129*(1), 211–223.

Pardeck, J. T. (1990). Bibliotherapy with abused children. *Families in Society, 71*(4), 229–235.

Pardeck, J. T. (1991). Using books to prevent and treat adolescent chemical dependency. *Adolescence, 26*(101), 201–208.

Pardeck, J. T. (1993). Literature and adoptive children with disabilities. *Early Child Development and Care, 91,* 33–39.

Pardeck, J. T., & Pardeck, J. A. (1993). *Bibliotherapy: A clinical approach for helping children,* Vol. 16. Langhorne, PA: Gordon and Breach Science.

Pardeck, J. T., & Pardeck, J. A. (1998a). An exploration of the uses of children's books as an approach for enhancing cultural diversity. *Early Child Development & Care, 147*, 25–31.

Pardeck, J. T., & Pardeck, J. A. (1998b). *Children in foster care and adoption: A guide to bibliotherapy.* Westport, CT: Greenwood Press.

Pehrsson, D.-E. (2007). Fictive bibliotherapy and therapeutic storytelling with children who hurt. *Journal of Creativity in Mental Health, 1*(3/4), 273–286.

Pehrsson, D.-E., Allen, V. B., Folger, W. A., McMillen, P. S., & Lowe, I. (2007). Bibliotherapy with preadolescents experiencing divorce. *The Family Journal, 15*(4), 409–414.

Pehrsson, D.-E., & McMillen, P. (2005). Bibliotherapy evaluation tool: Grounding counseling students in the therapeutic use of literature. *The Arts in Psychotherapy, 32*, 1.

Pehrsson, D.-E., & McMillen, P. (2006). Competent bibliotherapy: Preparing counselors to use literature with culturally diverse clients. *Vistas 2006.* Alexandria, VA: American Counseling Association.

Pehrsson, D.-E., & McMillen, P. (2007). Bibliotherapy: A review of the research and applications. *American Counseling Association Digest (Charter series).* Alexandria, VA: American Counseling Association.

Pehrsson, D.-E., & McMillen, P. S. (2010). A national survey of preparation and practices of bibliotherapy by professional counselors. *Journal of Creativity in Mental Health, 5*, 412–425.

Pehrsson, D.-E., & Pehrsson, R. S. (2006). Bibliotherapy practices with children: Cautions for school counselors. *The Journal of Poetry Therapy, December, 19*(4), 185–193.

Pehrsson, D.-E., & Pehrsson, R. S. (2007). Language fantasy approach: A therapeutic group intervention by creating myths with children. *The Journal of Poetry Therapy, January, 20*(1), 41–49.

Rapoport, J. L., & Ismond, D. R. (1996). *DSM-4 training guide for diagnosis of childhood disorders.* New York, NY: Brunner/Mazel.

Rawls, W. (1998). *Summer of the monkeys.* New York, NY: Bantam Books.

Robbins, J. M., & Pehrsson, D.-E. (2009). Anorexia nervosa: A synthesis of poetic and narrative therapies in the outpatient treatment of young adult women. *Journal of Creativity in Mental Health, 4*(1), 42–56.

Rubin, R. J. (1978). *Using bibliotherapy: A guide to theory and practice.* Phoenix, AZ: Oryx Press.

Shechtman, Z. (2000). An innovative intervention for treatment of child and adolescent aggression: An outcome study. *Psychology in the Schools, 37*(2), 157–167.

Shechtman, Z. (1999). Bibliotherapy: An indirect approach to treatment of childhood aggression. *Child Psychiatry & Human Development, 30*(1), 39–53.

Shannon, D. (1998). *No, David!* New York, NY: Blue Sky Press/Scholastic.

Sharkey, P. B. (1998). Being adopted: Books to help children understand—Update 3. *Emergency Librarian, 25*(4), 8–10.

Shrodes, C. (1950). *Bibliotherapy: A theoretical and clinical-experimental study* (Doctoral dissertation, University of California, Berkeley, 1950). *Dissertation Abstracts Online.*

Shrodes, C. (1955). Bibliotherapy. *The Reading Teacher, 9*, 24–30.

Silverstein, S. (1974). *Where the sidewalk ends.* New York, NY: Harper Collins.

Todahl, J., Smith, T. E., Barnes, M., & Pereira, M. G. A. (1998). Bibliotherapy and perceptions of death by young children. *Journal of Poetry Therapy, 12*(2), 95–107.

Tway, E. (1989). Dimensions of multicultural literature for children. In M. K. Rudman (Ed.), *Children's literature: Resource for the classroom* (pp. 109–132). Norwood, MA: Christopher-Gordon.

Zaccaria, J. S., & Moses, H. A. (1968). *Facilitating human development through reading: The use of bibliotherapy in teaching and counseling.* Champaign, IL: Stipes.

# Integrating Cognitive-Behavioral Play Therapy and Adlerian Play Therapy Into the Treatment of Perfectionism

## 13

### Chapter

## *Jeffrey S. Ashby and Christina Noble*

## Introduction

> *In a parental consultation describing the client, Emily's mother looked up and said, "Emily seems like the* perfect child *in lots of ways; clean room, good marks in school, usually comes when she's called . . . but she doesn't seem happy . . . and lately we've noticed some differences . . . like it's hard for her to relax and just enjoy things. She just doesn't seem happy at all."*

This description of "Emily" is consistent with the way that perfectionistic children are often described. Kottman and Ashby (2000) noted that "perfectionistic children and adolescents are easy to recognize" (p. 182) due to characteristic patterns of behavior. Perfectionistic children usually come to the attention of play therapists because they seem a little "too serious" about schoolwork or other tasks. For instance, they complain that their drawings are "not good enough" (resulting in numerous crumpled pieces of paper). At school they may give up prized recess or playtime with friends to finish an assignment or task that they feel must be done perfectly. Ashby, Kottman, and Martin (2004) noted that these children are "easily frustrated when things do not go just as they would like . . . or they may be hesitant to engage in activities that might result in a 'mess' of some sort (e.g., baking or finger-painting)" (p. 36).

Perfectionistic children are often brought to play therapy because they exhibit extremely self-critical behavior or evidence psychological symptoms as anxiety or depression (Flett, Hewitt, Oliver, & Macdonald, 2002). A growing body of empirical research has investigated the association between perfectionism and a number of psychological constructs and concerns in children and adolescents. For instance, the results of various studies suggest a relationship between childhood perfectionism and academic achievement and academic confidence (Nounopoulos, Ashby, & Gilman, 2006), academic motivation (Accordino, Slaney, & Accordino, 2000), life satisfaction and clinical maladjustment (Gilman & Ashby, 2006), depression and suicide (Hewitt, Newton, Flett, & Callender, 1997), and headache pain (Kowal & Pritchard, 1990).

Despite the apparent pernicious effects of perfectionism in children, perfectionistic children are somewhat of an enigma. In contrast to other presenting problems children in play therapy might exhibit, perfectionism appears to have some clear rewards. Perfectionistic children typically engage in fewer acting-out behaviors that require discipline referrals. They are often praised for keeping their rooms and school workplaces neat and orderly and for attending diligently to schoolwork and other tasks. In academic settings, perfectionistic children often get good grades and are high achievers.

These observations are consistent with earlier theoretical work (e.g., Hamachek, 1978) and later empirical work (e.g., Slaney & Ashby, 1996) delineating differences between adaptive and maladaptive forms of perfectionism. This literature supports the distinction between the adaptive perfectionist (i.e., a child engaged in the pursuit of perfection but not consumed by that pursuit to the point that self-esteem or well-being is compromised in the process) and the more maladaptive perfectionist (i.e., a child who is excessively concerned with meeting unrealistic goals and never feeling "good enough" in that pursuit). Gilman and Ashby (2006) summarized the empirical research investigating perfectionism in children and noted that, despite the significant evidence supporting the problematic nature of maladaptive perfectionism, "perfectionism is not wholly synonymous with distress and can result in a number of positive outcomes as long as flexibility is maintained in concordance with high standards" (p. 310). In intervening with perfectionistic clients, like Emily, the first task of the play therapist will likely be to determine which aspects of the client's perfectionism are adaptive—and may contribute to the child's well being (e.g., striving to do one's very best)—and, conversely, which aspects are clearly maladaptive and causing the client distress.

In addressing the maladaptive aspects of a client's perfectionism, play therapists might do well to consider integrating cognitive-behavioral and Adlerian play therapy techniques. Each of these theoretical conceptualizations offers helpful frames for the distinction between adaptive and maladaptive perfectionism. In addition, research with adults and adolescents (e.g., LoCicero, Ashby, & Kern, 2000; Rice, Ashby, & Slaney, 1998) has illustrated the conceptualization of maladaptive perfectionism from each of these theoretical perspectives. For instance, the results of empirical studies have supported the relationship between maladaptive perfectionism and the Adlerian concept of inferiority (Ashby & Kottman, 1996). Similarly, results of additional studies have supported the relationship between the cognitive-behavioral concept of dysfunctional attitudes and maladaptive perfectionism (Ashby & Rice, 2002). Given the theoretical similarity between Adlerian and cognitive-behavioral theories noted by several authors (e.g., Freeman & Urschel, 2003) and the research findings supporting each theory's conceptualization of perfectionism, an integration of Adlerian and cognitive-behavioral play therapy approaches to perfectionism might arguably be a best practice for therapists. Each of these specific approaches is described in the following sections.

## Cognitive-Behavioral Play Therapy

Cognitive-behavioral play therapy is an adaptation of cognitive and behavioral therapy that incorporates play therapy techniques in order to provide age-appropriate, therapeutic interventions for young children with emotional and thought-related difficulties (Knell, 1998). Cognitive-behavioral play therapy (CBPT) emphasizes the behavioral construct that behavior is learned, reinforced, and maintained by a variety of factors that can be discovered and changed (Knell & Dasari, 2006). CBPT also shares some commonalities with Beck's (1976) cognitive therapy, including the three ideas that (1) beliefs and thoughts influence behavior and emotion; (2) beliefs influence the interpretations and perception of a person's environment; and (3) most people experiencing psychological distress have errors in logic, cognitive distortions, or maladaptive beliefs (Knell, 2009).

Knell (1994) identified six specific characteristics important to the understanding and efficacy of CBPT:

1. In CBPT, the child is an active participant in the therapy process.
2. CBPT is focused on the child's environment, thoughts, feelings, beliefs, and fantasies. It is not exclusively focused on any single domain.
3. CBPT emphasizes strategies for the development of adaptive thoughts and behaviors.
4. CBPT is directive, structured, and goal-oriented.
5. In CBPT the therapist uses techniques that have been empirically validated (e.g., modeling; Bandura, 1977).
6. CBPT allows for and emphasizes the empirical examination of treatment by using techniques that can be readily evaluated.

The process of CBPT has four stages: assessment, introduction/orientation, middle stage, and preparation for termination. In the assessment stage of therapy, the therapist uses a variety of means to assess the child's current level of development and level of functioning, as well as the child's and parents' perceptions of the presenting problem (Knell, 1998). These means may include observation, parent report, interviewing, play assessment, psychological tests, and therapist-assigned tasks. During this stage, the therapist may assess baseline frequencies of current behaviors so that behavioral change can be evaluated over the course of treatment. Play therapy clients may be employed with the task of monitoring their own behaviors and reporting back to the therapist. Changes in behaviors can be graphed over time, creating a visual representation of the child's behavioral shifts. Knell (1998) notes that, in addition to assessing current behavior, the assessment stage of CBPT emphasizes the identification of the client's "cognitive distortions and deficiencies" (p. 30).

In the introduction/orientation stage, the therapist prepares the child for therapy by setting the stage for the experience. The therapist may use a variety of means, including parent consultation, bibliotherapy, and structured tasks to facilitate the child's understanding of the therapy process. For instance, Knell (1993) developed the puppet sentence-completion task as a developmentally appropriate and structured way for clients to gain understanding about the process of CBPT. In this exercise the therapist and client each use puppets to ask and respond to a variety of sentence stems. In this activity the task of disclosure and exploration is introduced by and modeled by the use of puppets, helping the client understand what therapy may be like and grow more comfortable with it.

In the introduction/orientation stage of therapy, the treatment and therapeutic goals are also identified (Knell, 2009). In addition, the role of parents and other significant adults is clarified during this stage. Parent work can be an integral part of the assessment and treatment of the child. The therapist may work directly with parents to help them modify parenting interaction to assist with the goals of the treatment plan. Knell (1994) notes that even if the majority of the work of CBPT is with the child, the therapist continues to meet regularly with parents for ongoing assessment and consultation.

As CBPT treatment progresses, the middle stage of therapy is focused on interventions to assist the child in developing adaptive responses to problems, circumstances, and stressors (e.g., modeling, role-playing). Interventions during this stage are often aimed at shifting negative thoughts and beliefs and adopting positive self-statements. These traditional cognitive interventions are adapted to use several different mediums that are not dependent on the use of language, such as art, bibliotherapy, and semi-structured play with puppets (Knell, 1998). The child may draw pictures about her feelings or tell stories about a child or animal who shares similar fears. The child can receive modeling of helpful behaviors and coping skills through a story character or an interactive dialog with a puppet (voiced by the therapist), who shares the child's presenting concerns. The therapist and client can work to examine the fears and anxieties shared by the puppet and child, and to develop positive coping statements and behaviors that the child can utilize in times of distress. Change can then be assessed by the therapist through changes in the child's adaptive coping in these various play mediums.

In addition to these play-based interventions, cognitive-behavioral techniques such as systematic desensitization are sometimes used to reduce anxiety and fear responses in children. One key difference is that, whereas relaxation is commonly used for adults, play is used as the competing response in children. Systematic desensitization can occur through behavioral interventions, art, and story. Knell states that play is an ideal, mastery-related task that breaks down the child's association between stimulus and response (1998). Contingency management is often used to modify specific behaviors that are causing difficulties for the child or the family. This can include the use of positive reinforcement, the shaping of behavior, and extinction (Knell, 1994). A primary focus of this stage is assisting the child to generalize what is learned in therapy to the other settings in the child's natural environment. A part of this generalization process may be a form of relapse prevention (Meichenbaum, 1985). To maintain change over time, CBPT posits that both parents and children need to be prepared for the possibility of relapse, and the child should possess some coping strategies to prevent a return to old, maladaptive patterns of thinking and behaving.

The fourth stage of CBPT includes preparation for termination. During this stage, the therapist reinforces changes the child has made and may arrange for additional practice in generalizing learning from play therapy to other settings. The therapist may phase therapy with intermittent appointments over time to ease the transition to termination and reinforce the learning the client has done (Knell, 1994).

Neither cognitive theory nor CBPT places an emphasis on personality development. Rather, CBPT is directive therapy focused on the maladaptive assumptions, beliefs, and thoughts that lead to difficulty for the client. Knell (2009) notes that "Cognitive distortions in very young children may be developmentally appropriate, yet maladaptive" (p. 119). CBPT is focused on shifting those maladaptive beliefs and cognitive distortions and boosting adaptive thinking and behavior.

## Adlerian Play Therapy

Adlerian play therapy (APT) is the integration of the theoretical concepts of individual psychology with the techniques of play therapy (Kottman, 2009). APT is based on several theoretical tenets, including the following:

1. People are socially embedded and have a need to belong.
2. People are creative and self-determining.
3. Behavior is goal-directed.
4. Reality is experienced subjectively. (Kottman, 2003)

Based on these theoretical principles, APT is generally conceptualized as including four phases (Kottman, 2003). The first phase is building an egalitarian relationship with the client. Kottman suggests that the relationship between the child and the therapist must be an egalitarian one that is based in trust and equal sharing of power. The goal of this phase is to build a partnership with the client moving forward in therapy. In this initial phase of therapy, the therapist is usually nondirective and intentionally sharing power with the client. The Adlerian play therapist uses this phase to demystify the counseling process for the child, answer any questions, return responsibility to the child, and set any necessary limits. Initial sessions focus on tracking the child's behavior, a technique that allows the child to feel that his or her play is being attended to and respected. Similar to tracking, the therapist restates the content of the child's speech to show the child that he or she is being heard and understood. Reflecting surface-level feelings and deeper feelings also serves an important role in building the therapeutic relationship in this first phase. Encouragement is another technique often used in Adlerian play therapy to help children become aware of their strengths and progress (Dinkmeyer, Pew, & Dinkmeyer, 1979). Kottman (1994) notes that encouragement should be positive in nature, focus on joy in the process of doing and not the end result, emphasize progress instead of perfection, and empower the child in her ability to do things for herself.

In addition to utilizing these techniques with the client, Kottman suggests that this first phase of therapy also include an initial meeting with only the client's parents present. During this meeting, the therapist builds an alliance with the parents, explains the process of play therapy, and gathers information about the child (Kottman, 1994). The therapist will dialog with the parents to gather information relevant to an Adlerian conceptualization of the client, including the child's position in the family constellation, how he or she gains a sense of belonging, and the child's functioning in different settings. This additional information aids the therapist in discovering the goals of the child's behavior and possible sources of discouragement (Dreikurs & Stolz, 1964).

The second phase of Adlerian play therapy is exploring the client's lifestyle. Adlerian play therapy understands the client's lifestyle as the client's unique approach to life (Kottman, 2003). From observing self and others, each person develops a set of assumptions about self, others, and the world and patterns of behavior based on these views. Because, from an Adlerian perspective, individuals view reality subjectively, clients move through life as if these early lifestyle assumptions are accurate. During the second phase of Adlerian play therapy, the therapist uses a variety of directive and nondirective techniques to gain an understanding of the client's lifestyle. This formation of a theoretical conceptualization of the child can be organized around several ideas, including the client's assets, family constellation and atmosphere, goals of misbehavior, Crucial Cs, and private logic. Assessment of the client in these areas naturally leads to a treatment plan that guides the therapist in later phases.

In the exploration of the client's lifestyle, the Adlerian play therapist is typically careful to not overlook the assets the client may have. Consistent with the assumption that people are creative and self-directive, the play therapist in this phase is attempting to observe clients' strengths and resources. How have clients found a way to belong in the family, school, neighborhood, or other social context they are in? The answer to this question often points to the assets and strengths the client utilizes.

Adlerian theory suggests that clients are socially embedded and have a need to belong. Children typically find their first place in the world in the context of their family. As a result, the examination of the child's family constellation (Are there brothers and sisters? Stepbrothers and sisters? Are they older or younger?) helps the therapist assess what roles the client may have taken on to fit in the family. The combination of family constellation and atmosphere (the tone, structure, rules, etc. of the family) help the therapist to see what strategies clients may have used to belong in their families.

As noted previously, Adlerian theory posits that people are motivated by their desire to move toward goals and choose behaviors as a means to accomplish these goals (Mosak, 1995). The Adlerian play therapist assesses clients' behaviors and speech in the playroom, along with information from parents and teachers, to discover the underlying goals of behavior. Adlerian play therapists are interested in deemphasizing negative behavior by addressing the goals motivating the behavior. Dreikurs and Soltz (1964) identified several goals of misbehavior, including attention, power, revenge, and proving inadequacy. Kottman (2009) has noted that attention-seeking children are seeking to belong by being the center of attention. Power-seeking children are seeking significance and belonging by dominating others and maintaining control. Revenge-seeking children may have come to believe that hurting others is a normal way to gain significance or belong. Children whose goal is proving inadequacy may believe that they are failures and can't gain significance or belong.

Adlerian play therapists are also interested in assessing how effective children are at attaining positive goals. Lew and Bettner (1998) have identified four Crucial Cs that all children need:

1. Connecting with others (the goal of cooperation)
2. Being Capable (the goal of self-reliance)
3. Counting or being significant (the goal of contribution)
4. Having Courage (the goal of resiliency).

During the exploring the client's lifestyle phase of Adlerian play therapy, the therapist is assessing how strong or weak the client is in each of these positive goals. The therapist is also simultaneously using the results of this assessment to determine which interventions might be utilized to help the client move toward these positive goals.

One additional lifestyle assessment is the identification of private logic or mistaken beliefs. This private logic or mistaken beliefs are convictions that children have developed from the interpretations they have made of their environments. Mostly outside of awareness, these guiding beliefs naturally lead to feelings, thoughts, and behaviors that are unhelpful to the child. During this second phase of Adlerian play therapy, the therapist can see expressions of the client's lifestyle in the patterns of the child's play. The job of the therapist is to try and understand and value the client's subjective experience, with an eye toward how the therapist might help the child challenge any faulty convictions or private logic in later phases.

The third phase of Adlerian play therapy is helping the client gain insight into his or her lifestyle. During this phase, the therapist may continue to use a combination of directive and nondirective techniques. The therapist begins to share observations regarding the child's lifestyle with the child and utilizes metaphors to help the child to expand these observations to his or her life outside of the playroom. The therapist uses metaphor, interpretation, and metacommunication to help the client gain insight and make connections between playroom behavior and the outside world.

The fourth phase of the approach is reorientation and reeducation. During this final phase of the therapy, the therapist's goals are to help the child generate new behaviors outside of the playroom, teach and practice new behaviors for outside of the playroom, and encourage the child. This phase may include a variety of teaching strategies, such as modeling, role-playing, and therapeutic metaphors designed to help the client learn skills and alternate behaviors to be used outside of the playroom.

In a more fulsome description of the Adlerian approach, Kottman (2009) notes that "Parent consultation is a critical component of Adlerian Play Therapy" (p. 69). In each phase of the therapy, the therapist attempts to engage the parents of the client in a process parallel to the child. Consistent with the phases of therapy, the therapist attempts to develop an egalitarian relationship with the parents, understand their lifestyles and their perceptions of their child's lifestyle. The play therapist will also help the parents gain insight about their child's lifestyle, help them learn ways to be nurturing and structured in their interactions with their child, and assist them in acquiring parenting skills and approaches to support their child's new repertoire of behavior and skills.

## Integration of Theories

Although not all play therapy approaches are easily integrated, cognitive-behavioral and Adlerian play therapy can be more easily integrated than many other theories. This is partly because of their numerous overlapping assumptions and similarity of interventions. For instance, while both theories value the therapeutic relationship, neither sees that relationship as a sufficient medium for successful intervention. Both approaches allow the therapist to be planful and intentional in choosing techniques. While cognitive-behavioral play therapy may be more consistently directive than Adlerian play therapy, both approaches allow the therapist to be active and directive in choosing play therapy interventions and techniques. Indeed, both approaches may include a teaching component in the latter phases of therapy.

Another advantage of combining cognitive-behavioral and Adlerian approaches is their similarity in the conceptualization of pathology or distress. While Adlerian therapists might describe the client as discouraged rather than in more pathological terms, both cognitive-behavioral and Adlerian approaches would see thought patterns and beliefs about self, others, and the world as related to clients' distress. Whether labeled "dysfunctional thoughts" or "mistaken beliefs," both theories may target these assumptions, beliefs, and thoughts that may be outside of awareness as the best avenue to change. Both theories would hold that if the play therapist can help clients shift these thoughts in more functional and helpful directions, positive change will occur.

The ready integration of cognitive-behavioral and Adlerian play therapy is apparent in the similarity with which each identifies the phases or course of therapy. While CBPT does not identify a specific phase of developing a relation-ship, as APT does in its first phase (Kottman, 2003), CBPT does highlight the importance of a sound therapeutic relationship as a necessary condition of therapy (Knell, 1998). In the assessment phase of CBPT, the task of "ascertaining the individual's self-statements, attributions, beliefs, and assumptions" (Knell, 1998, p. 30) is very similar to APT's second phase of exploring the child's lifestyle. What CBPT identifies as the intervention stage of therapy seems consistent with APT's third and fourth phases of helping the child explore lifestyle and re-orientation and reeducation. Though not identified as a specific phase of therapy, CBPT does emphasize the need for the client to come to some insight and for the therapist to actively lead the client through verbal interpretations and other means (Knell, 1993). CBPT's active intervention phase with an emphasis on positive reinforcement, shaping, modeling, and coping are con-sistent with many of the techniques identified in APT's fourth phase of re-education/reorientation. Finally, both approaches also identify the importance of consultation with parents. While APT has a somewhat formal approach to parental consultation (e.g., Kottman, 2003), Knell (2003) noted that "parents should be involved in both the assessment and intervention phase" of CBPT (p. 39).

While cognitive-behavioral and Adlerian approaches to play therapy are similar in numerous ways, there are also some clear distinctions. For instance, the Adlerian approach includes more of an emphasis on the child's personality or lifestyle and how that lifestyle has developed with the client's family of origin. The cognitive-behavioral approach has a significant focus on behavior that results from cognition and, as a result, utilizes more behavioral techniques (e.g., systematic desensitization) than the Adlerian approach would typically use. Despite these and other differences between the theories, an integration of the two approaches does not result in significant contradictions in the underlying assumptions of each theory.

## Case Example

When Emily comes to the playroom for the first time, she initially appears somewhat anxious and spends a good bit of time inspecting the various toys, art supplies, and puppets that are placed around the room. The care with which Emily appears to be choosing a toy or puppet to play with is consistent with Emily's parents' descriptions of her behavior at school and at home. "Emily is a careful, almost cautious child in some ways," her mother said. "She rather needs everything to be 'just so'."

Emily is the 6-year-old only child of two professional parents in their early forties. Emily's father is an attorney, and her mother works in marketing. They have been married for 12 years. They dealt with infertility issues for two years before Emily was born. They do not have plans to have other children but have talked at times about the possibility of international adoption. Emily is a second-grade student at a public elementary school in an upper-middle-class neighbor-hood. She attends a private daycare center during the week after school, staying until approximately 6 p.m. each evening when her parents pick her up. Despite her young age, she was placed ahead a grade because of her emotional maturity, her intellectual curiosity, and her precocious abilities in reading.

Emily's parents were prompted to bring her to play therapy because "she just seems so stressed, and not happy." Her parents described a recent episode when Emily did not score a perfect grade on a spelling test as she usually does. Upon receiving the grade, she became agitated and tearful, crying uncontrollably until she had to be taken to the school counselor's office. Emily has largely excelled at school and has a reputation from her current and past teachers as a perfectionist in her work. The week before Emily's first appointment, she refused to take a math pop quiz because she did not think she could get a perfect score.

Recently, her parents have observed her rewriting her homework assignments several times until they look "just right." Her current teacher has noted that Emily consistently stays in the classroom at recess to read so she won't "get behind." Emily practices the violin for more than an hour per day. Her parents note that they can hear her talking to herself during practice, saying repeatedly that she is "horrible" and unable to "ever do anything right." She was very frustrated with her parents for not allowing her to bring her violin on a recent vacation, because she was afraid she would "forget everything" and have to "relearn everything" until it was right again.

Emily appears to have few friends. Feedback from her preschool and kindergarten teachers was that she was "a little bossy" with "strong opinions" about how things should be done. She appears to have some difficulty with peers, because she clearly thinks there are right ways to play games and play with toys and has difficulties when other children do not adhere to the correct way of doing these things. Emily's mother reports that Emily has been crying regularly at bedtime, claiming that "no one likes me, I'm not good enough."

Emily's parents were both present in the initial consultation about Emily and agreed to "do whatever we need to do to be helpful." They reported being very concerned about Emily and have been "racking their brains" about where all the pressure she feels can be coming from. They indicated that they have thought carefully about whether they've put pressure on Emily or have had too many expectations. They report feeling guilty that she is "so stressed . . . and only six." They have tried to help her lighten up and enjoy things but are aware that they have done this out of frustration and confusion about her behavior and so "she probably sensed their exasperation and didn't take their suggestions to heart."

In early play therapy sessions, Emily consistently played with the dolls and no other toys. When asked about this she responded, "I know how to play with dolls. I'm not sure of how to play with some of these other things." When invited to paint a picture, Emily got very frustrated with the runny paint, the consistency of the brushes, and the texture of the paper. After starting and restarting several pictures multiple times, she finally gave up, proclaiming, "I just can't get it right. I'll never try and paint again. I can't do anything right." Throughout early sessions, Emily was scrupulous about cleaning up as she went along. On several occasions, she paused to carefully and painstakingly arrange sandtray figures and other toys that she had not played with but wanted to fix because they "just weren't right."

## Theoretical Conceptualization of the Client

In an integrated approach to the client Emily, the therapist will be primarily interested in the cognitive distortions (CBPT) or mistaken beliefs (APT) that may result from Emily's early experiences in her family (APT) and how those patterns are reinforced in a variety of ways (CBPT). From the patterns described by Emily's parents and the themes observed in early sessions in the playroom, Emily appears to have strong maladaptive perfectionist tendencies. The described and observed themes of concern over making mistakes, great concern over being less than perfect, and overgeneralizing the making of any mistake to conclude that she is a failure are all consistent themes identified in the literature (e.g., Ashby et al., 2004) as indicative of maladaptive perfectionism.

Emily appears to have several cognitive distortions that are impacting her behaviors and emotions. She is clearly prone to black-or-white or all-or-nothing thinking, seeing herself as a complete success or a complete failure. As a result, any effort that does not result in a product that is consistent with her high standards (e.g., painting a picture) is inadequate and indicative of her worthlessness as a person. She is quick to overgeneralize her perceived failures to all other endeavors and to conclude that she can't do anything right. These distortions or mistaken beliefs may be inadvertently reinforced by parents who do not have other children and may model high standards and a critical attitude toward self and others. The therapist might view this reinforcement through the lens of Emily's family constellation and atmosphere.

As an only child, Emily is the primary focus of both of her parents' attention, and she spends a good bit of time among adults who are more proficient than she is at most tasks. Emily may well use her parents' and other adults' abilities and accomplishments as a metric in the development of her own high standards. She may have tried to develop skills and strategies to gain approval of the adult world, resulting in developmentally inappropriate and excruciatingly high standards for performance.

In addition, Emily is the single product of extended infertility treatments. As a result, she may perceive pressure to be all that her parents wanted and may even have caught some anxiety and insecurity from them. Without the distraction of another child, Emily may misinterpret all of the attention she receives from her parents as indicative of unarticulated, impossibly high expectations and pressure to perform to a particular standard.

Because of Emily's private logic and distorted thinking, she finds herself in a continuous loop of discouragement. With each incident where she does not see herself as meeting her standards, her sense of failure and not measuring up to her parents' imagined standards is reinforced. She loses the opportunity to see herself as important and valuable (a person who counts) and connected to others because she is hesitant to engage with other children ("Why would anybody want to play with me?"). Because of her tendency to see the world through this private logic of "I count/I don't count"–based performance, she is prone to interpreting reactions from others as negative feedback, further undermining her ability to connect.

Emily has several clear assets. She is of above-average intelligence and has a fairly extensive affective vocabulary. Emily possesses developmentally appropriate insight and has supportive and involved parents. These assets suggest a good prognosis for Emily's well-being and response to play therapy.

Given this conceptualization of the client, the following treatment goals might be appropriate. Specifically, treatment might be designed to help Emily (a) restructure/shift her cognitive distortions of all-or-nothing thinking and overgeneralizations; (b) learn to correctly interpret and moderate her reaction to perceived criticism; (c) recognize the self-defeating statements and play themes and begin to shift these; and (d) develop tolerance for mistakes and the performance of tasks that require less than perfect results.

## Treatment

Treatment of Emily in a play therapy context integrating CBPT and APT might include components of both theories and strategies and interventions that are very similar, though these interventions would be labeled differently by the different approaches. In this description, the reader will recognize numerous components of both approaches woven together throughout. Only the most specific techniques from each approach are referenced.

Following the basic stages/phases of CBPT and APT, the play therapist treating Emily would typically begin therapy by seeking to build a collaborative and supportive relationship with her. While building the relationship, the therapist would begin to explore her lifestyle and understand how her perceptions and interpretations of events are framed by her beliefs and assumptions. The therapist might utilize the puppet sentence-completion task (Knell, 1993) to facilitate the gathering of helpful information about themes in Emily's belief system (e.g., when Emily's puppet responds to sentence stems like "I am happiest when . . . " and "I am afraid of . . . "). Emily's completion of a kinetic family drawing (Kottman, 2003) would help the therapist explore her perceptions of her family constellation and atmosphere and assess how Emily sees her place in the family.

From the beginning of the therapy, the therapist using this integrated approach would seek to serve as a model for Emily directly and through play representation (e.g., giving voice to puppets or stuffed animals). This modeling might take the form of making mistakes and communicating self-acceptance despite the mistake made (e.g., the therapist saying, "Well, that's not what I wanted this picture I've painted to look like, but I think it's okay anyway"). Through metaphorical stories or structured play, the therapist can model positive self-statements and coping strategies for approaching and accomplishing tasks ("The bear says 'I want to do lots of things and they don't have to be done just right'").

As the therapist becomes clearer about Emily's cognitive distortions and private logic, the therapist might decide on some techniques to help Emily explore her lifestyle and see the maladaptive themes in her thinking and belief system. The therapist's choice of technique will largely rest on Emily's early response to specific play materials (e.g., bibliotherapy, puppets, sandtray, artwork).

Throughout the play process, the therapist might metacommunicate or make interpretations about Emily's play, attitudes toward play, actions, and verbalizations. The CBPT technique of identifying the maladaptive belief for Emily is similar to the APT technique of metacommunicating about the play theme. For instance, if the therapist notices a tendency of Emily's to ask very careful questions about what the rules are, the therapist might comment, "It seems like you ask me questions when you don't know what the rules are in here. I am guessing it is really important to you not to make a mistake." The therapist might also comment on how Emily is responding to the therapist by noting, "You seemed angry when I said that your picture didn't have to be perfect to be a picture you could feel good about," or "You get very quiet when I tell you that you can figure things out for yourself." This metacommunication or interpretation might also be in reference to Emily's play. For instance, if Emily has the mother in a puppet family get mad at the puppet children for not doing a job correctly "the first time," the therapist might say "I bet those kids are pretty scared they have to do everything right." Each of these interpretations and metacommunications are in the service of helping Emily become aware of her lifestyle themes, private logic, and underlying belief system.

During this intervention stage of therapy, the therapist might use therapeutic metaphors, role-playing, or structured play (e.g., puppet stories) to help Emily begin to shape her behavior and learn new skills in approaching tasks, dealing with challenges, and dealing appropriately with feedback she construed as negative or critical. For instance, the therapist might tell a story where a puppet who is fearful of making mistakes tries a new task, is not completely successful, expects very bad things to happen, but is surprised that other puppets are still accepting and acknowledge that "everybody makes mistakes and it is still okay." If the therapist were to communicate more directly with Emily about her need to avoid over-reacting, given her perfectionistic tendencies, she might likely perceive the feedback as highly critical and become defensive. Instead, using metaphors, stories, and role-plays will likely make intervention easier for Emily to respond to.

In the later stages of therapy with Emily, the therapist may want to help Emily consolidate the changes she has made and do some relapse prevention. Metacommunications and interpretations of Emily's verbalizations and play content can be shifted to become coping self-statements (e.g., "I can do my best and I'm okay no matter what"). Through structured play and/or discussion, the therapist can help Emily explore situations where she might be prone to falling back into dysfunctional thinking patterns or old private logic.

Throughout the stages of the therapy, the therapist would be meeting with Emily's parents for consultation. Helping the parents understand the themes of Emily's belief system and how they can help her shift to more adaptive helpful assumptions about herself and the world would be a priority for the therapist. In attempting to help Emily make some shifts, the therapist might suggest that the parents also take care to model imperfection without minimizing their desire to reach high standards (consistent with the distinction between maladaptive and adaptive perfectionism—see Ashby & Rice, 2002). Emily's parents might help her expand her tolerance for imperfection by engaging in playful mediums she might otherwise avoid (e.g., fingerpaints, mud pies, sand, or even shaving cream, which is clean but also messy). Playing games with Emily that have no clear winner or that have rules that shift at certain intervals might be somewhat difficult for her but might help her parents facilitate her ability to deal with lower structure situations where performance is harder to measure. All of these activities can reinforce for Emily that she counts and can connect without achieving anything or meeting any particular standard.

## Conclusion

Several authors (e.g., Kottman, 2001) have noted the trend of integrating theoretical conceptualizations into the treatment of clients. While some of these integrations would seem particularly challenging given the distinctly different assumptions and approaches of the theories, cognitive-behavorial and Adlerian play therapy approaches are complementary and would appear to benefit from integration. This may be particularly true in the treatment of perfectionistic play therapy clients. Some authors (e.g., Hamachek, 1978) have suggested that a cognitive-behavioral approach to the treatment of perfectionism may be particularly efficacious. Similarly, Adlerian theory offers a helpful conceptualization and empirically supported view of perfectionism (e.g., Ashby & Kottman, 1996). The integration of these two approaches may better help maladaptive perfectionistic clients become more adaptive by maintaining their striving for excellence but developing coping strategies to deal "more easily with life in all of its glorious imperfection" (Ashby et al., 2004, p. 52).

## References

Accordino, D. B., Slaney, R. B., & Accordino, M. P. (2000). An investigation of perfectionism, mental health, achievement and achievement motivation in adolescents. *Psychology in the Schools, 37*, 535–545.

Ashby, J. S., & Kottman, T. (1996). Inferiority as a distinction between adaptive and maladaptive perfectionism. *Journal of Individual Psychology, 52*, 237–245.

Ashby, J. S., Kottman, T., & Martin, J. (2004). Play therapy with young perfectionists. *International Journal of Play Therapy, 13*, 34–55.

Ashby, J. S., & Rice, K. G. (2002). Perfectionism, dysfunctional attitudes, and self esteem: A structural equations analysis. *Journal of Counseling and Development, 80*, 197–203.

Bandura, A. (1977). *Social learning theory*. Englewood Cliffs, NJ: Prentice-Hall.

Beck, A. (1976). *Cognitive therapy and the emotional disorders*. New York, NY: International Universities Press.

Dinkmeyer, D.C., Pew, W.L., & Dinkmeyer, Jr., D.C. (1979). *Adlerian counseling and psychotherapy*. Monterey, CA: Brooks/Cole.

Dreikurs, R., & Stolz, V. (1964). *Children: The challenge*. New York, NY: Hawthorn/Dutton.

Flett, G. L., Hewitt, P. L., Oliver, J. M., & Macdonald, S. (2002). Perfectionism in children and their parents: A developmental analysis. In G. L. Flett & P. L. Hewitt (Eds.), *Perfectionism: Theory, research, and treatment*. Washington, DC: American Psychological Association.

Freeman, A., & Urschel, J. (2003). Adlerian psychology and cognitive-behavioral therapy: A cognitive therapy perspective. In R. E. Watts (Ed.), *Adlerian, cognitive, and constructivist therapies: An integrative dialogue* (pp. 71–88). New York, NY: Springer.

Gilman, R., & Ashby, J. S. (2006). Perfectionism. In G. Bear & K. Minke (Eds.), *Children's Needs III* (pp. 303–312). New York, NY: National Association of School Psychologists.

Hamachek, D. E. (1978). Psychodynamics of normal and neurotic perfectionism. *Psychology, 15*, 27–33.

Hewitt, P. L., Newton, J., Flett, G. L., & Callender, L. (1997). Perfectionism and suicide ideation in adolescent psychiatric patients. *Journal of Abnormal Child Psychology, 25*, 95–101.

Knell, S. M. (1993). *Cognitive behavioral play therapy*. Northvale, NJ: Jason Aronson.

Knell, S. M. (1994). Cognitive-behavioral play therapy. In C. E. Schaefer & K. J. O'Connor (Eds.), *The handbook of play therapy, Volume II* (pp. 111–141). Hoboken, NJ: John Wiley & Sons.

Knell, S. M. (1998). Cognitive behavioral play therapy. *Journal of Clinical Child Psychology, 27*, 28–33.

Knell, S. M. (2003). Cognitive behavioral play therapy. In C. E. Schaefer (Ed.), *Foundations of play therapy* (pp. 178–191). Hoboken, NJ: John Wiley & Sons.

Knell, S. M., & Dasari, M. (2006). Cognitive-behavioral play therapy for children with anxiety and phobias. In H. G. Kaduson & C. E. Schaefer (Eds.), *Short-term play therapy for children* (2nd ed.). New York, NY: Guilford Press.

Knell, S.M. (2009). Cognitive Behavioral Play Therapy: Theory and Applications. In A. Drewes (Ed.), *Blending Play Therapy with Cognitive Behavioral Therapy: Evidence-Based and Other Effective Treatments and Techniques*. Hoboken, NJ: John Wiley & Sons.

Kottman, T. (1994). Adlerian Play Therapy. In C.E. Schaefer & K. J. O'Conner (Eds.).

*Handbook of play therapy, Volume 2: Advances and innovations* (pp. 3–26). Hoboken, NJ: John Wiley & Sons.

Kottman, T. (2001). *Play therapy: Basics and beyond*. Alexandria, VA: American Counseling Association.

Kottman, T. (2003). *Partners in play: An Adlerian approach to play therapy* (2nd ed.). Alexandria, VA: American Counseling Association.

Kottman, T. (2009). Adlerian play therapy. In K. J. O'Connor & L. D. Braverman (Eds.), *Play therapy theory and practice: Comparing theories and technique* (pp. 237–282). Hoboken, NJ: John Wiley & Sons.

Kottman, T., & Ashby, J. S. (2000). Perfectionistic children and adolescents: Implications for school counselors. *Professional School Counseling, 3*, 182–188.

Kowal, A., & Pritchard, D. (1990). Psychological characteristics of children who suffer from headache: A research note. *Journal of Child Psychology and Psychiatry, 31*, 637–649.

Lew, A., & Bettner, B. L. (1998). *A parent's guide to motivating children*. Netwon Center, MA: Connexions Press.

LoCicero, K. A., Ashby, J. S., & Kern, R. (2000). Multidimensional perfectionism and lifestyle approaches in middle school students. *Journal of Individual Psychology, 56*, 419–434.

Meichenbaum, D. (1985). *Stress inoculation training*. New York, NY: Pergamon Press.

Mosak, H. H. (1995). Adlerian psychotherapy. In R. J. Corsini & D. Wedding (Eds.), *Current psychotherapies* (5th ed.) (pp. 51–94). Itasca, IL: Peacock.

Nounopoulos, A., Ashby, J. S., & Gilman, R. (2006). Coping resources, perfectionism, and academic performance among young adolescents. *Psychology in the Schools, 43*, 613–622.

Rice, K. G., Ashby, J. S., & Slaney, R. B. (1998). Self-esteem as a mediator between perfectionism and depression: A structural equations analysis. *Journal of Counseling Psychology, 45*, 304–314.

Slaney, R. B., & Ashby, J. S. (1996). Perfectionists: Study of a criterion group. *Journal of Counseling and Development, 74*, 393–398.

# Integrating Play Therapy for Attachment Disorders of Children

## IV
### Section

# Playing for Keeps: Integrating Family and Play Therapy to Treat Reactive Attachment Disorder

## Kyle N. Weir

## Introduction

Playing marbles as an elementary school student is a vivid memory from my childhood. One of the greatest decisions was whether the group of children was going to "play for funsies" or "play for keeps." If students played for funsies it meant that at the end of the contest, each child picked up the same marbles he or she started with, and there was no permanent risk of loss of marbles in the game. Playing for keeps was more daring, however, because it was a mutually understood fact that the contest would continue until someone had won and another had lost their precious marbles. It took confidence in one's marble-playing skill and a dash of recklessness to gamble with the prized marbles you had daringly won in previous matches. But "nothing ventured, nothing gained" was the motto of the marble players who were willing to play for keeps.

A lot can be learned from such childhood marble contests that can be applied to treating reactive attachment disorder (RAD) in young children. Issues of permanence, risk, confidence, daring, skill, persistent and incremental accumulation of previous successes punctuated with occasional failures or setbacks, relationships (either between the marble players and their marbles or children with RAD and their families), and emotional attachments to the eventual outcomes are all involved in both the game of marbles and the treatment of RAD. Though at times parents of children with RAD may feel as if they are "losing their marbles," family-oriented play therapy can help the family overcome those difficulties and play for keeps in ways that will strengthen the permanence of and attachments within their family relationships.

## The Diagnostic and Clinical Definitions of Reactive Attachment Disorder

The DSM-IV-TR (American Psychiatric Association, 2000) defines Reactive Attachment Disorder (RAD) as having the following characteristics: "markedly disturbed and developmentally inappropriate social relatedness in most contexts, beginning before age 5 years" that can be characterized as either inhibited or disinhibited. Inhibited forms of RAD are characterized by social withdrawal (inhibition), hypervigilance, or "highly ambivalent and contradictory responses (e.g., the child may respond to caregivers with a mixture of approach, avoidance, and resistance to comforting, or may exhibit frozen watchfulness)." Disinhibited RAD may appear in the form of "diffuse attachments as manifested by indiscriminate sociability with marked inability to exhibit appropriate selective attachments (e.g., excessive familiarity with relative strangers or lack of selectivity in choice of attachment figures)." Furthermore, the DSM-IV-TR indicates that children with RAD must have received "pathogenic care" from their caregivers (usually in the form of abuse or neglect) or have experienced repeated changes of their primary caregivers (e.g., multiple placements in foster care) and that the pathogenic care led to the inappropriate social relationships and attachments. Finally, the DSM-IV-TR indicates that behavior is not better accounted for in some other type of disorder, such as a developmental delay.

A more clinical definition of RAD illustrating the detailed behaviors and feelings of children with RAD (and parents of children with RAD) stems from the extensive work of Hughes with foster and adoptive children in the Eastern United States. Clinically, Hughes (1997, 2007) describes some of the symptoms of common attachment-related behavioral problems in children as: poor response to discipline, aggressive or oppositional-defiant demeanor, social interactions that lack mutual enjoyment and spontaneity, increased attachment efforts by caregivers produce discomfort or resistance, poor planning/problem solving, ability to see only the extremes (all good/all bad), pervasive shame, clingy, poor eye contact, lying, gorging food, educational underachievement, school refusal, compulsion, indiscriminate friendliness, and/or social withdrawal. Furthermore, Hughes (2007) notes that problematic children's behaviors stem from attachment problems, and that to understand the root of these behaviors we have to look "under the behavior" to the feeling level. For children, Hughes suggests that some of the underlying feelings include:

> *sense that only self can/will meet own needs, not feeling safe, frequent sense of shame, sense of hopelessness and helplessness, fear of being vulnerable/dependent, fear of rejection, feeling "invisible," inability to self-regulate intense affect—positive or negative, inability to engage in the co-regulation of affect—positive or negative, felt sense that life is too hard, assumptions that parents' motives/intentions are negative, lack of confidence in own abilities, lack of confidence that parents will comfort/assist during hard times, inability to understand why self does things, need to deny inner life because of overwhelming affect that exists there, inability to*

*express inner life even if he or she wanted to, fear of failure, fear of trusting happiness, discipline is experienced as harsh or unfair, inability to be comforted when disciplined/hurt, and inability to ask for help. (Hughes, 2007, p. 129)*

Though lengthy, Hughes' list of the underlying feelings behind attachment-related behavior problems is the most comprehensive and descriptive found in the literature, and it matches the experience of children in my own clinical work.

Systemically, foster and adoptive parents who are not trained in attachment issues will tend to respond in ways that further encourage, maintain, and exacerbate the problem. Hughes (2007, p. 130) notes that parents lacking attachment savvy may respond with "chronic anger, harsh discipline, power struggles, not asking for help, not showing affection, difficulty sleeping, appetite problems, ignoring child, remaining isolated from child, reacting with rage and impulsiveness, lack of empathy for child, marital conflicts, withdrawal from relatives, anxiety and depression." Particularly, when social workers and other clinicians encourage behavioral approaches to correct behaviors in attachment-disordered children, the problematic behaviors from the child generally *increase*, which furthers the systemic cycle leading to the aforementioned parental behaviors. Correspondingly, under these parental behaviors are feelings that are the root of their parental behaviors. According to Hughes, these may include:

*desire to help child develop well, love and commitment for child, desire to be a good parent, uncertainty about how to best meet child's needs, lack of confidence in ability to meet child's needs, specific failures with child associated with more pervasive doubts about self, pervasive sense of shame as a parent, conviction of helplessness and hopelessness, fear of being vulnerable/being hurt by child, fear of rejection by child as a parent, fear of failure as a parent, inability to understand why child does things, inability to understand why self reacts to child, association of child's functioning with aspects of own attachment history, feeling lack of support and understanding from partner and other adults, difficulties addressing relationship problems with partner, felt sense that life is too hard, assumptions that child's motives/intentions are negative, belief that there is no other option besides the behavior tried. (Hughes, 2007, p. 130)*

It is important to understand these underlying feelings suggested by Hughes (2007) and not simply focus on the systemic, interactive dance of parent-child behaviors. As clinicians work to address these feelings, the behavioral cycles can change. My clinical experience with families of children with RAD has taught me that as I focus clinically on attachment, behaviors improve. That does not work in the converse. When I focus on behaviors, generally the behaviors do not improve and the attachment patterns and systemic, interactive relational feelings remain distant and frustrated. I think that is an important lesson for parents, as well as therapists. Focusing on improving the attachment and positive feelings in the relationship will lead to improved behavior quicker than the focus on behavior can improve behavior. The child will initially resist (often strenuously) positive affect, but a consistent, long-term course of tender (noncoercive) attachment-enhancing treatment will generally lead to the best long-term outcome.

Hughes' descriptions of the behaviors and underlying feelings of both children with RAD and their parents underscores why family systems approaches to therapy must be coupled with traditional play therapy in cases of attachment-disordered youth.

## Literature

The research literature has presented varied opinions about both the nature of RAD and appropriate treatments for the disorder. As attachment theory emerges and evolves, so does our understanding of treatment for attachment-disordered children and youth, but controversies have marred this field's history, including incidences where the death of children in specific treatment modalities has brought those treatments under scrutiny and unfavorable repute.

### Attachment Theory

John Bowlby's (1969/1982, 1988) work at the Tavistock Clinic in London, England, coupled with Mary Ainsworth et al.'s (1978) research, establishes the foundation for attachment theory. Briefly, attachment is a function of social interaction between an infant or child and his or her primary caregivers (usually parents). Attachment has been described as meeting the child's basic needs for protection, safety, and security in human relationships (Hornor, 2008; Weir, 2006). Though attachment patterns are generally formed in the child's younger years (beginning in the first year of life and established before age 5 years old), the socially learned attachment style has implications throughout the individual's life course (e.g., Susan Johnson's 2004 work with emotionally focused therapy [EFT] holds that attachment patterns have significant implications for marital relationships). Zeanah and Smyke (2009) suggest that attachment is a developmental process whereby the parent (or primary caregiver) responds to the child's sleeping, crying, eating, and attention needs—giving the child good eye contact and playful responsiveness (e.g., singing and cooing) matched to the temperament and interests of the child. Parents demonstrating such attunement to their children will have better parent-child relationships and facilitate healthier attachments.

As parents (or primary caregivers) show consistency and a balance of love, affection, warmth, connection, structure, and appropriate discipline, children grow feeling *secure* in their attachments to their caregivers. When parents are inconsistent and children do not know what to anticipate, they will form an insecure attachment known as *anxious-resistant* (or sometimes called *anxious-ambivalent*) attachment. If children consistently receive poor care from their parents, they will develop *anxious-avoidant* attachment patterns. These three patterns are largely measured through the use of the Strange Situation procedure developed by Ainsworth and her colleagues (1978), whereby children, their attachment figure, and a stranger were observed to determine how children would respond to a series of interactions and situations with and without their primary caregiver in the room with them. Main and colleagues (Main & Hesse, 1990; Main & Solomon, 1990) later used Ainsworth's Strange Situation procedure to identify a fourth attachment category, *disorganized attachment*, whereby the child demonstrates "aberrant behaviors and/or mixed strategies involving incoherent combinations of secure, avoidant, and resistant attachment behaviors" (Zeanah & Smyke, 2009).

Unfortunately, the DSM-IV-TR (2000) does not correlate the diagnosis of RAD (with its two subtypes of inhibited and disinhibited) with the four attachment patterns of Bowlby (1969/1982, 1988), Ainsworth et al. (1978), and Main and colleagues (Main & Hesse, 1990; Main & Solomon, 1990). Drisko and Zilberstein (2008, p. 477) suggest that is because:

> *The DSM diagnosis locates the disorder within the child, despite attachments being widely understood as interactions between specific people. The DSM diagnoses emphasize the child's general social behavior, but do not target attachment behavior specific to primary caregivers. Notably, attachment quality with a specific caregiver is not included in the DSM diagnostic criteria. This may be because the DSM seeks to be atheoretical and descriptive.*

Thus limited to only one single attachment disorder listed in the DSM, attachment-savvy clinicians may struggle to differentially diagnose when variations of attachment-disordered children and families present themselves for therapy. While a clinician may see attachment-related difficulties in a child or family, the diagnostic criteria may not lend itself easily to RAD. Future editions of the DSM should be expanded to better account for more relational etiologies and treatments of disorders (including systemic models).

Attachment theory has further progressed to include a biopsychosocial model of attachment pathology. Corbin (2007) posits that neurobiological components explain the psychological component of RAD stemming from the stress resulting from poor social interactions with primary caregivers. He states that RAD may be the result of the body's attempts in the "Hypothalamic-Pituitary-Adrenal (HPA) axis to regulate the body and brain's response to stress in a significant and enduring way" in response to early childhood trauma and neglect (Corbin, 2007). Drawing heavily from Trevarthen's (1998) work on infant intersubjectivity and Perry et al.'s (1995) research regarding the neurobiological adaptation of the brain to early childhood trauma, Corbin (2007) articulates a model that explains how RAD is a biopsychosocial disturbance of attachment. He posits a recursive process whereby the social elements of attachment, neurological process, and psychotherapy interact to explain RAD and proffer treatment suggestions:

> *We have learned that psychotherapy changes the brain by forming new neural connections through the concurrent processes of attachment and new learning.*

> *Neuroscience research lends hope and illuminates specific therapeutic techniques that alter and form a "counterbalance" (Lieberman et al., 2005, p. 507) for these complex functions in children with RAD. "The therapeutic setting should provide a protective sphere not only to explore painful events but also to retrieve and integrate experiences that promote self-worth" (p. 512). Psychotherapy should promote this integration of these "good" and "bad" parts of experience into a coherent sense of self and other (Fairbairn, 1954; Freud, 1923; Kernberg, 1976; Klein, 1932; Mahler et al., 1975; Winnicott, 1965). (Corbin, 2007)*

Corbin further gives examples whereby play therapy is effectively used to treat RAD and then concludes:

> *The neurobiological effects of early and enduring childhood neglect can be profound. The effects of these early toxic experiences, however, can be mitigated through appropriate systemic and therapeutic intervention. (Corbin, 2007)*

## Treatment for Reactive Attachment Disorder

Corbin's (2007) assertion that the treatment of RAD should involve both play therapy and systemic interventions lends support to the assertion of this chapter that integrating family therapy and play therapy is the preferred treatment modality for RAD, but such a position is not universally accepted. Several treatment modalities have claimed successful outcomes treating children with RAD, including behavioral approaches (including Behavioral Management Training [BMT], Dyadic Developmental Psychotherapy [DDP], Theraplay, Circle of Security, and coercive therapies (e.g., holding and rebirthing therapies).

It should be noted that the literature is bereft of empirical studies that would suggest which models meet the criteria of "empirically supported treatments" or ESTs (Sprenkle, 2002), so research about the effectiveness of treatment modalities has mainly focused on parents' perceptions of what worked during therapy (Drisko & Zilberstein, 2008; Wimmer, Vonk, & Reeves, 2010), with the exception of Wimmer, Vonk, and Bordnick (2009), who did a preliminary study about the effectiveness of attachment therapies in a pretest/post-test design. However, their preliminary study was limited in sample size (N=24), and a variety of attachment therapies mixed with traditional therapies were utilized as interventions: DDP, elements of Theraplay, narrative therapy, eye movement desensitization and reprocessing (EMDR), psychodrama, parent-training, neurofeedback, and gentle holding to facilitate good eye contact while discussing issues of past abuse and/or neglect (no coercive therapies, such as holding or rebirthing therapy, were utilized) (Wimmer, Vonk, & Bordnick, 2009). Their study gave preliminary credence to the effectiveness of attachment therapies in terms of clinical improvement in children with RAD.

Despite the paucity of rigorous, empirically designed research models verifying treatment effectiveness, there are good studies conducted by proponents of various treatment modalities that lend preliminary support for such models. There are also controversial treatment models lacking scientific scrutiny, but they have become clinically popular in some circles to the point that they warrant attention. A brief review of the major therapy treatments is required here.

## Coercive Therapies: The Source of Controversy With Attachment Therapy

Speltz (2002) accurately articulates a description, history, and critique of "corrective attachment therapies" known under the broad umbrella of attachment-based coercive therapies. Drawing on Zaslow and Menta's (1975) work with autistic children involving coercive holding (research that has since been repudiated with our greater understanding of the genetic etiology of autism), Welsh (1989) developed the concept of "holding time," which Cline (1991) utilized to create Holding Therapy, a treatment that is primarily conducted at the Attachment Center at Evergreen ("The Center"). Holding Therapy posits that attachment-disordered children and youth require a reconnection with their primal needs. Speltz (2002, p. 5) describes the process of Holding Therapy as follows:

> . . . *the following sequence of events is described: (1) therapist "forces control" by holding (which produces child "rage"); (2) rage leads to child "capitulation" to the therapist, as indicated by the child breaking down emotionally ("sobbing"); (3) the therapist takes advantage of the child's capitulation by showing nurturance and warmth; (4) this new trust allows the child to accept "control" by the therapist and eventually the parent. According to The Center's treatment protocol, if the child "shuts down" (i.e., refuses to comply), he or she may be threatened with detainment for the day at the clinic or forced placement in a temporary foster home; this is explained to the child as a consequence of not choosing to be a "family boy or girl." If the child is actually placed in foster care, the child is then required to "earn the way back to therapy" and a chance to resume living with the adoptive family.*

Despite the attachment-laden vocabulary utilized by Holding Therapy advocates, the process described has nothing in common with the warm, nurturing, and consistent attachment-enhancing processes described by Bowlby (1969/1982, 1988; see also Mercer, 2002 and Mercer, 2005, for excellent critiques of coercive attachment-based treatments). The notions that placement in temporary foster care should be used as a threat or punishment, that demeaning boot camp (Mercer, 2002) techniques should be employed in those foster homes as a behavioral incentive for change, and that children must "earn (their) way back to therapy" and their adoptive home is utterly absurd and emotionally abusive. It is at odds with the processes that we have learned from Bowlby (1969/1982, 1988), Ainsworth et al. (1978), and others (Main & Hesse, 1990; Main & Solomon, 1990) about promoting healthy parent-child attachments.

A similarly coercive attachment-based model is Rebirthing Therapy. This model purports to facilitate attachment through the figurative replication of the birthing process. Utilizing blankets, flannel sheets, and/or pillows, a child is forced into a simulated womb where they must exert themselves to get out (representing the birth canal). The therapist and parents and other adults (up to four or five adults may be utilized) hold the child down in the blankets, making it difficult for them to emerge. When the child, through strenuous effort, is able to extricate him or herself from the tangle of blankets, pillows, and adults, this figuratively represents a rebirth, and the child is then held by his or her adoptive mother and bonding is supposed to occur. This is the model utilized where young Candace Newmaker was tragically suffocated to death after 70 minutes in the womb of blankets (Mercer, 2002). Such reprehensible behavior by mental health professionals and adoptive parents is without the slightest empirical support and can only be construed as unethical.

Coercive therapies such as Holding and Rebirthing Therapies have been discredited, and nearly all of the respectable mental health profession associations and organizations (e.g., AAMFT, ACA, and APA) have warned against their use (Weir, 2006). While gentle, nurturing use of holding and appropriate use of touch in a noncoercive format is essential in any parent-child relationship (and any good attachment-based treatment), treatment for attachment-disordered children and youth should *never* include force or coercion. Ethically motivated clinicians should not utilize coercive therapies, and such treatments are illegal in some states (e.g., Colorado, North Carolina, and Utah). Such coercive treatments are strenuously discouraged.

## Behavioral Treatments

Barth, Crea, John, Thoburn, & Quinton (2005), in a scathing criticism of attachment therapies, vehemently warned against the use of attachment therapies with adoptive and foster families where children had RAD (it should be noted that their definition of attachment therapies is exclusively focused on coercive therapies). Barth et al. (2005) indicate that although attachment therapies are widely practiced among children's services practitioners, there is a lack of scientific support for their effectiveness. They also contend that while attachment therapies have intuitive explanatory power, the emphasis on the disorder arising from prior caregivers can undermine efforts to get foster and adoptive parents to examine their part in the current process of parenting as a factor. Barth et al. (2005) suggest that training parents to model appropriate behaviors and teaching them parent-child-oriented behavioral therapies with strong empirical backing is a more productive treatment modality for RAD. They specifically suggest The Incredible Years (Webster-Stratton & Hammond, 1997), Parent Management Training (Reid & Kavanagh, 1985), Multisystemic Therapy (Henggeler, Schoenwald, Borduin, Rowland, & Cunningham, 1998), Parent Child Interaction Therapy (Eyberg et al., 2001; Chaffin et al., 2004), and Functional Family Therapy (Alexander & Parsons 1997) as effective intervention strategies.

Buckner, Lopez, Dunkel, and Joiner (2008) illustrate a behavioral approach to treating RAD with an in-depth case study of a 7-year-old female child. Buckner et al. (2008), drawing from Barkley's (1997) manualized treatment for defiant children, expound the virtues of Behavior Management Training (implemented with precision and detail to the model) as being efficacious for treating RAD. BMT involves a 10-session manualized treatment program for caregivers of children with specific behavioral problems (such as defiance, aggression, and attention/concentration issues), and involves psychoeducation for caregivers to instruct them about childhood misbehavior, parenting skills, and behaviorally based disciplinary systems (including a home-based reward system for improved school behavior) (Buckner et al., 2008). It has been demonstrated to be effective in reducing these behavioral problems at schools in children ages 6 to 11 years old. Importantly, Buckner et al. (2008) report there have been "no reports of harmful outcomes for children participating in BMT." The contribution by Buckner and colleagues is that they applied BMT to a case involving a 7-year-old girl with RAD and demonstrated, based on assessments and the report of the child's caregivers (her grandparents), that the child's problematic behaviors significantly decreased.

In my clinical experience, this is unusual for behavioral approaches to be effective with cases of RAD. Although most children respond well to behavioral approaches, in general (hence the vast extent of empirical data of the effectiveness of behavioral approaches on other diagnosed disorders), attachment-disordered children and youth tend to exhibit the cognitive distortion of personalizing behavioral consequences and extrapolating them in relational terms rather than focusing on improving specific behaviors (e.g., the child thinks "My foster mom hates me" rather than "I shouldn't have done that" when given a behavioral consequence).

Chaffin (2008) comments on the implications of Buckner et al.'s (2008) findings, suggesting that they lend credence to attempting to apply previously successful models of evidence-based treatment for other diagnoses to RAD. In his commentary he argues against attachment therapies suggesting that:

> One of the opinions offered about these children is that regular treatments do not work and that therefore unconventional, highly intense, radical, risky, and coercive treatments are required to avoid dire outcomes. This clinical lore, almost completely untested, has been a foundational assumption legitimizing the use of concerning treatments. It is an opinion lacking in scientific support. (Chaffin, 2008, p. 313)

Earlier, however, Chaffin led a task force reporting on attachment therapy, RAD, and attachment problems to the American Professional Society on the Abuse of Children (APSAC) and reported greater distinguishing categories among attachment therapies that bear elucidating distinction (Chaffin et al., 2006). In that report, the task force made a key distinction between "accepted and noncontroversial attachment interventions" and "controversial theories of attachment disorder and corresponding controversial treatments" (Chaffin et al., 2006), noting that not all attachment therapies are alike. While the task force does not specifically mention particular treatment models by name, the descriptions given clearly indicate that parent-child models of behavioral treatments that are sensitive to attachment histories and concerns fall into the camp of "accepted treatments" and that coercive treatment models (Holding and Rebirthing Therapies) are in the "controversial treatment" grouping.

Taking Barth et al. (2005), Buckner et al. (2008), Chaffin (2008), and Chaffin et al. (2006) together, we see a clear delineation between the empirical support for parent-child-oriented behavioral models and the paucity of evidence for coercive therapies, but the aforementioned studies generally fail to distinguish coercive attachment-based treatments from noncoercive attachment-based treatments, either falsely implying a dichotomy that obscures the reality or lumping all attachment-based treatment approaches into the same controversial coercive treatment camp. We might be led to ask: "What of other attachment-based models that are neither behaviorally based nor coercive in their approach?" "What benefit is there to play therapy models and family systems approaches that have either a clear evidence base or show promise to do so as it applies to the treatment of RAD?" "Is there any scientific support not based solely on clinical lore for these moderate attachment-based, noncoercive play therapy and/or family-systems-oriented models?" I contend that there is a moderate position whereby integrating empirically based family systems theories with noncoercive, attachment-based play therapy approaches warrants significant merit in the clinical treatment of RAD.

## Moderate Models That Show Promising Practice

### Family Therapy

Family systems theory and many models within family therapy have become established as empirically supported within the mental health profession (Carr, 2000a, 2000b; Charles, 2001; Cottrell & Boston, 2002; Crane & Hafen, 2002; Larner, 2004; Pinsoff & Wynne, 1995; Sprenkle, 2002). For issues involving parent-child relationships (including attachment issues), a family systems approach has both prima facie and empirical support. Structural family therapy, Bowenian family therapy, attachment-based family therapy, multisystemic therapy, and many others have all been clinically tested and found significant scientific support for the assertion that they can improve parent-child relationships (e.g., Charles, 2001; Diamond, Siqueland, & Diamond, 2003; Henggeler et al., 1998; Vetere, 2001; Weir, 2007).

Of particular note is Diamond et al.'s (2003) study utilizing randomized control trials to treat depressed adolescents with attachment-based family therapy (ABFT). ABFT utilizes a brief, manualized treatment approach to "repair relational ruptures and rebuild trustworthy relationships" between adolescents and their parents. Their study would suggest that applying a family therapy model (in this case ABFT) that has empirical support could be extrapolated to families with RAD, much in the same manner that Buckner et al. (2008) followed Barkley's (1997) model to treat RAD from a behavioral perspective. In another study, Weir (2007) illustrated a case study integrating structural family therapy with elements of Theraplay and Hughes' DDP model, demonstrating the vital role family systems theory has to play in the treatment of RAD.

Barth et al.'s (2005) point that the current caregivers too often emphasize the role of the previous caregiver who perpetrated the pathogenic care in the etiology of RAD and undermine their own systemic role in the process further underscores that current caregivers need to be involved in family-systems-oriented family therapy to explore their own part in the process. Not that the current parents are part of the etiology of RAD, but living with a child with RAD can cause significant strain in even the best of families and marriages. As family difficulties increase in response to the child's RAD behaviors, family therapy is crucial to exploring family dynamics and preventing the maintenance and/or exacerbation of the RAD behavioral problems.

*Play Therapies and Other Attachment-Based, Parent-Child Relational Models of Merit*
Typically, in the United States most play therapists use some type of child-centered play therapy (CCPT) or variation thereof (for a good, detailed description of CCPT, see Landreth, 2002). Another impressive model of play therapy is ecosystemic play therapy developed by O'Connor (2000). Both of these models have much to offer a child in the way of personal growth, but because of the parent-child nature of attachment, these models would be lacking in the treatment of RAD as they both tend to treat children individually (Carmichael, 2006).

More specific to attachment are the play therapies developed by Ann Jernberg (Theraplay) in the late 1960s and Daniel Hughes (dyadic developmental psychotherapy or DDP) in the 1990s (Booth & Jernberg, 2010; Hughes, 1997; Hughes, 2007). Theraplay uses fun, safe, engaging play to build more secure attachments in the family and strengthen the parent-child bond. Specifically, parents are taught how to balance the critical dimensions of attachment-building in their relationships: structure, engagement, nurture, and challenge. The therapist models and then coaches the parents how to interact with their child in more attachment-savvy ways. Typically, the treatment is used with a population of children from birth to 12 years old, but it has been adapted to work with teens and even adults. Commonly, the treatment modality involves one or two parents and a pair of co-therapists working with an individual child, but it has been found to work effectively with groups and in school classrooms (Rubin & Tregay, 1989), in private practices with only one therapist (Weir, 2007), and in larger family contexts (Booth & Jernberg, 2010; Weir et al., n.d.).

Theraplay is an action-oriented model requiring therapists to take a directive position in therapy and use their personal presence or "self-of-the-therapist" as the primary instrument of change. The therapist directly relates to the child through a series of playful activities to model appropriate adult-child relationships. Then parents (who are taught and coached by the co-therapist), when they have learned this style of relating, are bridged into the play, and the therapist and co-therapist then support the play indirectly. While Theraplay therapists do use some materials, those materials are not expensive therapeutic toys or puppets, but rather, mostly household items such as cotton balls, straws, lotion, M&Ms, and toilet paper that parents will likely have at home without having to make special purchases. The goal is for the therapist to first model the correct use of the household objects through activities and games. After the parents play the games in session with the children, the family goes home and carries out the activities in their home settings as homework. Theraplay does incorporate appropriate touch (such as playing patty cake, imaginary face painting, or having parents hold the child while feeding a snack to foster nurturing). Touch is never used in a coercive or regressive manner. Theraplay allows the family to experience a different way of relating to each other in everyday tasks in the hope that, once learned in session, the interaction will carry on without the therapist present.

Theraplay is a play therapy model that has an emerging body of empirical support. Coleman (2010) provides an English-language synopsis of a study conducted in Finland by Makela and Vierikko (2004). Their study of Finnish foster children demonstrated through rigorous pretest, post-test, and follow-up testing at the six-month post-treatment mark that children with attachment issues made significant, positive behavioral progress upon completion of treatment and that the progress remained at the six-month post-treatment interval.

Wettig, Franke, and Fjordbak (2006) also conducted efficacy research of Theraplay with 319 children in Germany and Austria. Their findings are impressive. Not only did children demonstrate a significant reduction of problematic symptoms (e.g., noncooperation, oppositional defiance, aggression, shyness, social withdrawal, and social anxiety) by the completion of treatment, but children who received Theraplay continued to maintain these low levels of symptomatic behavior at the two-year post-treatment follow-up (Wettig et al., 2006). Having the parent-child dynamic change in the treatment sessions seemed to translate into their relationship at home, thus strengthening the child against relapse into former behaviors.

Additionally, Weir et al. (n.d.) concluded a pilot study testing the efficacy of Theraplay with adoptive families in preparation for a larger study with foster children to commence in the Fall of 2010. While the manuscript is still in preparation for submission and publication, our preliminary findings of the pilot study demonstrated that Theraplay made a statistically significant difference in the overall measure used to determine the children's behavioral outcomes (the Youth-Outcome Questionnaire described in Wells, Burlingame, Lambert, & Hoag, 1996), as well as one subscale (communication) on the systemic assessment we utilized (the McMaster Family Assessment Device or FAD; see Epstein, Baldwin, & Bishop, 1983). More will be addressed regarding this project later in this chapter, but it adds to a growing number of studies involving the efficacy of Theraplay (see also Franklin et al., 2007; Hong, 2004; Kwon, 2004; Siu, 2009). Theraplay is beginning to develop an emerging record of empirical evidence that shows promise and should not be ascribed as mere "clinical lore."

Another noncoercive form of attachment play therapy with a promising record of empirical support is dyadic developmental psychotherapy (DDP; Hughes, 2007), which emerged from Hughes' clinical work with foster and adoptive children in the eastern United States. Much like Theraplay, Hughes (2007) developed a directive, attachment-based style of play therapy that addresses a child's fundamental need for connection. DDP focuses on the reciprocal attunement of the parent-child dyad, whereby parents become more responsive to the child's subjective experience. Although puppets and other play materials are often incorporated, the focus is more on the therapist's and parent's ability to be attuned with the child and enhance their relationship during the play. The four crucial therapeutic stances of the therapist toward the child in DDP are found in the acronym PACE: playful, accepting, curious, and empathetic. By providing a therapeutic setting around these qualities, the therapist tries to get to the "feelings underneath the behaviors" (Hughes, 2007) in a way that facilitates attachment. Parents are taught to add the dimension of "Loving" to PACE in their interactions, forming the acronym PLACE. The DDP model may encourage a parent to hold a child who is emotionally dysregulated and in need of parental nurturance to feel a sense of safety, security, and containment, but such holding is never coercive, not intended to facilitate a negative emotional response, and should only be employed when less active means have been futile (DDPI, 2010).

DDP is beginning to show a promising empirical research base. Becker-Weidman (2008) conducted a study of 34 families receiving DDP and 30 families in a control group receiving other forms of treatment. The families receiving DDP treatment showed statistically significant improvement in terms of a decrease of symptoms as measured by the Achenbach CBCL and the Randolph Attachment Disorder Questionnaire. Moreover, four years post-treatment, families from the DDP treatment group reported that low levels of symptoms had been maintained. With the control group, the children's problematic symptoms increased and worsened, despite having received an average of 50 sessions during that time period. While more studies of DDP efficacy are clearly warranted, Becker-Weidman (2008) demonstrates that Hughes's model warrants the attention of clinicians treating RAD and is not based on mere clinical lore.

One further brief note is necessary. Psychoeducational programs such as Circle of Security (Powell, Cooper, Hoffman, & Marvin, 2009) can be useful adjuncts to treatment with RAD. Though this parent training model is best used to prevent attachment disorders from developing, it can be helpful in assisting parents to better understand the principles of attunement and the posture they must take to facilitate and maintain healthier attachments with their children. Specifically, the visual charts provided in the Circle of Security model may further reinforce parental understanding of other treatment models (such as Theraplay and DDP) if the learning style of parents is more visual than experiential.

## Whole Family Theraplay: An Integrative Model for the Treatment of Reactive Attachment Disorder

With so many available options to treat RAD, clinicians may struggle to determine how to best approach selecting a model. I recommend an integrative model called Whole Family Theraplay that I developed (in conjunction with the

Theraplay Institute) at Fresno Family Counseling Center (FFCC), a community mental health agency/student training clinic operated by the Marriage and Family Therapy faculty and master's degree students of the Counselor Education program at California State University—Fresno.

Lebow (1997) argues that integration of therapeutic models offers clinicians the benefit of drawing from the strengths of several models to meet the unique needs of individual cases, allowing for the needed flexibility clinicians must have to adapt to fit a family's idiosyncratic presentation. He further argues that integration, as opposed to eclecticism, allows the therapist to continue to utilize models in a considered, scholarly, and rigorous approach rather than from a hodgepodge of random assimilations of models applied indiscriminately. Crucially, Lebow (1997) also contends that any integrative model must include at least one systemic therapy model and then attempt to address how the multiple models employed mesh (or do not mesh) at the theory, strategy, and intervention levels.

As we at FFCC approached the idea of conducting a research project utilizing both Theraplay and family systems models to treat adoptive families struggling with attachment issues, we needed to find a way to treat whole families. So often Theraplay and other attachment-based models focus on parent-child interactions where one or two parents interact with a single child, but when the parents go home they must engage all of their children and may deviate from the healthy attachment style of parent interaction because they lack the knowledge of how to apply that approach to a larger group of children.

For example, I am the father of six adopted children. I learned early on that when I engage all of my children (as opposed to one-on-one interaction), I have to modify my parenting style and structure our interactions differently to facilitate family harmony and individual appreciation. My children like to play sports. Whenever I go out to throw the football with one or two of my children, inevitably several more will want to join. I learned that having competitive football games where I divide my children into teams never ends well in our family. So I began structuring a more collaborative interaction, much like a coach would set up practice drills, where each child takes a turn running a route with me throwing to them. As they line up and take turns running routes and catching passes, they all get to be involved, and each child gets an individual one-on-one experience when it is his or her turn. It has allowed us to enjoy much family play, yet avoid conflicts, with the large number of children involved.

This personal experience with my family helped me think about how we could restructure Theraplay to work with larger families and bring in the richness of sibling dynamics to support the attachment-enhancing processes of the parent-child relational dynamic. So often parents simply do not know how to interact with their children in large numbers in a manner that can still be attachment-enriching, particularly if they have adopted one or more children with attachment issues (as I have). I hypothesized that carefully considering how to use Group Theraplay elements (interactive play with large numbers of people) and parallel play elements from preschool-aged developmental research

(Campbell, 2002) in a structured way that would work for larger families might be effective. I began to develop a theory about integrating family systems theory with Theraplay to form Whole Family Theraplay (Booth & Jernberg, 2010; Weir et al., n.d.).

I was fortunate to associate with Phyllis Rubin, who developed Group Theraplay (Rubin & Tregay, 1989). Together we worked with the Theraplay Institute to develop a project testing the efficacy of Whole Family Theraplay with adoptive families. The Theraplay Institute provided an in-kind training grant valued at more than $20,000. To ensure reliability and validity, the Theraplay Institute sent trainers (Phyllis Rubin and Sandra Lindaman) to provide three-day trainings to my students and then, once the project commenced, we sent a sampling of recordings of the sessions along with recordings of my on-site supervision sessions to the Theraplay Institute for review by Certified Theraplay Supervisors. By the latter part of the study, the Theraplay Institute was confident in my ability to supervise, so I was awarded the status of University-Based Theraplay Trainer and Supervisor and was allowed to provide some of the trainings and much of the supervision of my students' Theraplay work.

We developed an abbreviated Marschak Interaction Method (MIM) to accommodate larger families involving only five family tasks: (1) Play with hats, (2) Teach your children a familiar game, (3) Stack hands, (4) Apply lotion to your children, and (5) Feed your children a snack. We were able to assess the four dimensions of structure, engagement, nurture, and challenge with these five tasks. Most MIM sessions lasted between 20 to 30 minutes. (See Appendix A of Booth & Jernberg, 2010, for a detailed review of the MIM tasks.)

For treatment sessions, two student-trainees would greet the family in the waiting room, enter the treatment room using a playful method (e.g., silly walk, making a train, and so forth), conduct a Theraplay session with the parents and all of the children residing in the household for about 30 to 35 minutes, and then one student would debrief with the parents while the other student continued to play with the children. All sessions were digitally recorded and observed by the supervising professor and other students not engaged in sessions. Families and students also had a midweek communication such as a phone call or e-mail so that parents could discuss items with the therapist that they may not wish the children to overhear, as well as follow-up to make sure the families were doing their homework by playing the games they learned in sessions at home.

Sessions were structured with activities (interventions) planned from all the four dimensions of attachment (Structure, Engagement, Nurture, and Challenge), but with a particular emphasis on those dimensions where the family's MIM indicated they needed improvement. We learned that the student-trainees needed to have a plan of activities (interventions) but also be attuned to the family's needs. They had to be attuned to how certain activities/interventions needed to be done in a whole family (group play) format, but other activities needed to be conducted in a parallel play format. For example, hand-stacking, playing Mother-May-I, Hot-Warm-Cold-Potato, Zoom-Erk, and Weather Report naturally tended toward whole family interactive play, whereas

Patty-Cake, Imaginary Face Painting, Measuring, Pop Cheeks, Beep-Honk, Cotton Ball Touch, Lotioning, and Feeding Snacks tended to best be done in parallel play, where each adult in the room paired off with a child to do the activity (in very large families we sometimes added a third student-trainee to assist the two parents and two other student-trainees). (See Appendix B of Booth & Jernberg, 2010, for an excellent description of Theraplay activities and games.) Some interventions such as Cotton Ball Hockey/Soccer and Keep-the Balloon-in-the-Air could be done either in whole family interactive play or parallel play format depending on the discretion of the therapist who is attuned to the family's needs.

Because of the family dynamics of the larger family systems in the room, student-trainees also had to attend to larger systemic issues, such as unhooking the identified patient, observing the impact of marital conflicts on children, balancing the sibling rivalries, helping the family genuinely interact in more emotionally open and enjoyable interactions, and supporting the hierarchical structure of the executive subsystem (parents) over the sibling subsystem (children). These strategies drew from family therapy models such as structural family therapy and experiential family therapy. Theraplay strategies included facilitating stronger attachments and helping parents be more attuned to their children's needs, which completely fit with the family therapy goals.

Not only were parent-child attachments a focus of treatment, but facilitating healthy sibling attachments were an additional focus of treatment. As siblings learned to participate in cooperative, mutually enjoying activities and games, their sibling bond grew. For example, one pair of brothers aged 9 and 5 years old had a strained sibling relationship. Through Whole Family Theraplay they grew closer. At one point the older brother got excited and hugged his little brother. Surprised by his demonstration of affection, he turned to his mom and said, "I accidentally hugged him." The benefit of strengthening sibling attachment is one of the most distinctive discoveries of Whole Family Theraplay.

Pedagogically, theoretical connections were formulated for student-trainees as they observed how the directive style of Theraplay meshed with Minuchin's (1974) use of the self-of-the-therapist in structural family therapy. In fact, the dimensions of Theraplay (especially structure and engagement) helped students better understand several concepts from structural family therapy, including hierarchy, boundaries, coalitions, scapegoating, and enmeshment/disengagement. From experiential family therapy, students integrated the concepts of the here-and-now temporal focus (Nichols & Schwartz, 2006), being attuned to the family's emotional needs (Napier & Whitaker, 1978), and understanding the roles individuals play in families (Satir, 1988) with Theraplay.

In some sessions, students were attempting to do Theraplay and the families were not as open to it that particular evening. One memorable moment came when student-trainees, attuned to their family, recognized that the mother, father, and two preteen girls were not as engaged in the Theraplay as they usually were. The students simply asked what was going on. The family proceeded to describe how they got into a fight in the car on the way to therapy. The student-trainees stopped trying to do Theraplay for the evening and engaged in more traditional family therapy to process the family's concerns. Once those issues were resolved by the conclusion of the session, the family returned next week ready to play. Such experiences exemplify that there are times when the play therapy needs to be briefly interrupted to utilize more traditional family therapy models.

In another family situation, it was clear that marital conflicts were affecting the Theraplay sessions, so it was arranged for the couple to receive couples counseling separate from, but concurrent with, the Theraplay sessions. This allowed the family to make significant progress by the conclusion of the Theraplay treatment course.

Because the treatment was part of a university-based project, the student-trainees were only involved in the Whole Family Theraplay project for the semester in which they took the university course. This resulted in the treatment course for families to range from 12 to 15 weeks. Typically, in the first two to three sessions the children were on their best behavior. This frustrated parents because they wanted the therapists to see the problematic behaviors the parents had to deal with at home. Parents also were still wondering how playing such simple, childish games would alleviate the significant behavioral problems their children exhibited. As supervisor, I would suggest my students use phrases like: "We've learned that as attachments are strengthened, behavioral problems diminish," "Trust us, there's a method to our madness," and "There's a magic to Theraplay, and if you just hold out a little longer, you'll see some significant changes."

By week four or five, the student-therapists and families had joined sufficiently that the children felt comfortable behaving more naturally. Parents seemed almost pleased that the student-trainees were finally seeing what they had to deal with at home. Student-trainees would come in from those sessions where the children felt comfortable enough to exhibit their problematic behaviors with eyes wide-opened and wondering what they had gotten themselves into. I would reframe it for the students as, "You know the attachments are forming when the kids can be their true selves with you," and I would remind them that when they took the MFT theories course with me, I taught them that theory helps you organize and know how to make order of the chaos. I would help them focus on specific strategies and interventions from both family therapy and Theraplay® that would most likely be effective with the behaviors exhibited. As they began to think about family therapy theory and the theories behind Theraplay they did discover they could focus on the important elements the family presented them with and ignore the rest of the family chaos in the room. This helped students better integrate family systems approaches and Theraplay at the theory, strategy, and intervention levels, as suggested by Lebow (1997). By the seventh or eighth session, we would typically hear parents reporting that the children's problematic behaviors were beginning to diminish at home (if not, we would inquire about homework, and usually the families who did not do their homework were the ones lagging in progress). Though there may be a small recurrence of the behavioral problems around the ninth or tenth session, by the concluding sessions (in weeks 12 through 15) parents generally expressed appreciation for the significant behavioral changes and improvements made by the children and the family as a whole.

To gather data, we administered measures at the beginning of treatment and again at the end of treatment. The family took the McMaster Family Assessment Device (FAD), each parent took the Outcome Questionnaire (OQ), and one of the parents (usually the mother) completed a Youth-Outcome Questionnaire (Y-OQ) for each child. Because of the small sample size of this pilot study [N=12 adoptive families; 22 adults (one family was a single parent and with another family the father never attended due to his work schedule); and 30 children], much of our findings were not statistically significant. While an article is in preparation for publication in a peer-reviewed journal that provides much more detail of the findings of the study (Weir et al., n.d.), we were pleased to discover that even with this limited sample size we still learned that Whole Family Theraplay made a statistically significant difference in improving the children's overall Y-OQ scores (measuring overall problematic behaviors) and that family communication was enhanced (as measured by the FAD communication subscale). As we prepare for the larger study with foster children, we will continue to use these measures (FAD, OQ, and Y-OQ), possibly add the Randolph Attachment Disorder Questionnaire (Randolph, 2000) or Disturbances of Attachment Interview (DAI) (Smyke, Dumitrescu, & Zeanah, 2002; Smyke & Zeanah, 1999), and significantly increase the sample size.

## Conclusion

It amazes me that playing together as a family can have such a powerful impact on family attachments, yet it consistently does. To me the phrase "playing for keeps" takes on a whole new level of relational meaning. It implies that parents and children can learn to relate to each other through play in ways that solidify family connections and attachments and further helps the children know that the adoptive parents are committed to keeping them in a permanent family relationship. As families learn to play for keeps by utilizing Whole Family Theraplay, they strengthen their attachments not only in parent-child relationships but also between siblings.

Children seem to intuitively understand the marble analogy at the beginning of this chapter. It does not take as much convincing of the children as it does the parents that such play can help them feel more secure in their family relationships, because play is the medium of communication or language of children (Carmichael, 2006). When children (and parents) learn that playing together in these specific attachment-enhancing ways strengthens the trust that the parents really want to keep their adopted children and develop a permanent connection with them, attachment-based problematic behaviors very quickly diminish. It is so important for parents to come down to the child's level of understanding through play. Parents who embrace the magic of Whole Family Theraplay and trust that such childlike playful interactions really have profound relational meanings will reap significant benefits in their relationships with their children.

For clinicians who are seeking an attachment-based model of treatment for RAD (particularly in cases where behavioral approaches have not been successful, as has been common in my experience), but who also want a treatment that is not ethically controversial, noncoercive, not based solely on clinical lore, and integrates evidenced-based family systems with an empirically promising play therapy (Theraplay), Whole Family Theraplay offers a model with merit. Such integration to treat RAD opens new opportunities for these children and families to heal and connect as they play for keeps.

# References

Ainsworth, M. D. S., Blehar, M. C., Waters, E., & Wall, S. (1978). *Patterns of attachment.* Hillsdale, NJ: Erlbaum.

Alexander, J., & Parsons, B. (1997). *Functional family therapy.* Monterey, CA: Brookes-Cole.

American Psychiatric Association. (2000). *Diagnostic and statistical manual of mental disorders* (4th ed., text revision; DSM-IV-TR). Washington, DC: American Psychiatric Association.

Barkley, R. A. (1997). *Defiant children: A clinician's manual for assessment and parent training* (2nd ed.). New York, NY: Guilford Press.

Barth, R. P., Crea, T. M., John, K., Thoburn, J., & Quinton, D. (2005). Beyond attachment theory and therapy: Towards sensitive and evidence-based interventions with foster and adoptive families in distress. *Child and Family Social Work, 10,* 257–268.

Becker-Weidman, A. (2008). Treatment for children with reactive attachment disorder: Dyadic developmental psychotherapy. *Child and Adolescent Mental Health, 13,* 52–60.

Booth, P. B., & Jernberg, A. M. (2010). *Theraplay: Helping parents and children build better relationships through attachment-based play* (3rd ed.). San Francisco, CA: Jossey-Bass.

Bowlby, J. (1969/1982). *Attachment [Vol. 1 of Attachment and Loss].* New York, NY: Basic Books.

Bowlby, J. (1988). *A secure base: Parent-child attachment and healthy human development.* New York, NY: Basic Books.

Buckner, J. D., Lopez, C., Dunkel, S., & Joiner, T. E. (2008). Behavior management training for the treatment of reactive attachment disorder. *Child Maltreatment, 13,* 289–297.

Campbell, S. B. (2002). *Behavior problems in preschool children: Clinical and developmental issues.* New York, NY: Guilford Press.

Carmichael, K. D. (2006). *Play therapy: An introduction.* Upper Saddle River, NJ: Pearson Education.

Carr, A. (2000a). Evidence-based practice in family therapy and systemic consultation. I: Child-focused problems. *Journal of Family Therapy, 22,* 29–60.

Carr, A. (2000b). Evidence-based practice in family therapy and systemic consultation. II: Adult-focused problems. *Journal of Family Therapy, 22,* 273–295.

Chaffin, M. (2008). Commentary on Buckner and implications for treatment selection among foster children with RAD. *Child Maltreatment, 13,* 313–314.

Chaffin, M., Hanson, R., Saunders, B. E., Nichols, T., Barnett, D., Zeanah, C., . . . & Miller-Perrin, C. (2006). Report of the APSAC task force on attachment therapy, reactive attachment disorder, and attachment. *Child Maltreatment, 11,* 76–89.

Chaffin, M., Silovsky, J. F., Funderburk, B., Valle, L. A., Brestan, E.V., & Balachova, T. (2004). Parent-child interaction therapy with physically abusive parents: Efficacy for reducing future abuse reports. *Journal of Consulting and Clinical Psychology, 72,* 500–510.

Charles, R. (2001). Is there any empirical support for Bowen's concepts of differentiation of self, triangulation, and fusion? *The American Journal of Family Therapy, 29,* 279–292.

Cline, F. W. (1991). *Hope for high-risk and rage-filled children*. Evergreen, CO: Author.

Coleman, R. (2010). Research findings that support the effectiveness of Theraplay. In P. B. Booth & A. M. Jernberg, *Theraplay: Helping parents and children build better relationships through attachment-based play* (3rd ed.). San Francisco, CA: Jossey-Bass.

Corbin, J. R. (2007). Reactive attachment disorder: A biopsychosocial disturbance of attachment. *Child & Adolescent Social Work Journal, 24*, 539–552.

Cottrell, D., & Boston, P. (2002). Practitioner review: The effectiveness of systemic family therapy for children and adolescents. *Journal of Child Psychology and Psychiatry, 43*, 573–586.

Crane, R. D., & Hafen, M. (2002). Meeting the needs of evidence-based practice in family therapy: Developing the scientist-practitioner model. *Journal of Family Therapy, 24*, 113–124.

Diamond, G. S., Siqueland, L., & Diamond, G. M. (2003). Attachment-based family therapy for depressed adolescents: Programmatic treatment development. *Clinical Child and Family Psychology Review, 6*, 107–128.

Drisko, J. W., & Zilberstein, K. (2008). What works in treating reactive attachment disorder: Parents' perspective. *Families in Society: The Journal of Contemporary Social Services, 89*, 476–486.

Dyadic Developmental Psychotherapy Institute (DDPI). (2010). *What is DDP?* Retrieved on July 28, 2010 from = www.dyadicdevelopmentalpsychotherapy.org/ddp.html

Epstein, N. B., Baldwin, L. M., & Bishop, D. S. (1983). The McMaster Family Assessment Device. *Journal of Marital and Family Therapy, 9*, 171–180.

Eyberg, S. M., Funderburk, B. W., Hembree-Kigin, T. L., McNeil, C. B., Querido, J. G., & Hood, K. K. (2001). Parent-child interaction therapy with behavior problem children: One- and two-year maintenance of treatment effects in the family. *Child and Family Behavior Therapy, 23*, 1–20.

Fairbairn, W. R. D. (1954). *An object relations theory of personality*. New York, NY: Basic Books.

Franklin, J., Moore, E., Howard, A., Purvis, K., Cross, D., & Lindaman, S. (2007). An evaluation of Theraplay using a sample of children diagnosed with pervasive developmental disorder (PDD) or mild to moderate autism. Poster presentation at the American Psychological Association Conference, San Francisco, CA.

Freud, S. (1923/1966). The ego and the id. In J. Strachey (Ed. & Trans.), *The standard edition of the complete psychological works of Sigmund Freud*. London, England: Hogarth Press.

Henggeler, S. W., Schoenwald, S. K., Borduin, C. M., Rowland, M. D., & Cunningham, P. B. (1998). *Multisystemic treatment of antisocial behavior in children and adolescents*. New York, NY: Guilford Press.

Hong, J. (2004). Effects of group Theraplay on self-esteem and interpersonal relations for abused children. Presentation at Sookmyung Women's University, Seoul, South Korea.

Hornor, G. (2008). Reactive attachment disorder. *Journal of Pediatric Health Care, 22*, 234–239.

Hughes, D. A. (1997). *Facilitating developmental attachment: The road to emotional recovery and behavioral change in foster and adopted children*. Northvale, NJ: Jason Aronson.

Hughes, D. A. (2007). *Attachment-focused family therapy*. New York, NY: W. W. Norton.

Johnson, S. (2004). *The practice of emotionally focused couple therapy: Creating connection* (2nd ed.). New York, NY: Brunner-Routledge.

Kernberg, O. (1976). *Object relations theory and clinical psychoanalysis*. Northvale, NJ: Jason Aronson.

Klein, M. (1932). *The psycho-analysis of children*. London, England: Hogarth Press.

Kwon, E. (2004). The effect of group Theraplay on the development of preschoolers' emotional intelligence quotient. Presentation at Sookmyung Women's University, Seoul, South Korea.

Landreth, G. (2002). *Play therapy: The art of the relationship*. New York, NY: Taylor & Francis Books.

Larner, G. (2004). Family therapy and the politics of evidence. *Journal of Family Therapy, 26*, 17–39.

Lebow, J. (1997). The integrative revolution in couple and family therapy. *Family Process, 36*, 1–17.

Lieberman, A. F., Padrón, E., Van Horn, P., & Harris, W. W. (2005). Angels in the nursery: The intergenerational transmission of benevolent parental influences. *Infant Mental Health Journal, 26*(6), 504–520.

Mahler, M., Pine, F., & Bergman, A. (1975). *The psychological birth of the human infant.* New York, NY: Basic Books.

Main, M., & Hesse, E. (1990). Parents' unresolved traumatic experiences are related to infant disorganized attachment status: Is frightened and/or frightening parental behavior the linking mechanism? In M. T. Greenberg, D. Cicchetti, & E. M. Cummings (Eds.), *Attachment in the preschool years: Theory, research, and intervention.* Chicago, IL: University of Chicago Press.

Main, M., & Solomon, J. (1990). Procedures for identifying infants as disorganized/disoriented during the Ainsworth Strange Situation. In M. T. Greenberg, D. Cicchetti, & E. M. Cummings (Eds.), *Attachment in the preschool years: Theory, research, and intervention.* Chicago, IL: University of Chicago Press.

Makela, J., & Vierikko, I. (2004). *From heart to heart: Interactive therapy for children in care. Report on the Theraplay project in SOS children's villages in Finland 2001–2004.* Finland: SOS Children's Village.

Mercer, J. (2002) Attachment therapy: A treatment without empirical support. *Scientific Review of Mental Health Practice, 1*(2), 9–16.

Mercer, J. (2005). Coercive restraint therapies: A dangerous alternative mental health intervention. *Medscape General Medicine, 7*(3), 6.

Minuchin, S. (1974). *Families and family therapy.* Cambridge, MA: Harvard University Press.

Napier, A. Y., & Whitaker, C. A. (1978). *The family crucible.* New York, NY: Harper & Row.

Nichols, M. P., & Schwartz, R. C. (2006). *Family therapy: Concepts & methods* (7th ed.). Boston, MA: Pearson.

O'Connor, K. J. (2000). *The play therapy primer.* New York, NY: John Wiley & Sons.

Perry, B. D., Pollard, R. A., Blakley, T. L., Baker, W. L., & Vigilante, D. (1995). Childhood trauma, the neurobiology of adaptation, and "user-dependent" development of the brain: How "states" become "traits" *Infant Mental Health Journal, 16,* 271–291.

Pinsoff, W. M., & Wynne, L. C. (1995). The effectiveness and efficacy of marital and family therapy: Introduction to the special issue. *Journal of Marital and Family Therapy, 21,* 341–343.

Powell, B., Cooper, G., Hoffman, K., & Marvin, R. S. (2009). The circle of security. In C. H. Zeanah (Ed.), *Handbook of infant mental health* (3rd ed.). New York, NY: Guilford Press.

Randolph, E. (2000). *Manual for the Randolph attachment disorder questionnaire* (3rd ed.). Evergreen, CO: Attachment Center Press.

Reid, J. B., & Kavanagh, K. (1985). A social interactional approach to child abuse: Risk, prevention, and treatment. In M. A. Chesney & R. H. Rosenman (Eds.), *Anger and hostility in cardiovascular and behavioral disorders.* Washington, DC: Hemisphere.

Rubin, P., & Tregay, J. (1989). *Play with them: Theraplay groups in the classroom.* Springfield, IL: Charles C. Thomas.

Satir, V. M. (1988). *The new peoplemaking.* Palo Alto, CA: Science and Behavior Books.

Siu, A. (2009). Theraplay in the Chinese world: An intervention program for Hong Kong children with internalizing problems. *International Journal of Play Therapy, 18,* 1–12.

Smyke, A. T., Dumitrescu, A., & Zeanah, C. H. (2002). Disturbances of attachment in young children: I. The continuum of caretaking casualty. *Journal of the American Academy of Child and Adolescent Psychiatry, 41,* 972–982.

Smyke, A. T., & Zeanah, C. H. (1999). The disturbances of attachment interview. Unpublished manuscript. Available at www.jaacap.com.

Speltz, M. L. (2002). Description, history, and critique of coercive attachment therapy. *The APSAC Advisor, 14,* 4–8.

Sprenkle, D. H. (2002). *Effectiveness research in marriage and family therapy.* Alexandria, VA: American Association for Marriage and Family Therapy.

Trevarthen, C. (1998). The concept and foundations of infant intersubjectivity. In S. Braten (Ed.), *Intersubjective communication and emotion in early ontogeny: Studies in emotion and social interaction.* Cambridge, England: Cambridge University Press.

Vetere, A. (2001). Structural family therapy. *Child Psychology and Psychiatry Review, 6,* 133–139.

Webster-Stratton, C., & Hammond, M. (1997). Treating children with early-onset conduct problems: A comparison of child and parent training interventions. *Journal of Consulting and Clinical Psychology, 65,* 93–99.

Weir, K. N. (2006). Repairing adoptive and foster attachments. *Family Therapy Magazine, 5,* 17–20.

Weir, K. N. (2007). Using integrative play therapy with adoptive families to treat reactive attachment disorder: A case example. *Journal of Family Psychotherapy, 18,* 1–16.

Weir, K. N., Lee, S., Canosa, P., Rodrigues, N., McWilliams, M., & Parker, L. (n.d.). Whole Family Theraplay: Integrating family systems theory and Theraplay to treat adoptive families. (Unpublished manuscript in preparation for submission to *Adoption Quarterly*).

Wells, M. G., Burlingame, G. M., Lambert, M. J., & Hoag, M. J. (1996). Conceptualization and measurement of patient change during psychotherapy: Development of the Outcome Questionnaire and Youth Outcome Questionnaire. *Psychotherapy: Theory, Research, Practice, & Training, 33,* 275–283.

Welsh, M. (1989). *Holding time: How to eliminate conflict, temper tantrums, and sibling rivalry and raise happy, loving, successful children.* New York, NY: Fireside Books.

Wettig, H. H. G., Franke, U., & Fjordbak, B. S. (2006). Evaluating the effectiveness of Theraplay. In C. E. Schaefer & H. G. Kaduson (Eds.), *Contemporary play therapy: Theory, research, and practice.* New York, NY: Guilford Press.

Wimmer, J. S., Vonk, M. E., & Bordnick, P. (2009). A preliminary investigation of the effectiveness of attachment therapy for adopted children with reactive attachment disorder. *Child & Adolescent Social Work Journal, 26,* 351–360.

Wimmer, J. S., Vonk, M. E., & Reeves, P. M. (2010). Adoptive mothers' perceptions of reactive attachment disorder therapy and its impact on family functioning. *Clinical Social Work Journal, 38,* 120–131.

Winnicott, D. W. (1965). *The maturational processes and the facilitating environment.* London, England: Hogarth Press.

Zaslow, R., & Menta, M. (1975). *The psychology of the Z-process: Attachment and activity.* San Jose, CA: San Jose State University Press.

Zeanah, C. H., & Smyke, A. T. (2009). Attachment disorders. In C. H. Zeanah (Ed.), *Handbook of infant mental health* (3rd ed.). New York, NY: Guilford Press.

# Integrating Attachment Theory and Nondirective Play Therapy to Treat Children With More Serious Attachment Problems

| 15 |
| :---: |
| Chapter |

## *Jessica Jäger and Virginia Ryan*

## Introduction

The application of attachment theory and research to clinical situations is a much sought-after goal. However, clinicians have argued that the usual attachment classifications do not sufficiently account for the complex range of problems encountered in their practice (Crittenden, 2010). Two different models that extend attachment theory to encompass a wider range of clinical issues have been developed, those of Crittenden (1995, 2005) and Heard and Lake (Heard, 1982; Heard & Lake, 1997). Both models have taken decades to build up, and they both attempt to provide practical frameworks for interpreting clinical material provided by practitioners. This chapter intends to apply Heard and Lake's extended attachment theory to nondirective play therapy (NDPT) practice. The chapter's goal is to demonstrate that play therapists can increase their understanding of underlying relationships and changes within these relationships during interventions, in more informed ways by using this extended attachment theory framework.

The chapter begins by providing a brief summary of both extended attachment theory and NDPT, arguing that applying attachment theory to nondirective play therapy cases assists decision making both in designing treatment interventions and in enhancing therapists' understanding of process issues during interventions. Practice considerations using an extended attachment theory framework at the assessment stage, during the intervention, and at the end phase of NDPT are described. The influences of the child's, carer's, and therapist's attachment styles on the process are also delineated. These applications of extended attachment theory are illustrated later in the chapter with a case study of a child with serious attachment problems in kinship care.

The chapter concludes that understanding the therapeutic process from an attachment perspective can be particularly beneficial, and arguably essential, when working with children who have more serious attachment difficulties and with children who are embedded within more complex family and professional systems. This chapter, therefore, concentrates on exploring attachment-related practice considerations. Other frameworks, and in particular trauma and resiliency frameworks, also are essential for understanding and responding to these children's therapeutic needs. These frameworks will be alluded to where needed, but an extended discussion is outside the scope of this chapter.

## Rationale for the Integrative Approach

### Description of Nondirective Play Therapy (NDPT)

NDPT, often known as child-centered play therapy (CCPT) in the United States, is based on Rogerian person-centered psychotherapy, a humanistic approach utilizing the core conditions of empathy, congruence, and unconditional positive regard (see Rogers, 1951). At the center of this approach is the relationship that therapists form with clients. Mearns and Thorne (2000, p. 83) impress that the core conditions of the humanistic approach are an "attitudinal expression of a belief system about human nature and development, and about the healing qualities of relationship." These core attitudes place primary emphasis on therapist-client relationships. Therefore, attachment theory and research, examining primary relationships and their development, are highly relevant to person-centered practice.

It is well known that Axline (1989) proposed eight principles of NDPT, which detail the type of relationship the nondirective play therapist strives to develop with children in order to provide the responsive and accepting environment thought to be conducive to self-growth. These principles encompass warmth, acceptance, permissiveness, respect, patience, and allowing the child to lead, with therapists setting only those limits necessary to anchor the therapy in reality. This chapter argues that attachment theory provides a framework for further understanding these features of relationships that play therapists aim to foster with children to promote their growth and healing.

The second author, along with Wilson (see Wilson and Ryan, 2005), has previously set NDPT within the broader developmental frameworks of children's mental development. In particular, Piaget's theory of cognitive development, Erikson's theory on emotional and social development, and Bowlby's attachment theory are applied to NDPT. Attachment theory also has been applied extensively to deepen the understanding of the therapeutic relationship (for example, see Ryan and Wilson, 1995; Ryan, 2004a, 2004b). In this chapter, further application of attachment concepts to NDPT are discussed and illustrated in the case study. First, a brief overview of general attachment theory and concepts is provided, along with a description of developments in NDPT practice that relate to an attachment perspective.

## Description of Attachment Theory and Extended Attachment Theory

Bowlby's (1980) and Ainsworth's (Ainsworth, Blehar, Waters, & Wall, 1978) original works on attachment theory are the foundation of the vast literature in this area. Bowlby described the bond that develops between mother and children. He focused on when separations occur in this relationship and formulated the important concept of a goal-corrected behavioral careseeking system. That is, children seek care and protection from their carers when they become distressed. If the goals of care and protection are met by carers, children return to a less distressed condition (see Bowlby, 1988).

A further key theoretical concept developed by Bowlby was the internal working model. Bowlby asserted that individuals build a set of mental representations built on their experiences with caregivers, which act as templates for future relationships (see Bretherton and Munholland, 1999, for a full discussion). Heard and Lake (1997), in their extended attachment theory which builds on Bowlby's original conceptualizations, have latterly described these as internal working models of the experience of relationships (IMERs) to reflect the possibility of having more than one template for the varying experiences humans have, even within the same relationship, which then act as guides for the future.

Ainsworth identified qualitatively different patterns in mother-child dyads when the careseeking system was activated through her well-known Strange Situation experiments. Ainsworth introduced the concept that the carers are a secure base for the child, from which the child can explore. Ainsworth's Strange Situation assessed the level of security infants experienced with their carers in a stressful environment. Three attachment patterns were identified: insecure-avoidant (a); secure (b); and insecure-ambivalent (c) (Ainsworth et al., 1978).

Both Main and Crittenden have extended Ainsworth's classifications. Main and Solomon (1986) identified a fourth category: insecure-disorganized. In contrast, Crittenden, in her dynamic-maturational model of attachment (Crittenden, 1995, 2005), conceptualized attachment classifications as a continuum whereby each of Ainsworth's categories has three subcategories ranging from compulsive Type A strategies to obsessive Type C strategies. These classifications encompass both adaptive and maladaptive behavior.

## Extended Attachment Theory: Dynamics of Attachment and Interest Sharing Model

Heard and Lake's (1997) aim was to encompass findings from more recent attachment-related research and clinical findings of psychotherapists that were not explained by attachment theory. They hoped that their extended theory could be used as a tool to enhance therapists' understanding of their clients.

Bowlby argued that these goal-corrected systems for attachment were motivational, that they were activated by specific cues that would lead to behavioral outcomes, rendering the system quiescent (Heard and Lake, 2001). Heard and Lake used this concept as a base but moved away from the one-dimensional approach and formulated five interrelated behavioral systems, which they then termed the Dynamics of Attachment and Interest Sharing (Heard & Lake, 2001). They identified three specific areas in which clients experienced difficulties, which were hitherto not fully explained. These were: (1) peer relationships, (2) sexuality, and (3) how clients coped with unresponsive or rejecting care.

This formulation was based on their observations within the context of adult psychotherapy, and to a lesser extent child psychotherapy. The five systems are as follows:

1. The interpersonal *attachment or careseeking system* (as described by Bowlby)
2. The interpersonal *parenting system*. This includes Bowlby's *caregiving* component, where the adult provides protection from danger, but also includes physical care, comfort, and soothing when in psychological distress, including emotional regulation.
3. The *exploratory interest-sharing system* with peers. This includes an interpersonal component, where understanding is enhanced, competencies are discovered, and skills are developed because of sharing an interest and the enjoyment of this interest with others (e.g., soccer, dressing up), and an intrapersonal component, where an individual experiences curiosity and creativity in a solitary activity.
4. The *sexual/affectional system*. An interpersonal system developed with peers.
5. The *personal self-defense system*. Essentially an intrapersonal system, activated when the individual experiences fear of abandonment, shaming, and/or dismissive or angry care, in order to minimize discomfort (Heard & Lake, 1997, 2001).

Heard and Lake argue that when the goals of all five systems are reached, a person is able to relate cooperatively, enabling satisfactory adaptation to change. However, when the goals of systems are not being met satisfactorily, the functions of the systems change to seeking personal survival through dominant or compliant behavior towards others (Heard and Lake, 2001). If the careseeking or caregiving system is activated, the other systems are inhibited. If the personal defense system is highly activated, the exploratory system is inhibited. McCluskey (2005, p. 241), who has researched these concepts with adults, has clarified that Heard and Lake and other attachment theorists argue that the goal of careseeking is not to achieve proximity to the caregiver, as Bowlby had originally proposed. Rather, an effective response by the caregiver is required, to assuage the careseeking of the careseekers and allow them to "get back on track and deal more competently with the world."

Empirical research and theoretical application to practice examples has begun on the ways in which the five systems interrelate in therapeutic encounters (e.g., Heard & Lake, 2001; Hunter, 2003 unpublished; Jäger, 2010 unpublished; McCluskey, 2005; McCluskey, Hooper, & Miller, 1999; O'Sullivan & Ryan, 2009; Ryan, 2004a; and Wilson, 2006). In this chapter, Heard and Lake's dynamics of attachment, along with other relevant attachment concepts, are applied to the composite NDPT case set out as follows. The discussion of this case illustrates the ways in which application of this model can enhance play therapists' understanding of process issues from an attachment perspective during an intervention.

## Nondirective Play Therapy Sessions: An Optimal Environment

Kaufman (1989, cited in Schore, 1994, p. 445) argues that "psychotherapy must mirror development by actively engaging the identical processes that shape the self." The second author has previously detailed the parallels between NDPT sessions and normal infant socialization with a sensitive carer (Ryan & Wilson, 1995). Arguably one of the aims of NDPT sessions is to provide children with emotional security along with physical safety. This outcome is facilitated when their therapists' generalized attitudes are ones of emotional availability and dependability toward the children and young people they help. These attitudes are necessarily conveyed to children through their therapists' use of emotive verbal and nonverbal messages, along with compatible motor actions, in play sessions.

In addition, play therapists promote face-to-face interactions with children, which are similar to those occurring in early, highly responsive infant-carer relationships. Therapists promote children's ability to move beyond more primitive child-adult or child-object-only interactions, where required, to more complex child-object-adult interactions, as has been observed in normal developmental studies. Arguably the play environment and responsiveness of their therapists heightens children's interest in exploration and helps foster a sense of personal competence. The combination of these conditions mirror those observed in optimal socialization patterns between an infant and a sensitive carer during normal development (Ryan & Wilson, 1995).

Such an environment has been lacking for children with serious attachment difficulties—the client group discussed here. Providing such an environment can arguably help these children rework their early experiences of relationships. Neurological theory and research supports these children's need to create new neural pathways through intensive, restorative relationships (e.g., Schore, 2003). For these seriously damaged children, it is important that every aspect of their lives, including therapy, home, and school, is optimal. Because these children have serious attachment deficits, this process of reconnection is necessarily lengthier and more arduous, with the risk that for some rare children, sufficient neurological repair and reworking of relationships may not be possible.

One aspect of attachment relationships that will need reworking for these children is to help them develop relationships with adults who are important to them. This leads to children beginning to care about their carers' reactions to their behavior, which is a necessary step in conscience formation. Within these significant relationships, children can begin to develop more empathy with their carers and start to want to follow their carers' rules. These positive changes also seem to occur within therapeutic relationships, which mirror attachment relationships in these respects. In terms of NDPT practice, a central issue that has been developed by Landreth (2002) and Guerney (2001) is the importance of therapists' understanding of therapeutic limit setting within the relationship in nondirective practice; the rationale and practice of setting limits has now been well explored and established. In addition, the second author and O'Sullivan have expanded the theoretical underpinning of therapeutic limit setting within NDPT through the application of attachment theory (O'Sullivan & Ryan, 2009). In that article the use of limits to provide emotional containment for children and promote emotional self-regulation is explored. In this chapter some of these arguments are revisited and applied to the composite case discussed as follows.

A second practice issue that has received considerable attention and development in the UK is the use of congruence in NDPT. The practice of congruence within play therapy has received little attention in the play therapy literature. However, it has been taught in depth in the UK within one of the central training programs (at the University of York). Ryan and Courtney, (2009) demonstrate the ways in which congruence can be expressed by play therapists verbally and nonverbally in both NDPT and filial therapy. Expressing congruence also seems to be essential in NDPT for children with serious attachment difficulties. Actively using congruence is particularly important for these children—similarly to younger children and those with learning disabilities—because they often have difficulty understanding others' inner thoughts and feelings. Often this cohort of children with deep-seated attachment problems has experienced serious maltreatment. Subsequently, they have developed distorted representations and expectations of adult responses. Therefore, therapists' verbalization of their thoughts and feelings during their interactions with children at key moments seems important in order to support children's understanding of normal adult responses in close relationships and to deepen their therapeutic encounters (see Ryan & Courtney, 2009). The ways in which therapists show transparency and genuineness, beyond indirect nonverbal communication with this group of children, will be discussed further later.

Another well-known form of therapy, filial therapy, also is highly relevant to working from within an attachment framework (see Guerney, 1964; Landreth & Bratton, 2005; VanFleet & Guerney, 2003; and VanFleet, Ryan, & Smith, 2005). While the focus is on *individual* NDPT in this chapter, the influence of filial play therapy on play therapy practice as a whole is important to acknowledge. There is a growing literature on including parents and carers in play therapy generally (see Crane, 2001, and Hill, 2005, for examples). This qualitative literature, along with quantitative outcome research (Bratton, Ray, Rhine, & Jones, 2005), suggests that there are significant advantages in terms of outcomes and process when parents/carers are included in therapeutic work with children. This is reinforced by child development findings and reflected in play therapy practice.

Many play therapists, including the authors, involve parents/carers to varying degrees during individual NDPT interventions. This may include consultations with the carers in addition to the carer(s) observing the last 10 minutes of the play therapy session, or more active involvement for a substantial part of the therapy session. These options are particularly chosen when there are contraindicators to filial therapy. The intervention may progress to joint play therapy, with both the carer and therapist actively involved in the entire session, and finally progress to a filial therapy intervention. The following example, however, focuses on a child's individual play therapy sessions with only brief references, due to space limitations, to ways the carers were involved in the intervention.

## Practical Implementation of This Integrative Approach

There are numerous ways in which attachment concepts can inform NDPT practice—from initial assessment to decisions regarding readiness to end therapy. Some of these issues are summarized here, and they are illustrated in greater detail in the case example to follow.

### Assessments

The two major international classification manuals, DSM-IV-TR (American Psychiatric Association, 2000) and ICD-10 (World Health Organization, 1992), describe attachment disorders with diagnostic criteria. These systems differentiate two types of disorder: inhibited and disinhibited. Children with attachment disorders have marked disturbance and are developmentally inappropriate in their social relationships. Both disorders are described as being pervasive across relationships and are likely to occur in relation to neglectful or abusive care. The age of onset is 5 years or younger. The inhibited subtype is characterized by fear and hypervigilance or highly ambivalent contradictory responses. Children persistently fail to initiate or respond in a developmentally appropriate way to social interactions. They may exhibit frozen watchfulness and avoid or resist comforting. The disinhibited subtype is marked by indiscriminate friendliness and lack of a specific attachment figure to whom children go for comfort. These diagnostic categories are considered during NDPT assessments and may inform play therapists' case formulation and treatment plan.

In addition to these broad classifications, several assessment methods may be used to gather information on children's attachment styles and to identify those with serious attachment difficulties. In addition to gathering comprehensive information from referrers and key professionals, along with interviewing carers and a home visit to the child, one or more of the following in-depth direct assessment measures is considered, by the authors, to be necessary with this cohort of children.

## Referral Information and Interview With Caregivers From an Attachment Perspective

For children who have very serious emotional problems, referral information often concentrates on these children's presenting problems. Focusing on these children's strengths and resilient factors during parent interviews and administration of standardized quantitative measures, such as the child behavior checklist (CBCL; Achenbach, 1991), is important. During the assessment period, a family history, including a social work chronology where available, is required to help play therapists understand the likely responses given to these children's careseeking needs as infants, along with any traumatic experiences these children have suffered. In the parental interview, it is important for play therapists to specifically ask parents to reflect on their children's behavior at times when their attachment system would usually be activated, including major transitions, separations, illnesses, and events evoking emotional distress.

### Home Visits

From an extended attachment theory perspective, children's exploratory systems are engaged and their defensive system deactivated in familiar and stress-free situations. Attachment-disordered children often rely on the safety of familiar routines and familiar surroundings more than most children, because they cannot adequately attach to their carers and have not developed IMERs that are positive ones to sustain them. In new situations all children need the support of their primary attachment figures or the capacity to be self-sufficient based on their IMERs. Even though playrooms are inviting for children in general, for children who have more serious attachment difficulties, the new situation of play therapy can be very anxiety-provoking. These children are likely not to have developed IMERs that are helpful to them in new situations with new adults. Therefore, it is useful for therapists to ensure that these children's attachment needs are met as optimally as possible. Home visits by therapists for the introductory meeting, with therapists aiming to fit into the children's routine lives and familiar environments, are potentially less anxiety-provoking. Home visits have the added advantage of helping children who have learned to separate and compartmentalize their relationships and experiences previously to immediately link their therapy with their home life (see Ryan, 2001).

### Story Stems

In addition to interviews and home visits, there are other assessment methods for both children and their carers that are clinically useful. Story stem assessments, originally developed for research purposes, have been adapted for use as a clinical tool in the UK with children and require play therapists to complete specialist training before their use. They seem particularly suitable for play therapists to use during assessment because of their use of figures and play scenarios, thus mirroring some of the activities children engage in during play therapy. The story stem assessment allows children to use both verbal and nonverbal means of communication to express their expectations and representations of attachment figures (see Hodges, Steele, Hillman, & Henderson, 2003). While such an assessment does not provide a categorization of attachment style, it does provide clinicians with helpful information regarding children's style of relating to others, which can inform the subsequent intervention. As Hodges et al. (2003, p. 352) argue, children's play narratives demonstrate the child's most basic scripts for human relationships—their "internal working model" (Bowlby, 1969).

The assessment battery used by the first author includes 13 stems used in Hodges et al.'s (2003) research. This battery is designed to elicit responses regarding parent-child relationships, including the security of attachment, in particular whether parental figures are aware of children's need for protection and comfort. Furthermore, responses regarding the likelihood that the parent will respond appropriately to these needs are also sought. Therapists begin the story, using dollhouse figures and furniture to enact what happens, and ask children to show and tell what happens next in the story using the figures. Both human figures and animal figures are used in the stems. Separations, exclusions, accidents, and dilemmas in friendships are all represented in the stems. All of these themes are likely to trigger children's attachment systems and provide play therapists with information on children's expectations within relationships. Story stems can be particularly informative when little is known regarding children's early history and can help identify the likelihood and intensity of a child engaging in traumatic play during the therapeutic intervention. This in turn is useful information for play therapists in assessing the appropriateness of filial therapy, joint play therapy, or individual play therapy for each case. If there is a high level of traumatic play, then individual play therapy may be indicated in the first instance.

## Attachment Style Interview

During NDPT assessments for children with serious attachment difficulties, it is helpful to gain an understanding of the current caregivers' style of relating in order to help them to meet these children's emotional needs more fully. Comprehensive and in-depth assessments, such as the Adult Attachment Interview (AAI; George, Kaplan, & Main, 1984), although rigorous and typically used in the study of parent-child relationships, are also cumbersome and time-consuming both in terms of training to administer and code the measure. However, the Attachment Style Interview (ASI; Bifulco, 2002), which was originally developed for research purposes to assess vulnerability in adults and has since been utilized in the field of adoption and fostering in the UK to assess and understand carers' support needs, provides a workable alternative. This hour-plus-long interview assesses carers' abilities to make relationships and their style of relating. The interview focuses on the carers' close relationships and their general attitude in relationships. These cover avoidant behaviors, specifically mistrust, constraints on closeness, fear of intimacy and overly high self-reliance, and anxious-ambivalent behaviors, namely a high desire for engagement, intolerance of separation, and anger.

Gaining information on the carers' style of relating, and both the presence of and their ability to use support, assists therapists' in their decision making regarding treatment and their understanding of current interactions between carers and their children. If a carer finds it difficult to access support and/or the ASI identifies that a carer has unresolved emotional issues, then filial therapy may not be the treatment of choice for a child with serious attachment difficulties in the first instance. Individual therapy for the child alongside carer consultations or joint play therapy, where the play therapist and carer undertake the therapy together, may be more appropriate.

## Family Play Observations

Observing the interactions during 20 minutes of free play between children and their carers and any siblings can provide important additional information about both the children's and carers' styles of relating *within the current family system* (VanFleet, 1999). Family play observation has previously been applied to the case of a child with an insecure attachment (Rye & Jäger, 2007). Puppets (Irwin, 2000; Ross 2000) or the collaborative drawing technique (Smith, 2000) also can be used to gather this information. From an attachment perspective, specific attention is paid by therapists to attuned and misattuned interactions (see Stern, 1985). Carers' responses to children's defensive strategies can be identified and provide a baseline for therapists and families to talk about everyday family interactions.

## Case Formulation and Chosen Treatment Approach

The use of assessments of both children and their carers based on attachment concepts provides a guide for the direction of treatment. Case formulation and treatment options are shared with the family to jointly decide what to offer. This will be illustrated in the case described later. The ways in which extended attachment theory can be used to inform therapists of the progress of therapy will be discussed in general terms first.

### During the Intervention

During the play therapy intervention, it is recommended that attachment concepts be used to track themes and progress across sessions. Particular changes in attachment behaviors need to be attended to; for instance, transitions at the beginning and end of sessions, and children's ability to seek and receive comfort. Extended attachment theory is usefully applied to the interactions in the play therapy sessions and in the wider system to help therapists understand and respond nondefensively to the systems around the children they are helping. Extended attachment theory posits that if the careseeking or caregiving systems are activated, the other systems are inhibited. If the personal defense system is activated, then the exploratory system is inhibited.

Here we detail behavior descriptors of the five interrelated systems adapted from Heard's (1982), Heard and Lake's (1997), and McCluskey's (2005) work in the adult psychotherapy context and applied to the context of play therapy. The following behaviors are considered to be indicative of each system being activated in a play therapy context for children. This list is not intended to be exhaustive; instead, it is intended as an indication of what kinds of behaviors fit within each system. It is also important to note that play therapists may convey careseeking, caregiving, interest-sharing, or defensive messages to the children and families they are helping by the behaviors listed as well. Therapists' own attachment styles also are important to understand, as discussed further shortly.

Careseeking behaviors:

- Indications of *tiredness or discomfort* (including sighs, yawns, frequent fidgeting, heavy body language, verbal/nonverbal requests for comfort such as food or drink)
- *Uncertainty, mild fear, or distress* (including facial expression and/or tone of voice)
- *Seeking interaction* (including nonverbal and verbal requests to play)
- *Stating concerns* (e.g., making a verbal statement about worries or asking for help)

Caregiving behaviors:

- *Verbal statements that incorporate empathy*: statements conveying that the meaning and feeling of a careseeker's communication has been understood
- Cross-modal nonverbal attunement:

  *"the therapist must be experienced at being in a state of vitalizing attunement to the patient, that is, the crescendos and decrescendos of the patient's affective state must be in resonance with similar states or crescendos and decrescendos, cross modally, of the therapist. (E.S. Wolf, personal communication, 1991, cited in Schore, 1994, p. 449)*

- *Providing comfort or actively relieving children's discomfort*: this includes physical and psychological comfort; for instance, providing a drink or providing structure by initiating breaks, regulating the overregulated child by setting limits in a calm manner; all *in response* to a child's careseeking cues.

Exploratory system/interest-sharing system activated (Note: interest sharing can be individual or realized together with the therapist):

- Sharing of views, experiences, or interests
- Engaging in play behavior
- Exploring the playroom environment
- Expressions of *pleasure, joy* (verbal and nonverbal, e.g., laughter, smiling)

Defensive behaviors:

- *Angry responses,* such as throwing toys around the room, challenging and breaking limits, verbal expressions of anger
- *Fearful behaviors,* such as tensing of body, trembling, hiding
- *Withdrawn responses,* including a lack of motivation to play
- *Distressed behaviors,* such as crying, self-soothing, increased chewing, etc.

Sexual system:

- Sexualized behavior
- Sexual talk

Within play therapy sessions, play therapists try to be responsive caregivers who are accepting and nondefensive. Thus play therapists try to provide optimal care to children in all contexts, including in response to children's defensive and careseeking systems being activated. Therapists intend that children will learn that their therapists will not react defensively when children's defensive systems are active and that their therapists are available to offer comfort and support when needed. With children who have serious attachment difficulties, their defensive system is likely to be highly active much of the time and their careseeking behaviors either indiscriminate or weakly expressed. As therapy progresses, it is hoped that a reduction in the frequency, intensity, and duration of their defensive systems being active will occur. This in turn will lead to an increase in children's appropriate careseeking behavior and greater activation of their exploratory system subsequently.

## Play Therapist's Attachment Style

The role of therapists' attachment styles is beginning to be acknowledged and researched (for example, see Meyer & Pilkonis, 2002; Rubino et al., 2000). As mentioned previously, therapists who use attachment-related concepts, particularly when working with children who have more serious attachment difficulties, will need to have an in-depth understanding of their own attachment-related behaviors and strategies. It is essential while writing up process notes and during clinical supervision that play therapists reflect on the five interrelated systems of the attachment dynamic and the presence or absence of the aforementioned behavior indicators in both the child they are helping and in themselves. For instance, how active the child's defense system was during the session is important to reflect on. This may take the form of the child avoiding the need for comfort. For example, a child may engage in a very active and challenging ball game with the therapist for much of the session, never following the therapist's increasingly strong suggestions to have a rest period, although the child seems exhausted. Therapists may usefully reflect on their own response to this defense within the interaction, being aware of their own attachment style. This is likely to include therapists' underlying personal reasons for their own strong emotional reactions in this situation, or it may evoke emotional detachment in this and other difficult interactions with children. Increased understanding may be gained through therapists' personal therapy and/or through further assessment of their own attachment style, including undertaking the ASI themselves. Clinical supervision and reflection using the dynamics of attachment also can assist therapists in maintaining a much-needed, nondefensive, collaborative stance.

## Applying Extended Attachment Theory to Working With Caregivers and Other Professionals

Working in partnership with carers is seen as an essential aspect of working therapeutically with children who have serious attachment difficulties. These children often try to create some measure of control over their lives and over adults with power over them by compartmentalizing their worlds into separate boxes. Psychopathological patterns easily extend to professional and care systems, if adults are not aware of these patterns, because the needs of these children are complex and not easily assuaged. Child therapists have an important role in helping carers understand and respond appropriately to children's disturbed attachment behavior (Ryan, 2004a).

Extended attachment theory can inform everyone's responses and decision making in these cases. For example, play therapists may be able to understand and respond more fully to carers' activation of their own defensive attachment behaviors with these children, without therapists having their own defensive or careseeking systems becoming activated with carers. By therapists meeting caregivers' careseeking needs, including using verbal statements incorporating empathy and nonverbal cross-modal attunement, play therapists will then be able to help carers to deactivate their defensive systems. This enables companionable relating along with exploratory and interest-sharing agendas to take precedence.

Beyond the child's immediate family system, working together with other professionals in the system around these children seems essential. This may include social workers, school staff, and fostering social workers. Applying the dynamics of attachment to these interrelated roles can help foster supportive companiable patterns of relating; see Ryan's (2004a) presentation of Delroy, a child with serious attachment difficulties.

Developing negotiating skills in the professionals and carers of children first is an essential element of helping children with serious attachment difficulties. Children need their carers to scaffold these skills for them, because their previous experiences of attachment relationships have been that they have had to highly activate their personal defense systems due to repeated experiences encompassing fear of abandonment, shaming, and/or dismissive or angry care. The function of their entire attachment system often has changed, due to these very destructive experiences, to seeking personal survival through either extremely dominant or compliant behavior toward others. Helping carers to compromise within the children's capacities and let go of confrontation and dominance/submission patterns is therefore essential and helpfully explained within extended attachment theory. In addition, establishing and increasing positive experiences children have is important both by providing the accepting and playful environment of NDPT and encouraging carers and schools to provide children with both structured and unstructured play experiences. Again extended attachment theory helps therapists understand that a high level of positive playful, exploratory experiences are needed by these children in order to help them activate their exploratory systems, which were previously dampened down and thwarted by extremely negative attachment experiences.

Helping carers to manage and contain conduct problems and hostile acts toward self and others also is often an important task in the therapeutic process. High levels of aggression can easily activate the carers' defense system, namely fear or anger. This is also a task within the therapy sessions themselves, along with helping children take the risk of communicating their needs. Therapists need to look for opportunities for closeness that children will allow and also promote this in carers' interactions with children. In NDPT there is a focus on what children see as important, which helps disconfirm children's feelings of low self-worth. The intent is to help children to deactivate their defensive systems and to engage in exploratory behavior, once their careseeking needs are allowed to be appropriately met.

## Ending NDPT

As previously argued (Ryan, 2004a), the aim of psychotherapy can be seen as the restoration of harmonious functioning of the five interrelated systems posited by Heard and Lake. A sense of well-being, an ability to care for self and others, and an ability to enjoy creative and intimate relationships is present as the goals of the five systems are met. Tracking the levels of activation of each system throughout the therapy process can help highlight when it is appropriate to end the therapy intervention. Positive changes in relationship themes, and in particular children's ability to relate in supportive-companiable ways, rather than dominant-submissive patterns the majority of the time, are clear indicators. As detailed earlier, during the intervention therapists aim to reduce the activation of the child's defense system and increase activation of their careseeking system, particularly for those children who fit the inhibited subtype, and their exploratory system. Readministering the story stem assessment procedure can provide further information on any changes to the child's internal working model and highlight remaining areas of difficulty. Decisions regarding whether it is possible to transfer to filial therapy to further enhance children's attachment relationships are also relevant to consider here.

## Case Example

The following case example illustrates how an effective individual NDPT intervention can be designed and carried out with a child who has significant attachment problems, using extended attachment theory to inform practice. The case illustration is based on a composite of a few of the first author's cases with similar characteristics, particularly with regard to their attachment styles and behavior. (All names and some circumstances have been altered to protect anonymity.)

## Background

Callum was referred for therapy by his school when he was 7 years old. His birth parents had separated when he was young. He and his older brother lived with their mother until Callum was 5. Callum's birth mother misused drugs and alcohol; a history of neglect along with exposure to violence and acrimony in adult relationships was documented. There were periods of abandonment, and on one occasion his mother went missing for several days. Callum was found by social workers hungry and disoriented, locked in a bedroom with his brother in the family home after two days. Both Callum and his brother were placed in kinship care, in separate family units. In Callum's placement with his aunt were three other cousins under the age of 5.

Callum was of great concern to his new family and to his school, where he was displaying very poor attention skills and overly high motor activity levels. He could be suddenly defiant and bullying toward other children and at other times withdrawn and inhibited with a fixed smile. His relatives also were very concerned, describing him as talking frequently but with little real content in his communication. Callum expressed superficial emotions and didn't cry. He gorged on food, licking and sucking up drinks from the cup and frequently stored away food and rubbish in his bedroom. He suffered from secondary enuresis. He self-harmed by hitting his head on the floor or wall regularly and had frequently expressed a wish to die to his aunt. Other intake information also showed that Callum was overly self-reliant and unable to express his feelings to his aunt, Mary, when situations arose that would have been highly anxiety producing (e.g., hurting his finger badly in a car door). Signs of trauma were also present.

It was apparent from the therapist's first meeting with Callum's carers, Mary and John, that they were overwhelmed by meeting the needs of their large family. Whilst Mary spoke warmly and fondly about Callum, it was clear that the demands on her were high. Callum's uncle, John, was the breadwinner of the family and was largely absent due to working long hours.

## Assessment: Home Visit

During the therapist's home visit to meet Callum, she observed that he was expressionless, and sat quietly. He appeared to want the therapist's and aunt's attention, but he quickly withdrew into picking at his nails when interrupted by his younger cousins. Mary was warm and encouraging to Callum during the visit. However, she was preoccupied with the needs of the younger children, and John was present for only part of the visit, seemingly exhausted from his day's work. He returned intermittently to ask Mary about arrangements for the evening meal and other matters. The therapist had brought along photographs of the playroom to help familiarize Callum with the play therapy environment. He took only fleeting glances at these and appeared disinterested. The therapist left them for Callum to look at in his own time with his relatives.

## Story Stem Assessment

Because there was only limited information about Callum's experiences while in his mother's care, it was useful to undertake this type of assessment at the beginning of the therapy intervention. The first author is trained in administering and rating this battery of story stems using Hodges et al.'s (2003) rating manual. It was decided that the assessment would take place in Callum's home because he was so inhibited during the initial visit. His therapist assessed it as unlikely that he would engage in the task at the clinic base.

Despite being in familiar surroundings, Callum was highly anxious at the beginning of the story stem assessment. He employed several avoidance maneuvers throughout the assessment, for instance, prematurely ending the stories before any resolution to the presented dilemma was indicated. Callum would often finish the story with a fixed smile and a formulaic statement that "they all lived happily ever after." He often asked the therapist what she thought happened next or simply replied that he "wasn't sure." For instance in the little pig stem the therapist enacted the little pig going for a walk, past all the other animals, and then realizing he was lost. The therapist asked Callum what happened next, but Callum said he didn't know. After prompting, Callum said the little pig did a somersault and then found a muddy puddle to roll in. Callum cut off from the story and began talking about school. The therapist directed him back to the story and asked if any of the other pigs knew he was missing. Callum shook his head and said, "Oh, but then he remembered the way and they all lived happily ever after."

Adults were represented as often being unaware of the child's needs, and there was an absence of affection and comfort from parent figures. There was a sense of helplessness in Callum's stories, and the child figure was unable to solve problems that arose in a realistic way. Representations of anger and aggression were almost entirely absent, and there was a theme of self-blame with a strong need to please others.

## Application of Extended Attachment Theory to Callum's Assessment

Callum's careseeking system seemed to be deactivated much of the time. On occasion he sought interaction with his aunt or the therapist in the home visit. However, this was easily disrupted, and he withdrew when his younger cousins interrupted. Thus his careseeking behavior was quickly overridden by his defense system. During the home visit, his therapist could see that despite being in Callum's own surroundings, his anxiety levels and therefore defense system was too highly activated for him to engage in exploratory behavior and look at the photos the therapist had brought with her. Therefore, she left the photos with Callum and his carer to enable them to look at them together when Callum was less anxious.

Further assessment of family interactions with a family play observation was not undertaken, partly because of resource constraints and the family's schedule. However, the home visit enabled the therapist to observe family interactions in an informal way. Mary's caregiving system was highly activated by the needs of her younger children and, while she was encouraging toward Callum, she was distracted and preoccupied by others' needs. John's care-seeking system appeared to be active due to being tired from work, and he too made demands on Mary. Thus both Mary and John were unavailable to Callum when his defensive system was activated, and he withdrew from interactions.

Callum's story stem assessment suggested that he was a child who was constricted and inhibited. He appeared to utilize avoidant defenses to keep himself safe and to ensure he did not become overwhelmed by emotion. The representation of the child figure was one of high self-reliance who did not expect adults to be aware of his needs or meet them with affection or comfort. The information from Callum's story stem assessment, along with information gathered from the referrer and carers, suggested Callum had a Type A style of relating or avoidant attachment style (Ainsworth et al., 1978). This and other intake information correlated with the DSM-IV category of attachment disorder of the inhibited type. Clearly there were indicators of trauma, and Callum's experiences could be analyzed through a trauma lens. While the effects of trauma in Callum's early years were considered during the assessment and intervention, as stated previously, for the purposes of this chapter the focus is on analyzing the case from an attachment perspective.

There were some indicators that Callum's exploratory system could be activated in play therapy because he was able to engage in the story stem task and enact what happened in some stories. However, this was often overridden by Callum's defense system as he avoided and withdrew from the story. A deactivated careseeking system was also apparent in the story stem assessment. Here the child figure was portrayed as not seeking care or help from adults when hurt, injured, or lost. Instead Callum withdrew from the stories, adding falsely positive endings, which again indicated an activated defense system.

It was clear from the assessment that Callum would need help expressing a full range of emotions appropriately, because his emotional expressions seemed confined to fixed smiles, increased activity levels when aroused emotionally, and hurting himself when distressed (James, 1994; Pearce & Pezzot-Pearce, 1997). Crittenden (2005) suggests that individuals with a Type A style of relating are likely to benefit from interventions that are focused on feelings and somatic representation of feelings. And one of the values of working in NDPT with highly avoidant children is that the children set their own pace for increasing their emotional involvement with their therapists, thus minimizing their fearful and withdrawing responses. It was hoped that

NDPT, with its focus on children's affect states and attention to understanding and integrating children's experiences on a bodily level, would provide an optimal environment for Callum to develop new, healthier ways of relating to adults in close relationships. In our experience for avoidant children like Callum, concentrating first on nonthreatening positive affects in a low-key manner is important (e.g., "You have a little smile about that.").

Filial therapy (see VanFleet, 1999) or some form of joint play therapy may have allowed Callum to develop stronger attachment relationships in his new family, while he processed earlier traumatic events and learned new ways of relating to adults. It was apparent from the therapist's assessment that such an approach was not emotionally and practically possible for the family system to engage in. Mary was overwhelmed with meeting the careseeking needs of all four children. In addition, some of the traumatic experiences Callum may have begun to work through in play therapy may have been overwhelming emotionally for her to witness. It was likely that Callum may have begun to exhibit out-of-control behaviors as he connected with his inner experiences.

The ASI was not administered with Mary because of resource constraints and her own lack of opportunity. However, some of the questions from the ASI were incorporated by the therapist into the initial carer interview. This suggested that, although Mary had some practical support from her husband John, her emotional support system was limited. The therapist thought it was likely that Callum's defensive maladaptive behaviors in therapy would activate Mary's own defense system. With significant demands on Mary's caregiving system, and low levels of support to meet Mary's own careseeking needs, the therapist assessed that Callum's needs would be best met in individual therapy. A fairly high level of contact with the carers to support them with Callum's behavior and to help them understand and respond to his attachment needs outside of the therapy sessions was also indicated.

## Treatment Plan

Unfortunately, Mary and John felt unable to commit to additional trips to the therapy center on a regular basis for face-to-face consultations. Therefore, long-term weekly individual therapy for Callum, alongside biweekly fortnightly telephone consultations with Mary were agreed upon. These consultations would include helping Mary to understand Callum's attachment difficulties, developing her responses in order to increase attachment behavior in Callum, and fostering activities to engender attachment between Mary and Callum. In addition, the therapist planned to hold bimonthly meetings with Mary, and John where possible, along with school staff and Callum's social worker. Mary talked with Callum about this plan, and in Callum's first session, the therapist also told Callum that she would be talking to Mary on the phone to share ideas about how to help him at home. Longer term the therapist still hoped it might be possible to move from delivering individual play therapy to involving Mary more actively in the intervention.

*Initial Play Therapy Sessions (First Four Months)*

Callum had appeared cut off from his feelings and bodily sensations during the assessment. This was borne out in his initial therapy sessions, where he repeatedly said he could not feel any pain or denied being hurt when he banged himself as he darted around the playroom. His therapist frequently made empathic reflections that Callum was telling her that he was brave and strong, while congruently expressing concern for Callum and reflecting on how fast and rough he was with his body. She set limits to ensure that Callum did not seriously injure himself.

Callum was highly active in these initial sessions, seemingly unable to relax and flitting from one activity to another, anxious that he would miss out on something if he did not move on. Even though his aunt waited in the nearby waiting room during his sessions, Callum frequently mentioned that his carer would have wanted to go out to the shops while he was having his session, appearing emotionally flat and matter of fact when talking about this. During a telephone consultation with Mary, the therapist discussed this with Mary. Mary interpreted Callum's communication as an indication that he did not need her and saw it as an opportunity to go to the local shops. The therapist was warm and caring in her response to Mary, acknowledging the potential rejection Mary felt after the effort she was making to wait nearby for Callum. The therapist impressed on Mary the importance of her waiting in the waiting area near the room for the entire session, in order to help Callum to begin to expect that she would be available for him physically and emotionally, unlike the earlier care he had experienced. The therapist requested that Mary sit in the same place each week, specifically the sofa opposite the glass door through to the long corridor down to the playroom. This would enable Callum to see her immediately when he came out of his session, and if he needed to use the toilet. The therapist highlighted the importance of this transition period and explained to Mary that this increased predictability and concrete availability of his primary attachment figure was likely to help him to relax. Mary was open and accepting of this request, understanding more fully the reasons behind this request.

To begin with, Callum engaged in child-object interactions in a rather perfunctory way. He used objects such as the soccer ball but did not engage with his therapist. There was a lack of playfulness and a seriousness in his manner. Callum would pick up things in the playroom, briefly look at them curiously, and then quickly reject them. His therapist took these opportunities to not only reflect Callum's uncertainty, but also to respond playfully. For instance, Callum picked up a toy tea cup, and his therapist said, "Hmm, tea for us to drink. I'll have two sugars." She proceeded to add pretend sugar to another cup and took a sip. Callum looked at his therapist, still uncertain, and she stopped this play, saying "But you can choose most things to do here." This comment seemed to allow Callum to move onto drawing a pattern over and over again on his paper. However, the following week Callum showed further curiosity in the tea set, and a couple of weeks on, he handed the cup to his therapist and smirked slightly as his therapist pretended to take a sip and mentioned that Callum was enjoying this play a bit.

Issues highlighted in the story stem, such as a high level of self-reliance, alongside a sense of helplessness, were evident early on in the play therapy intervention. These two themes seemed highly contradictory. On the one hand, Callum would determinedly set about tasks that required adult help, for instance, moving furniture in the playroom. On the other hand, he would sit at the art table appearing listless and heavy, seeming helpless and requesting that his therapist choose what he did, or insisting she draw a circle as he was sure his own would not be good enough.

While Callum began to engage in some joint play in his early sessions, this initially only centered on soccer. In his 12th session, there was a turning point. A student therapist was observing the session through the one-way mirror, as Callum and the adults had agreed. As the therapist made reflections about them both trying hard to keep their soccer goals safe, Callum initiated making a den where they couldn't be seen or heard and would "feel safe." His therapist was responsive to this opportunity for closeness, looking into the den and showing an interest in it. Callum subsequently invited his therapist to crawl inside. Callum related to his therapist in a conspiratorial and caring manner, and his therapist had the distinct feeling she was likely to be playing Callum's brother, hiding from the student who was embodying the birth mother in Callum's imagination.

At home Callum's enuresis continued. During telephone consultations, the therapist learned that Mary was punitive toward Callum's behavior. She felt that the behavior was purposeful, believing that he was old enough to control himself, particularly as she experienced him as so self-reliant in other respects. The therapist empathized with Mary's situation and the amount of practical caretaking tasks she had with three younger children along with Callum. The therapist helped Mary to see that Callum's enuresis was likely to be anxiety based. Mary immediately identified that she was increasing Callum's anxiety through her responses, and she became committed to responding in a non-punitive way when enuresis occurred and to providing additional structure to support Callum with toileting.

Mary also found Callum's level of hyperactivity very difficult to deal with, and her concern for her younger children's safety was evident. With Callum's therapist, Mary was able to explore this fear and the subsequent impact this had on her responses to Callum. This enabled Mary to think of ways to allow Callum space to "run off energy" and set limits for him in a calm, rather than angry, manner. The therapist also concentrated on how to deal with Callum's self-harming behaviors and suicidal ideation in these early consultations. She advised Mary to be proactive in her caregiving of Callum when he was hitting his head, despite messages from Callum that what he was doing did not hurt. Mary learned to provide cushions to keep Callum safe and to direct him to squeeze and throw soft balls instead. Callum frequently said he wanted to die in a forlorn voice, and he occasionally drew explosions or planes crashing, saying that he was dead in the picture. At these times, Mary told Callum not to say horrible things and told him not to draw things that weren't nice. The therapist provided Mary with a space to explore her own feelings and the fears these drawings evoked in her. In particular, Mary's sense of responsibility for Callum was compounded by the fact that he was not her biological son. Mary recognized that she tried to cope with Callum's "big feelings" by shutting them out. She tried to avoid them for fear of them happening, if she allowed Callum to talk about them. Mary resolved to attend to Callum when he expressed these feelings and become proactive in explicitly expressing her care and love for him.

*Discussion and Application of Extended Attachment to Callum's Early Sessions*
His high level of anxiety and dissociation during initial sessions suggested that Callum's defensive system was activated much of the time. His therapist was proactive in asserting and expressing verbally and nonverbally her wish for caregiving by congruently sharing her concern for him despite his messages that he was fine. Callum was not able to relax enough or experience a sense of security that would enable exploration. His emotional self-defense system seemed to be highly activated all of the time. Despite Mary waiting nearby, Callum appeared unable to use Mary as a safe base. Initially Mary felt that Callum did not need her. Mary's defense system seemed to be activated by his behavior, and her own avoidant tendencies seemed to lead to her disconnecting from her own feelings of rejection.

The therapist's caregiving toward Mary enabled Mary to explore her feelings with the therapist. Mary's defense system was acquiesced, and her exploratory system was activated. The therapist raised Mary's awareness of Callum's needs for predictability and consistency, despite the lack of careseeking cues from Callum to indicate this need. This activated Mary's caregiving system, and she consistently showed Callum that she was available to him during that time by her readiness to respond to him whenever he left the playroom. Consultation regarding Callum's behavior in the home setting seemed to provide Mary with the support she needed (therapist caregiving), and to thereby lessen her defensive responses of fear, anger, and withdrawal toward Callum, and instead activate her caregiving system. The therapist also was able to prevent Callum from engaging in hostile acts in the playroom (e.g., attempting to kick the ball as hard as possible at the therapist) and to teach Mary how to do this also without becoming punitive. The therapist achieved this herself in the playroom by taking responsibility for her own care needs and those of Callum, and by role modeling self-respect and keeping safe.

Children with attachment difficulties often have difficulty in engaging in child-object-therapist interactions. In NDPT therapists are trained to respond quickly and appropriately to even a slightly playful overture initiated by children, conveying by their manner that they are ready to enter into the playful spirit at children's discretion (Newson, 1992). When Callum displayed a small amount of curiosity in his play, the therapist recognized that Callum's exploratory system had become active to engage playfully. However, his un-certain expression indicated that he could not maintain exploration. The therapist interpreted this as a careseeking cue and actively tried to relieve Callum's discomfort by emphasizing that it was his choice what to do in the playroom. His subsequent engagement in repetitive drawing, rather than exploration, appeared to be self-soothing. Over time, Callum started maintaining engagement of his exploratory system for longer periods, with the therapist being mindful of proceeding at Callum's pace.

When Callum interacted directly with his therapist, he seemed to engage in dominant/submissive relating (Heard & Lake, 1997) rather than a companionable style. He was either submissive and helpless, as demonstrated in the previous example, or domineering in taking on the adult role. In later sessions during competitive games, Callum became fiercely determined to win and to be the strongest and most powerful. It was important that the therapist remained consistently available during this play, but she did not take up a submissive role during these games or assume the dominant role by rescuing Callum when he acted helpless. It became clear that developmentally Callum had a strong sense of inadequacy, which led the therapist to revise her treatment goals to include Callum increasing both his competence and his sense of self-worth (Denham, 1998); both features are thought to be inherent in an NDPT approach (e.g., Josefi & Ryan, 2004).

With children who have serious attachment difficulties, particularly the inhibited type, actively looking for opportunities for closeness by therapists and carers is crucial, as is being highly attuned to the level of affect such children can tolerate. Callum's construction of a den provided one such opportunity for connection, and the therapist appropriately showed her interest in this new play. It appeared that Callum felt safe enough with his therapist at this point that he risked inviting her into the den. However once she was inside, Callum became highly agitated and unable to relax (defense system activated), perhaps being reminded of some of his previous, highly traumatic experiences.

*Middle Sessions (5 to 15 Months)*
Callum would frequently become annoyed with himself during this phase in play therapy. If Callum felt he had done something poorly, he would hit himself over the head with a hard object. His therapist set therapeutic limits on this behavior, telling Callum that she could see he was frustrated, but that she needed to keep him safe. Callum would deny the hits hurt him and repeat these hostile acts, saying "It doesn't matter, it's only my head." His therapist remained consistent in setting limits on this behavior and ensured he did not come to any harm. She congruently shared that he didn't care about his head but she did, and she needed to look after all of him. At other times, Callum would delight in throwing balls to the therapist. He made this game more and more challenging and requested that the therapist close her eyes as he threw a hard, bouncy ball for her to catch. The therapist again set limits on this behavior and reflected that she cared about herself and did not want to get hurt.

Callum was also hypervigilant to any changes in the playroom; even a miniature on the shelf being placed an inch to the left from one session to the next would attract Callum's attention and comment. To increase Callum's sense of security, his therapist took particular care over maintaining a consistent atmosphere. But the therapist also was congruent when small changes occurred despite her efforts, helping Callum to recognize his feelings of discomfort and to find his own solutions to her imperfections in his eyes. Callum soon began personalizing the room on each visit, rearranging the furniture to his preference. As the sessions progressed, Callum would take either a toilet break or a break to get a drink from the water cooler in the waiting room, seemingly to check on his carer's presence. The therapist noticed, and pointed out to Callum that he always appeared to return to the playroom with a smile, and was a little more relaxed in his body, once he had seen Mary.

Callum frequently engaged in drawing or painting during these sessions, repeatedly denigrating his efforts. His therapist reflected how he wasn't pleased with what he had done, even though he had been concentrating hard and done his best. Some weeks Callum did not draw or paint but spent his time pouring out the paints and mixing them. He expressed pleasure and excitement at the paint changing color, which was the strongest positive emotion he had expressed in his sessions to date. Another source of positive feelings was his sense of competence at soccer, recognized and reflected by his therapist as they played together.

Callum remained hyperactive and impulsive in his play during these sessions, and he often sped down the corridor back to Mary at the end of the session. The therapist decided to introduce 5 minutes of quiet time at the end of his therapy sessions, with Callum still afforded play choices, albeit more limited ones, within this time. The therapist told Callum that in quiet time there was no fast, messy, or noisy play. It was hoped that this formal structure would help Callum to regulate his emotions before returning to Mary. At first Callum found it impossible to slow down during this time. The therapist persisted and had to offer a range of suggestions for play during this time to him. Over time Callum showed more and more interest in working out together with his therapist whether certain types of play were fast, noisy, or messy and taking pleasure in the one he chose to end his session.

Callum also began to acknowledge bumps to his body when they happened in the playroom and even began showing his therapist grazes on his elbows and knees that he had received playing soccer at school. However, initially Callum would deny that the scrapes caused him any pain, and he fervently carried on the game of soccer with a bright and cheery demeanor. Subsequently, following the therapist's own supervision described more as follows, she was able to persistently acknowledge Callum's hurts and her own vulnerabilities, such as being too tired to carry on playing a physical game. The therapist began congruently communicating her need for a rest by both verbally articulating this and expressing this on a bodily level. Slowly Callum allowed himself to rest at the same time as the therapist, although he remained hyper-alert. He would lie down on the floor but spring up at the slightest sound. The therapist continued reflecting how hard it was for him to let his body relax, that he liked his body going fast because it made him feel safe and in charge of what happened next. The therapist reflected how her body felt when they had been playing fast games, commenting on her fast heartbeat and hot red cheeks, using gestures to accompany her verbal articulation. She also described how she relaxed her body, when Callum started watching her responses, saying that first of all she let her arms go limp, again modeling for him the ways in which her mind actively ensured that her body relaxed. At first Callum denied any changes happening to his body, simply stating that his heart always went fast. Keeping to Callum's pace, his therapist did not stress relaxation techniques and only mentioned them when Callum appeared to be noticing her responses.

Playfully creating dens increased for Callum during these middle sessions. For a long period, separate dens were made as army bases, and Callum wanted to have battles, with his therapist playing the other army. Callum would gather all the best weapons for his den. His therapist gathered medical supplies and food and drink as well as leftover weapons, reflecting that she thought she might need these things to look after herself. Callum rejected any need for these objects himself, preferring to emphasize his strength instead. As the weeks progressed and Callum allowed his army to own being hurt, his therapist commented that it looked like they needed some extra supplies to take care of them, offering some of her food and medicine. It seemed a breakthrough once again, when Callum accepted these from her. This later developed into Callum inviting his therapist to help him make his den stronger, and subsequently to join him in his den, and fight together against the army "out there."

Callum also began processing his traumatic experiences through play during this period. Some weeks the dens were not army bases but a place to hide. In the den Callum would cower and then want to keep busy. The therapist seemed to have been put in the sibling role, playing games inside the den with Callum, but remaining hypervigilant to sounds outside. The den was bare to begin with, but after several enactments the therapist wondered aloud if there were things she could take in there to help them feel safer. Slowly Callum decided to add things to the den, including cushions, blankets, books, and food.

However in other behaviors and play, Callum showed that he was unable to regulate himself and unable to accept caregiving. For example, his therapist provided Callum with a biscuit and drink every week. At first Callum would gobble up the biscuit as fast as possible and lapped up his drink with his tongue. He would hide both his own and his therapist's drink in safe places in the playroom. In his imaginative play, Callum would harm the baby doll, kicking it or telling it to shut up. The baby was left alone crying in a corner of the playroom. The therapist reflected Callum's angry feelings toward the baby, while congruently sharing worried feelings about the baby, and the need for a mommy to look after the baby. Callum would shout out: "He don't need no one! He can look after himself!" The therapist commented: "Baby is just small. You don't think he needs anyone. He's stopped crying now and wants to look after himself. I think he really needs a mommy, somebody big, to look after him. But I don't see any mommy there for him." Eventually, to the therapist's inner delight, Callum allowed his therapist to hold the baby, and she was able to model caring and appropriate responses to the baby.

At home during this period, Callum's angry feelings toward his younger siblings became more overt and he began purposefully kicking and hitting them. Callum also was becoming more defiant toward Mary and John, shouting and throwing things, alternating with helpless, regressed behavior, such as asking Mary what to do next at each stage of getting dressed for school in the morning. The therapist reframed this defiance as Callum becoming less avoidant and more able to show his feelings. The therapist explored with Mary ways to help Callum negotiate more effectively and harness this ability to express his feelings in a healthy way. At this time there was also a productive meeting with Callum's social worker and class teacher to explore ways of helping Callum.

*Application of Extended Attachment to Callum's Middle Sessions*
As suggested in Ryan and Courtney (2009), Callum seemed to benefit from his therapist being open and transparent in articulating her genuine feelings. It was helpful for the therapist to hold in mind the reasons for the falsely upbeat avoidant style that Callum exhibited and to discuss the effects of Callum's history of neglect, his need for self-reliance, and possible dissociation from pain and care needs in order to respond in the most helpful way during interactions in the playroom. Furthermore, exploration of the therapist's own attachment style and her own tendency toward self-reliance strategies, which developed at the same age as Callum, highlighted the potential she had to minimize Callum's careseeking needs. Callum was fast and unrelenting in his play. It was physically demanding for the therapist and hard for her to keep up with Callum's demanding expectations of himself. The therapist's supervisor undertook a caretaking role, encouraging the therapist to reflect to Callum that she could see that she had to look after herself. This led the therapist to deciding to take breaks during physical play, despite her inner drive to keep going (therapist's defense system), and to reflect to Callum that she was resting, because she could see that Callum would just keep going and going. This slowly enabled Callum to take breaks also, although at this stage his defense system would not allow him to truly relax. He remained hypervigilant, which seemed to highlight his persistent, underlying level of fear. When Callum's defense system was acquiesced momentarily, the therapist took these small opportunities to describe her own bodily sensations and perhaps bring to Callum's awareness the potential for his own body to relax. However, Callum could not tolerate too many comments; his defense system (fear) would reactivate, because he seemed to need to maintain a fast-paced body in which he could feel in control of any unexpected event.

As argued at the beginning of this chapter (see Ryan & Wilson, 1995), the consistency offered by the play environment mimics the normal child's stable atmosphere and is conducive to promoting a sense of security. To begin with, even this high level of consistency was not enough for Callum. However, through repeated reflection of Callum's discomfort in the room, this anxious careseeking behavior began to reduce. Callum began moving things around himself, activating his exploratory system more frequently and a little more freely. In addition, the therapist disconfirmed Callum's feelings of low self-worth by concentrating on what seemed important to Callum (e.g., the changing paint color, his soccer skills), thus sharing interest with Callum based on what he perceived as important. Here Callum's exploratory system could remain active without being inhibited by his defense system, which still became active when drawing or painting, as he became overwhelmed by a sense of inadequacy.

The importance of Callum's attachment to his brother, which first became evident in Callum's den play, became clearer in these further play sequences. The therapist talked to Callum about her intended feedback to his carers and social worker at a review meeting, regarding the importance of maintaining contact with his brother. Callum allowed the therapist to share this need to see his brother, which helped inform decisions regarding contact arrangements. Working together with carers and professionals in children's lives is essential in helping children with attachment difficulties. These meetings enabled the therapist to share attachment concepts and reframe Callum's changing behavior to others. Working in this collaborative manner enabled the adults around Callum to maintain an accepting and nondefensive attitude toward the changes in his behavior. His teacher, social worker, and carers were galvanized to promote ways of negotiating and compromising.

*Later Sessions (16 to 24 Months)*

Dens appeared again in these later sessions; however, the armies had disappeared, and shared play with the therapist inside the den became more frequent. For one session, Callum brought a puppet from home, which seemed important for his therapist to accept and allow into the session. During this session, Callum said they were to pretend that the puppet was mum. After pounding on the puppet, Callum threw it out of the den and curled up next to his therapist, stroking the soft blanket against his cheek. His therapist was asked to read him a bedtime story, which he'd brought into the den himself. This play became part of Callum's routine, and each week Callum would return to the den and suggest things he'd like in the den to feel "safe and comfy."

Callum's ability to self-regulate and allow his body to relax also became more evident. He would initiate quiet time himself, often 10 minutes before the session ended. Finding his own preferred activity in this time seemed important. Callum chose to sit at the art table mixing paints in an interested and engaged manner; this seemed to have a soothing effect on Callum. Callum commented himself on how calm he was now when drawing. He excitedly told Mary about this at the end of one of his sessions, and the therapist talked with Mary and with Callum's teacher about how they could incorporate drawing time for Callum at home and school. The therapist highlighted that although this was a method Callum had discovered at this stage, he needed adults to structure this time and be proactive in making it available to him, especially when he could become agitated.

Callum was more creative when he played games during sessions, initiating imaginative and playful elements into the games, such as both he and his therapist becoming frogs or crabs trying out different walks, a game they both found funny. The focus of the games shifted from a powerful desire to win and be the strongest to developing skills; the theme of competence and skill building began to be most prevalent. Callum shared new soccer tricks, creative new rules for games, and dance routines with his therapist. He spent increasing amounts of time in these activities. His ideas for play in quiet time continued to increase, and he developed a wide repertoire to draw from. Callum developed ritualized games together with his therapist in the playroom, such as hide-and-seek, playing guessing games such as hiding objects behind their backs, or tracing a letter on one another's backs. A favorite game was Grandmother's footsteps. The therapist had to play grandma sleeping with her back to Callum, while he tried to creep up behind grandma. The third week of playing this, Callum threw his arms around grandma when he arrived and said "That was so much fun!" with a wide smile.

In these later sessions, Callum confidently walked around the room in a relaxed fashion with his eyes closed. He occasionally stopped just inches away from chairs or tables and proudly stated "I know this room like the back of my hand." The therapist noticed that she too felt relaxed on a bodily level, very unlike earlier sessions where the therapist had noted strong tension in her body as Callum hurtled around the room, seemingly uncaring of any potential injury to himself. During active play Callum would now take breaks, flopping down and enjoying his therapist getting a cushion and blanket for him to fully relax. In one of these later sessions, Callum turned off the lights and closed the curtains in the playroom, making it darker than usual. He lay down on his back, resting his head on his therapist's shin, and closing his eyes. His therapist commented that she could see he wanted to be close to her and was trying to get comfy, but she knew her shins were hard for his head. She offered to put a cushion under his head or have him sit next to her. He chose to move up lying flat on his back with the therapist's thigh as his cushion, he closed his eyes, and he began breathing slowly and rhythmically. His therapist commented that he felt safe even though it was darker and that she felt glad that she was there looking after him.

Callum seemed to have made a good deal of progress in his therapy sessions. Discussion with Mary and Callum's school highlighted that he had made significant progress at home and at school. They reported a decrease in defiant and oppositional behavior, discontinuation of self-harm and suicidal ideation, and his peer/sibling relationships had improved, although there were still some difficulties there. His therapist decided it would be helpful to readminister the story stem assessment to record any change in a more systematic manner. Pleasingly this revealed that Callum was able to represent figures expressing anger and aggression, and these representations were mainly in a coherent manner rather than at the extreme. Adult figures were now represented as being more aware of a child's needs and able to offer help and protection. The child figure was shown to receive help from other child figures and was more able to problem solve. These all pointed to a more secure style of relating than Callum had at the beginning of the intervention. However, in the story stems there was still a very low level of adults actively showing comfort and affection to a child.

Readministering the story stem assessment reinforced the therapist's decision to bring therapy to an end. However, it also highlighted Callum's need to change his relationship with Mary into one that was more intimate and satisfying for both of them. At this point his therapist decided that involving Mary in Callum's final set of sessions was likely to help Callum generalize to everyday life the advances he had made within the therapeutic relationship. And importantly, it would support Mary directly in actively responding to Callum's relatively weak careseeking cues. Despite Mary's willingness, in the consultation sessions, to try putting the therapist's suggestions into place at home, the stronger careseeking demands of the other children and Mary struggling to read Callum's small invitations meant that this was not cultivated.

Therefore, the therapist spent time preparing Mary for taking part in Callum's sessions and provided her with in-the-moment cues to respond to with Callum in the playroom. The therapist had to arrange childcare and provided Mary with debriefing sessions following each joint session with Callum, but Mary was now able to make this time commitment because she had been very encouraged by Callum's progress and because it was to be a time-limited committment. As a result of these final sessions, Mary developed a greater capacity to respond supportively to Callum, since Callum's defensive strategies had greatly reduced. Callum's therapist also helped Mary work out when in the day she was able to give 10 minutes of special one-to-one time to Callum, once his therapy had ended, while consultations for Mary with his therapist continued for a time.

*Application of Extended Attachment to Callum's Later Sessions*
Callum seemed much more attuned to his own careseeking needs in these later sessions. He could allow himself to be tired and request care from the therapist by bringing in stories for the therapist to read in the den, and he was able to overtly show a need for closeness with his therapist. The therapist was highly responsive to these cues and was active in caregiving, accepting Callum's need for closeness and making him comfortable both physically and emotionally. She used a soft, warm voice during these moments, which seemed to reassure him that she was there while he had his eyes closed. The games Callum developed in quiet time all promoted face-to-face interactions, eye contact, positive safe touch, and play-fulness in interactions (Ryan & Wilson, 1995), most of which were created by Callum, with his therapist following his lead. There were also clear indicators that Callum's exploratory system was active more frequently during these later sessions. As described, games such as soccer shifted in focus from dominant/ submissive themes to skill building, competence, and mutual and companion-able interest sharing (Heard & Lake, 1999).

The therapist continued to collaborate with other important adults in Callum's life during this period and encouraged them to maintain active care-giving for Callum. The therapist was aware of the importance of enhancing Callum's attachment relationship with his primary caregiver and ensuring that this was not undermined by the relationship he had built with her. Mary, as his carer, would be able to have direct guidance in responding to Callum's attach-ment overtures, because her caregiving system would not be activated with any of her other younger children during sessions. The ultimate goal of inviting Mary into the last play therapy sessions was to enable her to meet Callum's needs appropriately in the child-carer relationship. The therapist was able to take on a caregiving role toward Mary and help her to notice opportunities to meet Callum's careseeking needs.

## Conclusion

Callum's case has been used in this chapter to illustrate the demanding, and many times rewarding, features of play therapy with children who have serious attachment difficulties. The suggestions given in this chapter for working with such children in NDPT by integrating attachment theory show that attachment thinking needs to be applied from the outset, helping to inform therapists' thinking and practice throughout complex interventions in NDPT. In particular, application of extended attachment theory provides greater understanding and clarity of the complex intra- and interpersonal dynamics of the child, therapist, carer, and professionals involved with the child. Taking into consideration the activation of not only the child's but also the adult's attachment systems and how they interact arguably enhances the effectiveness of the therapeutic intervention. This is not only applicable to complex cases with children who have serious attachment problems.

Indeed, for all NDPT practice, as argued at the outset, relationships are at the heart of therapy, and attachment theory and extended attachment theory can usefully be integrated with informed and sensitive NDPT practice. However, it is recognized that the need to work from an attachment framework in collaboration with carers and professionals is essential when working with children with serious attachment difficulties, because their disturbed attachment behavior and patterns of relating easily extend to the system around them. As Callum's case has illustrated, play therapists need to create an optimal environment of sensitive caregiving, not only within the playroom but *beyond*, thereby encompassing important figures in all areas of the child's life.

## References

Achenbach, T. M. (1991). *Manual for the Child Behaviour Checklist 4-18 and 1991 Profile.* Burlington: University of Vermont, Department of Psychology.

Ainsworth, M. D. S., Blehar, M. C., Waters, E., & Wall, S. (1978). *Patterns of attachment: A Psychological study of the Strange Situation.* Hillsdale, NJ: Erlbaum.

American Psychiatric Association. (2000). *Diagnostic and statistical manual of mental disorders* (4th ed., text revision; DSM-IV-TR). Washington, DC: American Psychiatric Association.

Axline, V. (1989). *Play therapy.* London, England: Churchill Livingston.

Bifulco, A. (2002). Attachment style measurement: A clinical and epidemiological perspective. *Attachment and Human Development, 4,* 180–188.

Bowlby, J. (1969). *Attachment and loss: Attachment* (Vol. 1) London, England: Pimlico.

Bowlby, J. (1980). *Attachment and loss: Loss, sadness and depression.* London, England: Pimlico.

Bowlby, J. (1988). *A secure base: Parent-child attachment and healthy human development.* Oxon, England: Routledge.

Bratton, S. C., Ray, D., Rhine, T., & Jones, L. (2005). The efficacy of play therapy with children: A meta-analytic review of treatment outcomes. *Professional Psychology: Research and Practice, 36*(4), 376–390.

Bretherton, I., & Munholland, K. A. (1999). Internal working models in attachment relationships: A construct revisited. In J. Cassidy & P. R. Shaver (Eds.), *Handbook of attachment: Theory, research, and clinical applications* (pp. 89–114). New York, NY: Guilford Press.

Crane, J. (2001). The parents' part in the play therapy process. In G. L. Landreth (Ed.), *Innovations in play therapy: Issues, process, and special populations* (pp. 83–98). Philadelphia, PA: Bruner-Routledge.

Crittenden, P. M. (1995). Attachment and psychopathology. In S. Goldberg, R. Muir, & J. Kerr (Eds.), *John Bowlby's attachment theory: Historical, clinical and social significance* (pp. 367–406). New York, NY: Analytic Press.

Crittenden, P. M. (2005). Attachment theory, psychopathology, and psychotherapy: The Dynamic maturational approach. *Psicoterpia, 30,* 171–182.

Crittenden, P. M. (2010). Preface: Pathways forward. *Clinical Child Psychology and Psychiatry, 15*(3), 299–302.

Denham, S. A. (1998). *Emotional development in young children.* London, England: Guilford.

George, C., Kaplan, N., & Main, M. (1984). Adult Attachment Interview Protocol. Unpublished manuscript, University of California at Berkeley.

Guerney, B. (1964). Filial therapy: Description and rationale. *Journal of Consulting Psychology, 28*(4), 304–310.

Guerney, L. (2001). Child-centered play therapy. *International Journal of Play Therapy, 10*(2), 13–31.

Heard, D. (1982). Family systems and the attachment dynamic. *Journal of Family Therapy, 4,* 99–116.

Heard, D., & Lake, B. (1997). *The challenge of attachment for caregiving.* London, England: Routledge.

Heard, D., & Lake, B. (1999). The attachment dynamic: Core concepts. Paper presented at the Dynamics of Attachment Conference, The University of York, England.

Heard, D., & Lake, B. (2001). Empathic attunement and the attachment system: The contemporary relevance of attachment theory.

Paper presented at the First International Attachment Network, London, England.

Hill, A. (2005). Patterns of non-offending parental involvement in therapy with sexually abused children. *Journal of Social Work, 5* (3), 339–358.

Hodges, J., Steele, M., Hillman, S., & Henderson, K. (2003). Mental representations and defenses in severely maltreated children: A story stem battery and rating system for clinical assessment and research applications. In R. N. Emde, D. P. Wolf, & D. Oppenheim (Eds.), *Revealing the inner worlds of young children: The MacArthur story stem battery and parent-child narratives* (pp. 240–267). Oxford, England: Oxford University Press.

Hunter, J. (2003 unpublished). *An attachment perspective of the relationships within filial therapy.* University of York, England.

Irwin, E. C. (2000). The use of a puppet interview to understand children. In K. Gitlin-Weiner & A. Sandgrund (Eds.), *Play diagnosis and assessment* (pp. 682–704). New York, NY: Wiley.

Jäger, J., (2010 unpublished). *Experts in play: Exploring the development and use of play-based evaluation methods in facilitating children's views of non-directive play therapy.* Doctoral dissertation, The University of York, England.

James, B. (1994). *Handbook for treatment of attachment-trauma problems in children.* New York, NY: Lexington Books.

Josefi, O., & Ryan, V. (2004). Non-directive play therapy for young children with autism: A case study. *Clinical Child Psychology and Psychiatry, 9*(4), 533–551.

Landreth, G. L. (2002). Therapeutic limit setting in the play therapy relationship. *Professional Psychology: Research and Practice, 33*(6), 529–535.

Landreth, G. L., & Bratton, S. C. (2005). *Child-Parent Relationship Therapy (CPRT): A 10-session filial therapy model.* New York, NY: Routledge.

Main, M., & Solomon, J. (1986). Discovery of a new, insecure-disorganized/disoriented attachment pattern. In T. B. Brazelton & M. Yogman (Eds.), *Affective development in infancy* (pp. 95–124). Norwood, NJ: Ablex.

McCluskey, U. (2005). *To be met as a person: The dynamics of attachment in professional encounters.* London, England: Karnac.

McCluskey, U., Hooper, C., & Miller, L. B. (1999). Goal-corrected empathic attunement: Developing and rating the concept within an attachment perspective. *Psychotherapy, 36*(1), 80–90.

Mearns, D., & Thorne, B. (2000). *Person-centered therapy today: New frontiers in theory and practice.* London, England: Sage.

Meyer, B., and Pilkonis, P. A. (2002). Attachment style. In J. Norcross (Ed.), *Psychotherapy relations that work: Therapist's contributions and responsiveness to patients* (pp. 367–382). New York, NY: Oxford University Press.

Newson, E. (1992). The barefoot play therapist: Adapting skills for a time of need. In D. Lane & A. Miller (Eds.), *The handbook of child and adolescent therapy* (pp. 89–107). Berkshire, England: Open University Press.

O'Sullivan, L., & Ryan, V. (2009). Therapeutic limits from an attachment perspective. *Clinical Child Psychology and Psychiatry, 14*(2), 215–235.

Pearce, J. W., & Pezzot-Pearce, T. D. (1997). *Psychotherapy of abused and neglected children.* London, England: Guilford.

Rogers, C. R. (1951). *Client-centered therapy.* London, England: Constable.

Ross, P. (2000). The family puppet technique for assessing parent-child and family interaction patterns. In K. Gitlin-Weiner & A. Sandgrund (Eds.), *Play diagnosis and assessment* (pp. 672–681). New York, NY: Wiley.

Rubino, G., Barker, C., Roth, T., & Fearon, P. (2000). Therapist empathy and depth of interpretation in response to potential alliance ruptures: The role of therapist and patient attachment styles. *Psychotherapy Research, 10*(4), 408–420.

Ryan, V. (2001). Home visiting and play therapists. In H. G. Kaduson & C. E. Schaefer (Eds.), *101 more play therapy techniques* (pp. 412–416). New York, NY: Jason Aronson.

Ryan, V. (2004a). Adapting non-directive play therapy for children with attachment disorders. *Clinical Child Psychology and Psychiatry, 9*(1), 75–87.

Ryan, V. (2004b). 'My New Mum': How drawing can help children rework their internal models of attachment relationships in non-directive play therapy. *British Journal of Play Therapy, 1*(1), 35–46.

Ryan, V., & Courtney, A. (2009). Therapists' use of congruence in nondirective play therapy and filial therapy. *International Journal of Play Therapy, 18*(2), 114–128.

Ryan, V., & Wilson, K. (1995). Non-directive play therapy as a means of recreating optimal infant socialization patterns. *Early Development and Parenting, 4*(1), 29–38.

Rye, N., & Jäger, J. (2007). Assessing families for filial therapy. *British Journal of Play Therapy, 3*, 32–39.

Schore, A. N. (1994). *Affect regulation and the origin of the self.* Hillsdale, NJ: Erlbaum.

Schore, A. N. (2003). *Affect regulation and the repair of the self.* New York, NY: W. W. Norton.

Smith, G. (2000). Assessing family interaction by the collaborative drawing technique. In K. Gitlin-Weiner & A. Sandgrund (Eds.), *Play diagnosis and assessment* (pp. 446–456). New York, NY: Wiley.

Stern, D. J. (1985). *The interpersonal world of the infant: A view from psychoanalysis and developmental psychology.* London, England: Karnac.

VanFleet, R. (1999). *Filial play therapy: Using parent-child play to strengthen families.* Boiling Springs, PA: Play Therapy Press.

VanFleet, R., & Guerney, L. (2003). *Casebook of filial therapy.* Boiling Springs, PA: Play Therapy Press.

VanFleet, R., Ryan, S. D., & Smith, S. K. (2005). Filial therapy: A critical review. In L. Reddy, T. M. Files-Hall, & C. E. Schaefer (Eds.), *Empirically based play interventions for children* (pp. 241–264). Washington, DC: American Psychological Association.

Wilson, K. (2006). Can foster carers help children resolve their emotional and behavioural difficulties? *Clinical Child Psychology and Psychiatry, 11*(4), 495–511.

Wilson, K., & Ryan, V. (2005). *Play therapy: A non-directive approach for children and adolescents* (2nd ed.). Oxford, England: Balliere Tindall.

World Health Organization. (1992). *The ICD-10 Classification of Mental and Behavioural Disorders: Diagnostic criteria for research.* Geneva, Switzerland: World Health Organization.

# Integrating Ecosystemic Play Therapy and Theraplay in the Treatment of Attachment Disorders[1]

## *Kevin O'Connor*

## Introduction

Over the past couple of decades, mental health practitioners have shown a steadily increasing interest in attachment disorders and attachment-related problems in their child clients. Problems that were once thought to be as the result of dramatic neglect akin to that experienced by the babies in Spitz's study (1946) are now known to occur in much more subtle circumstances. Especially at risk are children who are adopted and those who spend time in the foster care system (Hughes, 1997, 1998). Subtle disturbances in attachment range from excessively clingy to excessively distancing behavior on the part of the child toward the caretaker. At the severe end of the continuum are those children whose behavior meets the criteria for Reactive Attachment Disorder (American Psychiatric Association, 2000). While even subtle attachment problems have the potential to interfere with children's ability to develop healthy and satisfying interpersonal relationships later in life, the more severe symptoms most assuredly will.

Studies of attachment behavior have proliferated, yielding some findings that have significantly altered the way we think about the process and the long-term effects of children's early attachment experiences. Some of the initial

---

[1] This chapter contains material originally presented in three other publications:

O'Connor, K. (2005). Combining play and cognitive interventions in the treatment of attachment disordered children. In S. Brooke (Ed.), *Creative arts therapies manual.* Springfield, IL: C. C. Thomas.

O'Connor, K., & New, D. (2003). Ecosystemic play therapy. In C. Schaefer (Ed.), *Foundations of play therapy.* New York, NY: Wiley.

O'Connor, K. (2011). Ecosystemic play therapy. In C. Schaefer (Ed.), *Foundations of play therapy* (2nd ed.). New York, NY: Wiley.

conceptualizations of the attachment process roughly equated it with imprinting behavior in birds, failing to capture its very important role in determining the quality of children's relationships later in life. The psychobiological nature of children's attachment to their caretakers is now seen as a very complex process nicely summarized by Simpson and Belsky (2008), and by Polan and Hofer (2008). The caretaker's voice, facial features, scent, and touch are seen as essential building blocks in creating the child's initial bond. The degree to which infants come to see the interactions with their caretakers as both reliable and pleasurable, in turn, becomes the core of children's ability to view their caretaker as a secure base. For the very young child, the caretaker serves as the concrete, secure base that allows for successful individuation and exploration of the world and other interpersonal relationships (Mahler, 1967, 1972). Later in life children's early secure base experiences allow them to use relationships with other adults and peers as secure bases outside the home. This is easily observed in nursery schoolchildren, who will seek out their teacher when they become hurt or frightened.

Unfortunately, this reciprocal process of infant/caregiver attachment does not always go smoothly. Problems may arise because of individual, interactional, or systemic difficulties. On an individual level, either child or parent may present with problems, making both pragmatic and emotional transactions difficult. If a child is born with a medical condition, such as colic, the child is distressed more often than most and is more difficult to soothe. These children experience pain and, on some level, are aware of the caregiver's inability to soothe them. Unfortunately, young children do not have the cognitive sophistication needed to differentiate between the caregiver who is trying hard but is unable to find a way to soothe the infant and the one who is being intentionally neglectful. In either case, unmediated distress on the part of the infant or child has significant potential to interfere with the attachment relationship. Alternatively, caregivers may also experience individual problems, making it more difficult for them to be attuned to their infants. Again, infants and young children are not able to grasp the reason for the caregiver's unavailability; they only know their basic pragmatic and/or emotional needs are not being met.

Sometimes the attachment relationships of otherwise healthy and functional children and caregivers are disrupted by problems in their interaction. A common example of such interactional problems is the caregiver's use of inappropriate discipline. Many caregivers still use spanking or other forms of physical aggression to control children's negative behavior. Spanking is not attuned to children's pragmatic or emotional needs, nor does it help the child learn strategies for either emotional or behavioral regulation. Rather, it simply teaches the child aggression is a suitable means for getting others to suppress the expression of their needs and feelings.

Last, the attachment relationship may be disrupted by systemic factors. A sibling's medical crisis may require the caregiver to be away from the child more than is optimal. A job change may result in a highly disruptive change in residence. Or, something as catastrophic as a natural disaster may interfere with the caregiver's ability to meet the child's pragmatic and emotional needs. Regardless of the source of the interference, these disruptions in the attachment relationship often lead the child to develop pathologic (i.e., nonfunctional) behaviors.

Children whose early experience deprives them of a secure attachment to their caretaker later tend to generalize that deprivation to their interactions with other adults, making it difficult for them to establish any sort of secure base to anchor them in the course of their development. Because of this, children with more severe attachment problems can be very difficult to treat using traditional play therapy methods. This chapter discusses how a therapist might integrate two different models of play therapy—ecosystemic play therapy and Theraplay®—to maximize the chances of an optimal treatment outcome with this difficult population.

Before proceeding with a discussion of the integration of the two models, let us very briefly review each model separately.

## Ecosystemic Play Therapy[2]

Ecosystemic theory and the model for applying it to the practice of play therapy was developed in the 1980s and integrates elements of many psychological, social work, and systems theories, including Theraplay. The goal in creating an ecosystemic theory of play therapy was to encourage play therapists to take a very broadly systemic perspective in developing their case conceptualizations and treatment plans. Two aspects of ecosystemic play therapy are particularly relevant to this discussion. One is the emphasis placed on the importance of children's development in both understanding the origins and nature of their pathology as well as planning and implementing effective interventions. While ecosystemic theory shares some conceptual similarities with, and has adopted some terminology from, Urie Bronfenbrenner's (1979) ecological model, the way in which the two models conceptualize development is one point of distinction.

Human development was actually Bronfenbrenner's primary focus, and he was interested in the contribution of ecological systems to the process and its outcome. Ecosystemic theory considers individual development to be a chronosystem in and of itself. Development both affects and is affected by other systems. The rapid developmental progress children undergo across even very short periods of time becomes important for two reasons. On the one hand, it means even brief periods of stress or disruption can have significant negative effects on development. On the other hand, it also means the treatment methods a therapist uses may need to be adjusted frequently to accommodate a child's developmental progress even over the short term. The

---

[2] For a complete discussion of the theory and practice of ecosystemic play therapy, the reader is referred to:

O'Connor, K. (2000). *The Play therapy primer* (2nd ed.). New York, NY: Wiley

centrality of developmental issues to case conceptualization and treatment planning is a common thread in both Theraplay and ecosystemic play therapy.

The other aspect of ecosystemic play therapy important to this discussion is the emphasis it places on integrating experiential and cognitive-verbal interventions in children's play therapy sessions. The relative balance of experiential learning versus cognitive learning in the session is determined by the child's developmental level. Children functioning at lower developmental levels need sessions to include more experience-based interventions. They have trouble learning by just talking through a problem. Children functioning at higher developmental levels are better able to use hypothetical thinking and can solve problems conceptually without necessarily needing experience to reinforce their ideas. However, no matter what their developmental level, most children seem to respond best to a combination of both experience and language. Mothers do not wait until their babies can speak before speaking to them. Instead, they constantly narrate their interactions with their infants. The combination of maternal interaction with maternal language forms the foundation for the infant's subsequent development of language. At the same time, most mothers know it is one thing to get your teenagers to agree to something in the abstract and quite another to get them to follow through and do what they have agreed to. It seems both infants and teens benefit from both talking and doing.

# Theraplay[3]

Theraplay is a highly experiential play therapy method:

> [It] achieves its success by aggressively addressing four serious problems that face too many children and parents in our society today and that prevent the development of a secure attachment relationship that is essential to healthy development: inadequate structure in daily experience; too little personal engagement; insufficient empathic, nurturing touch; and failure to provide the right kind of challenge. (Jernberg & Booth, 1999, p. xxi)

Theraplay "treatment involves replicating as much as possible the range of experiences that are an essential part of the healthy parent-infant relationship" (Booth & Jernberg, 2010, p. 3). It can serve as a remarkable strategy for providing both child and adult clients with corrective attachment experiences. Structuring and Challenging activities serve an organizational function within the therapist-child or caretaker-child interaction. Structuring focuses on behavior, helping

---

[3] For a complete discussion of the theory and practice of Theraplay, the reader is referred to:

Booth, P., & Jernberg, A. (2010). *Theraplay: Helping parents and children build better relationships through attachment based play.* San Francisco, CA: Jossey-Bass.

provide children with ways of successfully approaching and interacting with their environment while remaining safe. Challenging focuses on cognition, providing children with a frame for successfully approaching and solving tasks and problems. Engaging and Nurturing activities tend to play more of a regulatory function. Like Structuring, Engaging is more behavioral. Children learn how to regulate interactions so as to make them pleasurable and gratifying. Nurturing is more emotional, as children get a sense of how the joy of having a positive connection with another person actually feels.[4] The younger the child, the more successful intervention relies on the interactive and experiential nature of Theraplay. With some older clients, this nature allows them to bypass their negative cognitive frame and actually *experience* an interaction. After completing a single Theraplay session and homework assignment with his father, one incredibly bright 19-year-old in treatment for depression secondary to disappointment in his relationship with his father said, grinning, "Our relationship is so much better suddenly. It is not like any of our history changed, but it just doesn't seem as important anymore."

## Integrating Theraplay and Ecosystemic Play Therapy

Ecosystemic play therapy combines experiential and cognitive-verbal interventions with a somewhat greater emphasis on the latter. Theraplay interventions are almost exclusively experiential. Both have been found to be effective in treating children with attachment problems. So what would motivate a play therapist to attempt to integrate these two specific models? Recent research data suggests combining a cognitive component with the child's experiences in therapy may make the intervention even more effective as both sides of the brain are engaged. This research has focused less on the individual's actual bonding or attachment experience and more on the ways in which they come to understand and make sense of those experiences (Siegel, 1999; Siegel & Hartzell, 2003). One of the most stunning evolutionary capacities humans have developed is their ability to cognitively override and reorganize experiences. Good experiences can be reframed as disastrous and disastrous experiences reframed as good. The capacity to do the latter seems to be a key element in predicting a person's resiliency or ability to withstand stress and trauma.

Similarly, this reframing is the basis of solution-focused and constructivist techniques that emphasize helping people change the meanings they attribute to their experiences (e.g., Anderson & Goolishian, 1992; Eron & Lund, 1996). Thus, for older children and adults, it is not necessarily their actual caretaker and their experience with that person that serves as a secure base but the internalized model of the caretaker and their reframed and recalled view of their attachment

---

[4] This conceptual classification of structure and challenge as behavioral vs. cognitive organizing functions and engaging and nurturing as behavioral vs. emotional regulatory functions was developed by Sue Ammen, PhD, RPT-S, and obtained via personal communication.

to him or her. For older children, this internalized model serves as the foundation for their peer relationships. For adults, their model is not only the foundation of their peer and spousal relationships but also the frame for the relationship they create with their own children. In all cases, the coherence of the person's recalled attachment history, as well as his or her ability to integrate the emotions associated with that history, are excellent predictors of the quality of their current attachments (Fonagy, Steele, Steele, Moran, & Higgitt, 1991; Hesse, 1999). Based on this research, it would seem the combination of Theraplay experiences with the language-based work described in ecosystemic play therapy should prove highly effective in addressing even very severe attachment-based problems.

Somewhat ironically, integrating elements of ecosystemic play therapy and Theraplay is a bit difficult, not because the models are so different but, because ecosystemic theory and the way in which it has been applied to the practice of play therapy has integrated so many Theraplay concepts and practices since it was first developed in the 1980s. Only a few key differences remain between the two models. The rest of this chapter is organized using the headings most often employed when describing the theory and practice of ecosystemic play therapy. Within this frame, the similarities and differences between the two models are highlighted. Along the way, the implications for the treatment of attachment-disordered children are discussed and, finally, illustrated with case material.

## Basic Concepts

Most of the major models of psychotherapy in general and play therapy in particular include certain key elements: an underlying philosophy, a way of conceptualizing personality, and a way of conceptualizing psychopathology. Consistent with its emphasis on the importance of experiential versus cognitive interventions in the treatment process, most of the Theraplay literature focuses more on practice than on theory. Consistent with its emphasis on the value of adding a cognitive component to all interventions with even the youngest children, the ecosystemic play therapy literature focuses quite heavily on theory. In the remainder of this section of this chapter, we will review the basic theoretical and conceptual elements underlying ecosystemic play therapy and relate those to the practice of Theraplay as appropriate.

## Underlying Philosophy

Ecosystemic theory is grounded in phenomenology, a philosophy based on the notion there are no absolute, right and wrong answers, but rather, all knowledge and its value are relative. When phenomenology serves as the basis for a treatment model, it has two effects. One effect is the therapist consistently assumes the information provided by each of the people involved in a given case is accurate. When two people's stories differ significantly, the therapist does not assume one or the other is mistaken or lying. Instead, the therapist begins by assuming each person perceives the situation very differently based on his or her experience and understanding. The other effect of working within a phenomenologic frame is that a person evaluates right and wrong only in context.

Phenomenology is also subject dependent (Giorgi, 1983); we can never really know how another individual perceives the world, but we can attempt to come to such an understanding by considering the client's life and those experiences the client has had. When working with children, this also means trying to understand how their developmental level makes their experiences and worldviews radically different from those of adults. Subject dependency applies to us all, therapists included. Therapists' own experiences and world-views affect how they understand children and their problems. This creates interplay between therapists' and children's subject-dependent perspectives. Therapy becomes a dance in which therapist and child learn to move between each other's worlds in search of ways to improve the child's quality of life.

> *Humanism (Herrick, 2005) is another philosophical perspective underlying eco-systemic theory. A significant aspect of humanism is the way in which it evaluates the 'rightness' or 'wrongness' of behavior. Unlike a fundamentalist or orthodox position, humanism does not maintain absolute standards of right and wrong across situations. Rather, all behavior must be evaluated in context. Behaviors with a positive or even neutral impact on the self and/or others are usually considered 'right' while those with a negative impact are usually considered 'wrong' or pathologic. An ecosystemic play therapist will examine the impact of children's behavior on the children themselves and those around them in order to determine if the behavior is problematic enough to warrant being the focus of therapy. To illustrate the differences in fundamentalist and humanistic perspectives let us consider hallucinations in children. From a fundamentalist perspective hallucina-tions are seen as inherently pathologic; a symptom requiring treatment. From a humanistic perspective treatment would only be necessary if the hallucinations cause the child distress or if they cause him or her to behave in ways that endanger others (O'Connor, 2005). (Schaefer, 2011, pp. 255–256)*

## Personality

In the ecosystemic model, *personality* is defined as the "sum of intra- and interpersonal characteristics, attributes, cognitions, beliefs, values, and so forth that make a person unique" (O'Connor, 2000, p. 90). The basic motive driving personality is thought to be the desire to maximize the rewards obtained in daily life while avoiding negative consequences (O'Connor, 1993). The egocentricity of this motive is tempered by the early attachments motivating children to see rewards in interpersonal and reciprocal relationships. In Theraplay, primacy is given to the attachment motive. "The Theraplay approach assumes that the primary motivating force in human behavior is a drive toward relatedness. Personality development is essentially interpersonal. The early interaction between parent and child is the crucible in which the self and personality develop" (Bundy-Myrow & Booth, 2009, p. 318).

Both models agree the parent-child relationship is the most potent organizer of personality. We now know this relationship actually shapes the hardwiring of the child's brain (Gerhardt, 2004), particularly with respect to how the child will expect the world to react to him or her (Siegel, 2002). As the relationship develops, the caregiver helps provide not only for the child's biological needs but also for the critical regulation of the child's affect. One of the caregiver's primary responsibilities is to be attuned to infants' external cues as well as their emotional states (Schore, 2001; 2005; Schore & Schore, 2008). When infants are distressed, the caregivers respond and attempt to soothe them. In so doing, infants learn to count on others to get their basic needs met as well as to self-soothe. When infants become bored or withdrawn, the caregiver attempts to keep them engaged, thereby taking responsibility for maintaining the relationship. Beyond simple soothing and engaging, healthy caregivers encourage happiness and delight in infants by engaging them in fun and games such as peek-a-boo and tickling. These interactions help infants see others as a source of emotional satisfaction and pleasant stimulation (Booth & Jernberg, 2010).

Both ecosystemic play therapy and Theraplay also place considerable emphasis on the importance of child development. In both models, developmental, as opposed to chronological, age is considered central to both the conceptualization of the child's problems and the interventions to be used. It is also important to note that significant differences between a child's developmental and chronologic ages can create additional problems. A very good intervention plan can be designed for a child whose capacity for attachment is consistent with that of a 2-year-old, irrespective of the child's chronological age. However, if the child is chronologically only 4 years old, the caretakers and the environment are not likely to experience 2-year-old attachment behavior as particularly problematic. On the other hand, if the child is chronologically 12 years old, such behavior is far less likely to be tolerated by others. The 4-year-old is much more likely than the 12-year-old to get the kind of nurturance and support he or she needs to move on without heroic efforts to engage those around him or her. An extensive discussion of various developmental models and the functioning of children at different ages as incorporated into ecosystemic theory and is presented elsewhere (O'Connor, 2000; O'Connor & Ammen, 1997).

## Pathology

Consistent with the model of personality just presented, pathology—when viewed from an ecosystemic play therapy perspective—is conceptualized as involving one or more of three factors. First and foremost, pathology is defined as occurring in children who are "unable to get their needs met at a level they consider to be satisfactory, or those who are unable to get their needs met in ways that do not substantially interfere with the ability of others to get their needs met" (O'Connor, 1997, p. 241). Essentially, they have been thwarted in their attempts to satisfy their basic drives. This first factor is often inextricably linked to a second factor, the disruption of children's attachment relationships. By the time children are brought to therapy, it is often difficult to tell which came first—the failure to get basic needs met or the disruption of the attachment. Similarly, the first two factors are highly related to the last one. Consistent inability to get their needs met and/or disruption of important attachments can interfere with children's developmental progress. The disruption in children's behavior or pattern of reinforcement or the sheer energy required by children's attempts to cope with life can leave them without the resources necessary to continue to develop normally. Temporary disruption in the ability to get needs met happens frequently and is not necessarily problematic—much less pathological. In ecosystemic play therapy, true pathology is conceptualized as occurring when a child "repeatedly engages in behavior that does not get his or her needs met and is unable to generate alternative behavior or to engage in effective problem solving" (O'Connor, 1997, p. 241). In the Theraplay model, psychopathology and attachment difficulties are nearly synonymous:

> *Psychopathology is the outcome of early and ongoing unresponsive, neglectful or abusive care. Such failures lead to insecure attachment of varying degrees of severity (including disorganized attachment) and a negative or inadequate sense of self. . . . Many behavior problems of older children can be traced back to their beginnings in insecure or disorganized attachment and in the consequent dysregulation and negative views of themselves and the world. (Bundy-Myrow & Booth, 2009, p. 322)*

Ecosystemic play therapy and Theraplay differ slightly when it comes to conceptualizing how children may come to the point where they are manifesting pathology. Ecosystemic play therapy posits individual, interactional, and systemic factors as each having the potential to both disrupt attachment and cause pathology. As seen in the previous paragraph, Theraplay emphasizes interactional (specifically parent-child) factors. The Theraplay model does recognize the role individual and systemic factors may play in disrupting the parent-child relationship, but it does not give these as much weight as does the ecosystemic model.

Individual factors children carry with them may make it difficult for them to get their needs met and/or to get them met appropriately, no matter the context. Children with neurologic, severe medical, developmental, or other conditions certainly fall into this category. These children's needs are simply not similar to those of other children and, therefore, they demand more of those around them. Consequently, they are likely to experience more frustration, have more disrupted attachments, and experience more developmental problems. Children may also come to manifest pathology because they are embedded in problematic interpersonal relationships. These children are basically able to function as are those around them, but their interactions are not mutually satisfying. One or both parties would like to improve the quality of the interaction but are unable to find a way to do so. Last, pathology may arise when children are embedded in pathogenic systems. The child has the capacity to function, but the system makes doing so difficult. No matter how well-intentioned, systems such as medical hospitals, foster care, and schools may create an environment in which children's needs are not adequately met, usually resulting in frustration and pain on the part of both the system and the children. These causes of pathology are by no means orthogonal, and often any two or even all three are operating at the same time, significantly complicating treatment.

## Conceptualizing Goal/Cure

As the ecosystemic play therapy conceptualization of pathology flows from its definition of *personality*, its definition of the goal(s) of therapy flows from its definition of *psychopathology*. Specifically, the goal of ecosystemic play therapy is to "maximize the child's ability to get his (her) needs met effectively and in ways that do not interfere with the ability of others to get their needs met" (O'Connor, 2000, p. 135). Simultaneously, the ecosystemic play therapist works to develop or enhance children's attachment relationships to ensure they have the resources they need to achieve a positive outcome. Additionally, good attachment relationships ensure the child does not become egocentrically or psychopathically invested in meeting his or her own needs at the expense of others. Finally, because children who are experiencing pathology have not made adequate developmental progress, ecosystemic play therapists work to ensure the child resumes normal developmental progress. The goal is to bring the child to a developmental level as close to age appropriate as possible and to even out the child's development across domains. The therapist works to have the child function equally well emotionally, cognitively, behaviorally, and socially, because more even developmental functioning across these dimensions will make it much easier for the child to get his or her needs met in daily life.

As with other aspects of the model, the goals of Theraplay treatment focus on repairing the parent-child relationship. "The goals of treatment are to 1) help parents establish a secure base and a safe haven, 2) attune to the child's needs for coregulation of affect, and, 3) interact in ways that change the child's representation of himself and others from negative to positive" (Bundy-Myrow & Booth, 2009, p. 323). These goals mesh nicely with the goals of ecosystemic play therapy and any or all of the treatment goals identified by either model could be addressed concurrently.

## Role of the Therapist

### Why Is the Therapist There?
As with most play therapy models, both Theraplay and ecosystemic play therapy emphasize the importance of the relationship between the child and the therapist. The Theraplay therapist is engaging and playful, interacting with the child in ways modeled after the healthy, attuned interactions of parents and their children. In both models, the relationship is the context in which the therapist creates therapeutic experiences for the child. Ecosystemic play therapy goes on to specify the therapist's primary task as being to help the

child "break set," thereby enabling the child to engage in new behavior, increasing the rate and intensity at which the child's needs are met. Here, *breaking set* is defined as helping children redefine their problems, thereby enabling creative problem solving. The very process of experiencing something differently or understanding different possibilities for getting their needs met can have a profound positive effect on clients (Elliott, 1984). Although this is the overarching goal, the therapist undertakes two other highly related tasks as needed. First, because children do not usually seek out treatment on their own, the therapist must help the child understand the nature of treatment and do most of the work of establishing the initial therapeutic alliance. And, second, the therapist actively helps the child engage in problem solving.

*How Much Direction Does the Therapist Provide?*
What differentiates both Theraplay and ecosystemic play therapy from most other types of play therapy is the degree of responsibility placed on the therapist for quickly establishing a growth-promoting relationship with the child. Theraplay therapists constantly interact with their child clients, refusing to let the child withdraw from the relationship. They strive to make every moment of the session meet the child's needs in fun and playful ways. Through the use of Structuring, Challenging, Engaging, and Nurturing activities, the Theraplay therapist provides children with experiences that build their sense of trust and pleasure in interpersonal interactions. These, in turn, help repair or even create the internalized secure base these children need. This base then allows children to be successful in their interactions with their environment and the people in it. This approach is often opposed in the play therapy literature by child-centered play therapists who believe children have an innate drive toward health and emphasize the importance of allowing children to work things out for themselves:

> The intensity of the opposition (between the two viewpoints) that sometimes gets expressed about this issue comes from each side having a somewhat distorted view of the other's approach. We (Theraplay therapists) oppose a laissez-faire, "leave it up to the child" approach that at its worst allows the child to flounder and fails to address essential relationship aspects of many problems. Our critics are opposed to an authoritarian, take-charge, nonempathic approach that fails to respect the child's potential for self-actualization. The true nature of each approach lies somewhere in between. Each approach has different goals to which it is well suited. (Jernberg & Booth, 1999, p. 39)

The approach advocated in ecosystemic play therapy truly lies in between the more therapist-directed nature of Theraplay and the more child-directed nature of child-centered play therapy. The ecosystemic therapist can be both active and directive in the session. He or she can also be a quiet observer of work done by the child. What determines the role to be taken is the child's developmental level. Just as in the world outside of the playroom, parents and other adults are more active and directive when interacting with younger children. It is safe to say, no one would allow toddlers to have the same level of control over their lives as one would allow teenagers. When the child's pathology is rooted in early attachment issues, a more interactive approach is developmentally appropriate. As the child makes developmental gains the therapist can step back, giving the child room to navigate the world on his or her own. The two approaches are not opposites, they are not in conflict, they simply reflect different points along a developmental continuum.

Having examined the principles and constructs underlying both ecosystemic play therapy and Theraplay and the ways in which the two can be integrated, let us now proceed to a discussion of how the integrated model would manifest in the course of a child's treatment.

*Role of Parents*

With respect to the role of parents in the treatment process, Theraplay has a great deal to contribute to an integrated Theraplay/ecosystemic model for treating attachment-disordered children. Theraplay engages parents in every step of the process. The interactions of the parent-child dyad are fully assessed before treatment even starts and serve as the foundation for planning the sessions. The parents observe the initial sessions and are coached and mentored about how to engage their child optimally. After an initial training-coaching period, parents are brought directly into the Theraplay sessions and gradually replace the therapist in conducting the interventions. This process has many benefits, but the most important one is the degree to which it results in children building primary attachments to the parent as opposed to the therapist. This ensures children have a positive attachment relationship and a secure base outside the playroom and facilitates generalization of the gains children make in therapy to their everyday lives.

# Pretreatment Process

## Intake

Both ecosystemic play therapy and Theraplay rely on a fairly comprehensive intake to obtain information to be used in conceptualizing the case. The multisystemic intake used by ecosystemic play therapists is presented in *Play Therapy Treatment Planning and Interventions: The Ecosystemic Model and Workbook* (O'Connor & Ammen, 1997). The Theraplay intake consists of four steps: (1) the completion of standardized questionnaires about the child's behavior and parents' attitudes, (2) an intake interview with the parents focusing on history and the current functioning of the family, (3) the assessment of the parent-child interaction using the Marschak Interaction Method (MIM; Marschak, 1960; Marschak & Call, 1966; Booth, Christensen, & Lindaman, 2005), and (4) a feedback session with the parents in which the MIM is reviewed, the need for treatment is determined, and the initial treatment plan is agreed upon.

## Assessment

Both ecosystemic play therapy and Theraplay make routine use of pretreatment assessment. Ecosystemic play therapists regularly assess the child's developmental level using any one of several instruments. One method for quickly assessing the child's current social-emotional developmental functioning is to use the Developmental Therapy Objective Rating Form (DTORF). It is a quick, semistructured interview in which the therapist gathers information from the caregiver and/or others who know the child well. Ratings are obtained in four domains: social, behavioral, academic, and communication. Additionally, because the items are worded as operationally defined objectives, the clinician has a list of six to eight specific therapy goals when the interview is completed. The DTORF can also be used to assess the child's progress as therapy proceeds. For direct access to the DTORF, the reader is referred to www.dtorf.com. The assessment method, as well as related intervention techniques, are detailed in *Teaching Responsible Behavior*, 4th edition (Wood, Quirk, & Swindle, 2007) and at www.fcs.uga.edu/dttp.

Theraplay therapists routinely assess the current parent-child relationship using the Marschak Interaction Method (MIM; Marschak, 1960; Marschak & Call, 1966; Booth, Christensen, & Lindaman, 2005). This is an observational method in which the parent is asked to complete seven to ten interactive tasks with the child. The activities are selected to sample the parents' ability to use the Theraplay dimensions of structuring, challenging, engaging, and nurturing as they interact with their child. One of the real strengths of the method is the fact that the parent or parent-child dyad are not expected to meet any external criteria. Consistent with phenomenology, there is no right or wrong way of completing the tasks. The quality of the sessions is evaluated based on the child's response to the parent's behavior. If the interaction is positive and the child is fully engaged, then the task is judged to have gone well even if the behavior might not be consistent with the therapist's notion of how he or she would have approached the task. The sessions are videotaped and reviewed with the parent, with the goal of identifying both strengths and weaknesses in the relationship. The observations also guide the therapist in determining the dimensions with which the dyad had the most difficulty, as well as the specific activities to be used in the sessions.

## Contracting

The overt establishing of a very specific treatment contract with the child at the outset of play therapy may be one of the ways in which ecosystemic play therapy most differs from other play therapy models, including Theraplay. By the end of the intake with the child, the therapist will present a potential treatment contract focusing on the child's unmet needs. From issues the child has discussed in the intake, the therapist selects the issue or issues that seem most distressing to the child and defines the purpose of therapy as trying to minimize these distressing issues and maximize the child's enjoyment of life. The contract is never about creating change simply to satisfy others; rather, the contract emphasizes change that will concretely improve the child's quality of life. This contract/goal is frequently referenced in sessions with the child over the course of treatment and serves as the measure of treatment efficacy. After all, it would be difficult to say play therapy has been effective because the child changed in ways that satisfied others if the child is still unhappy. A parallel contract can be made with the parents to help them focus on changing the child's problematic behaviors. When the contracts seem contradictory, which is not uncommon given a phenomenologic perspective, it is up to the therapist to help both sides see how mutual problem solving can result in both sides feeling happier and healthier and, best of all, having a better relationship.

The treatment contract forms the foundation upon which the ecosystemic play therapist then engages the child and/or the caregivers and/or those in the child's environment in active problem solving to ensure qualitative change. In this context, the term *problem solving* does not simply refer to a cognitive, rational exercise. Instead, the term is used more loosely to refer to all efforts at getting the child's needs met consistently and appropriately. An ecosystemic play therapist might help one child to better express emotion so others respond more appropriately, while helping another child develop specific strategies for coping with a bully at school. The problem-solving process might be overt, with the therapist training the child in basic problem-solving strategies, or the process might be entirely covert, with the therapist doing all of the problem solving and simply helping the child follow along.

## Room and Toys

The setup of the playroom and the way in which toys and other play materials are included in the session is another way in which ecosystemic play therapy and Theraplay are more similar to one another than to other models of play therapy. In most types of play therapy there is a great deal of emphasis on the therapeutic value of having the child engage in play, especially pretend play, with toys. For this reason a great many toys are usually included in the playroom, and the child is given free access to the toys and allowed to choose what to play with and when to play during each session.

In both ecosystemic play therapy and Theraplay the emphasis is on the interaction between the child and the therapist. The playroom is conceived of as a neutral container in which the relationship takes place. It is generally free from distractions and tends to be very simple and uncluttered to the point some might consider the room rather barren. The role of the toys is to support the interaction between the child and therapist. The number and complexity of toys is kept to a minimum, and the therapist controls the child's access to them. As a result, the child cannot use the toys to avoid engaging with the therapist in the therapeutic process.

At this point we have reviewed the conceptual underpinnings of both Theraplay and ecosystemic play therapy. We have looked at the way case information is gathered and the child's needs understood. We have also briefly looked at the pretreatment preparation in which the therapist engages. Once the therapist has formulated a case conceptualization, specific treatment goals are developed, a treatment plan is designed, materials and session activities are selected, and the actual treatment begins.

## Treatment Phases

The treatment phases described in ecosystemic play therapy were taken directly from the Theraplay model. The only modification made was the combination of the first two Theraplay phases into a single phase, Introduction and Exploration. Each phase will not be discussed in detail here, rather, some points regarding phase-specific issues in the treatment of children with attachment disorders will be presented.

### Introduction and Exploration

For children with attachment problems, the initial contact with the therapist can be a particularly daunting experience. For those children who are anxious or avoidant, the therapist represents exactly the type of social interaction they usually work hard to avoid. For these children the therapist must be very careful not to flood the child, making the session aversive. At the same time, if the therapist is too tentative, the child may interpret this as anxiety on the therapist's part and feel even less safe and secure. The therapist must simultaneously engage the child and provide a great deal of nurturing reassurance the child is safe. For those children who attach indiscriminately, the therapist needs to provide more structure and, potentially, even a little distance so as to demonstrate to the child the boundaries of healthy attachment. In both cases, the treatment contract can serve as a basis for providing the child with some cognitive reassurance about the nature of the process. Reiterating the contract frequently at the beginning of therapy reminds children that no matter how uncomfortable the initial sessions may seem, the ultimate goal is to help them feel less anxious in their everyday lives. It is also important for therapists to recognize the more severe the child's attachment disorder, the longer this phase may need to continue. Even if therapy seems to be proceeding very slowly at first, the secure base upon which all subsequent attachment behavior is based is being built. This critical process cannot be rushed.

### Tentative Acceptance

In this phase, children appear to have bought into the therapy process and into the notion of interacting with the therapist. On the surface they often look quite compliant and engaged. Yet, they will often attempt to distract the therapist from the process or, if content is introduced, avoid discussing it. In some ways it may seem as if not much is happening during this phase. However, under the surface children are learning about the therapist and the relationship and are gauging both the safety of the interaction as well as the therapist's ability to read and respond to their emotional cues and needs. When subtle struggle for control of these sessions occurs, it reflects children's fears of intimacy and needs to be identified and addressed by the therapist.

## Negative Reaction

Most therapists would agree that a negative reaction phase is part of every client's therapy, irrespective of the presenting problem. Clients come to therapy in the hopes of feeling better. They also hope the change will be easy and stress free. As they discover change will require them to think and react differently to the world around them, they fear giving up the beliefs and behaviors they have come to rely on to keep them safe in the world. This is true even when those beliefs and behaviors seem very counterproductive to an outside observer. As therapy progresses and clients are challenged to think and behave differently, they offer up some resistance. This is a sign therapy is progressing. In children with attachment difficulties these changes activate some very primitive fears they have about the inability of others to serve as a secure base and to provide for their emotional needs. When abuse or neglect are part of the child's history, these fears can be incredibly intense and lead to some fairly severe acting out in session. The therapist needs to provide enough structure to make sure the child continues to feel physically safe and enough emotional nurturing to help regulate the child's anxiety.

In providing a safe structure it is critical the therapist not end sessions as a way of managing severe acting out. Doing so provides the child with concrete proof the therapist is unwilling or unable to tolerate the child's anxiety and anger. It means the relationship is contingent on the child's behavior, not on the child's needs. As a result, it is unlikely children will go on to trust a therapist who sends them away when the going gets tough. Rather than ending the session,

> holding a child when he is angry has many benefits. He learns that you can keep him safe when he is out of control. He learns that you can accept and not condemn it, and that his anger does not drive you away. He learns you can survive his anger and still be there to hold and comfort him. Ultimately, he will be able to relax and accept your comfort. When this happens you have created a strong bond with the child. (Jernberg & Booth, 1999, pp. 131–132)

## Trusting, Growing, and Working Through

This is the primary phase in which the largely experiential approach central to the practice of Theraplay can be fully integrated with the cognitive, interpretive, and problem-solving approaches used by ecosystemic play therapists.

### Experiential Interventions
As we have previously discussed, Theraplay focuses on "active, physical, interactive play. There is no symbolic play with toys and very little talk about problems" (Jernberg & Booth, 1999, p. xxviii). Experience is the primary agent of change in the therapy process:

*Theraplay is geared to the preverbal, social, right-brain level of development. Because attachment is formed during the early months when the right brain is dominant and co-regulation is essential, efforts to change negative patterns must be direct, interactive, and emotionally focused. We use the language of the right brain—nonverbal face-to-face emotional communications involving touch, eye contact, rhythm, and attuned responses of pacing and intensity—to provide appropriate levels of stimulation to the areas of the brain that are involved in affect regulation. Activities are geared to the child's specific emotional needs and capacity to self-regulate rather than to the child's chronological age. Language is not a barrier to treatment because Theraplay relies so heavily on nonverbal communication. (Booth & Jernberg, 2010, p. 27)*

Structuring activities provide children with a sense of the predictability of the world and reassure them the therapist will do everything needed to keep them safe. Challenging activities promote growth and development. They also put children in situations that challenge their beliefs about the way relationships work. The therapist who is insistently engaged even when the child is angry challenges the child's belief that anger makes him or her unlovable. Engaging activities let children know the therapist wants to be with them, enjoys them, and sees them as valuable. And, nurturing activities allow children to experience the joys of being taken care of and supported as they make difficult changes in the way they interact with the world. Regardless of the dimension focused on in a given activity, it is important to remember activities "are geared to the child's current emotional level rather than to his (or her) chronological age" (Jernberg & Booth, 1999, p. 20).

One specific form of structuring, limit setting, directly relates to the child's motivation to engage in effective problem solving. If the child is not experiencing negative consequences for engaging in behavior that substantially interferes with the ability of others to get their needs met, he or she has little motivation to change. To establish such motivation, the therapist ensures proper limits are set in session and caregivers are setting appropriate limits as consistently as possible. When caregivers are able to successfully control their children's behavior, the children learn the extent and nature of the caregiver's and the environment's boundaries. In addition, they learn the caregiver is able to keep them safely within those boundaries. This same principle applies in the playroom (Landreth, 2002).

*Cognitive Interventions*
As previously stated, integrating a cognitive intervention with an experiential intervention such as Theraplay may increase the efficacy of both. While Theraplay emphasizes the power of experience to evoke change via right-brain-based emotional and social learning, ecosystemic play therapy emphasizes the benefits of simultaneously engaging both sides of the brain. It helps children find ways to benefit from new experiences while using the language and logic of their left brains to facilitate generalization of the gains to new and different experiences and interactions outside the playroom. Three cognitive interventions are of particular importance in the treatment of attachment disorders: identification

and expression of emotion, interpretation, and problem solving. It is important for the therapist to help children identify and express emotions in developmentally, socially, and culturally appropriate ways. After all, the child stands little chance of getting his or her emotional/affectional needs met if no one knows what those needs are.

One way of accomplishing this is through the use of fun, psychoeducational methods such as the Color-Your-Life Thermometer (O'Connor & New, 2003). This is a variation on the Color-Your-Life Technique in which children are taught to pair colors and affects so the colors become an indirect way of expressing and quantifying emotion (O'Connor, 1983). In this modification, children are given the outline of a thermometer at the beginning of the play session and asked to color in the feelings they have had since the last meeting. The therapist explains that just as medical personnel use body temperature to gauge the child's well-being, the play therapist uses feeling-temperature to gauge emotional well-being. This method encourages the children to focus on their emotional experience between sessions and to understand the degree to which the therapist is interested in their emotions and in helping them feel better.

Interpretation[5] is a useful strategy for helping children identify the cognitions and beliefs that interfere with their ability to get their needs met. For example, children whose early attachment experiences lead them to believe adults are simply not reliable will tend to approach all interactions expecting their needs to go unmet. For this reason, they may not express needs or do so only very indirectly. Interpretation is one way of bringing this counterproductive belief to the surface. Once identified, the ways in which the belief causes problems in the present can be explored. Problem-solving strategies can then be employed to develop ways of bypassing the belief and ensuring the child's needs are met. Interpretation is, therefore, not a freestanding intervention. It is used to prepare the child to engage in effective problem solving. The remainder of this discussion will focus primarily on how traditional interpretation strategies can be used to facilitate children's understanding (integration) of their emotions in Theraplay sessions and their use of what they learn in session in their daily lives.

The following six steps delineate how the interpretive process fits into the overall course of the child's treatment:[6]

---

[5] For a more detailed discussion of the use of interpretation in play therapy, the reader is referred to:

O'Connor, K. (2000). The play therapy primer (2nd ed.). New York, NY: Wiley.

[6] This discussion of interpretation is a slightly modified version of the one that appeared in both:

O'Connor, K. (2002). The value and use of interpretation in play therapy. *Professional Psychology: Research and Practice, 33*(6), 523–528.
O'Connor, K. (2005). Combining play and cognitive interventions in the treatment of attachment disordered children. In S. Brooke (Ed.), *Creative arts therapies manual.* Springfield, IL: C. C. Thomas.

1. Develop an initial, comprehensive case formulation that includes hypotheses about the underlying causes of the presenting problem and those factors maintaining the child's symptoms and/or behavior.

2. Develop a phenomenologically based treatment contract with the child specifying the way(s) in which the *child's* life will improve over the course of treatment. Simultaneously, therapists need to be clear with the child that such improvement will take work, including sometimes talking about things that make the child uncomfortable, sad, scared, etc. Therapists should stress their belief that the long-term gains the child will make will far outweigh the short-term discomfort.

3. Develop a series of interpretations that will be used to guide the child to a new understanding of his or her problems. This new understanding will be based on the hypotheses the therapist developed in Step 1.

4. Begin delivering the planned interpretations to the child as opportunities arise in the play, while observing the child's response so as to evaluate the accuracy of the hypotheses. If the child continually rejects the interpretations or does not begin to make behavioral changes, the therapist should revisit the original case formulation and rethink the hypotheses.

5. As the child gains insight, the therapist moves on to help the child use this new information to problem solve, developing alternative responses and behaviors.

6. Lastly, therapists repeat interpretive material as it applies to a variety of ongoing and new situations, so the children are able to use their new knowledge and skills outside the therapy session. This facilitates generalization.

By integrating interpretation and experiential activities such as those found in Theraplay, therapists can take events or emotions conveyed in the sessions and make meaning out of them, so the conflicts or problems they engendered can be addressed and resolved (Slade, 1994). However, therapists do not impose their a priori thoughts on the child. Rather, much as happens in traditional Theraplay, therapy becomes a delicate dance between the therapist and child. Therapists continuously offer their knowledge to the child, gauge the child's receptivity and response, adjust their thinking as needed, and reoffer these alternatives to the child. When all goes well, the play therapists' years of life and clinical experience are combined with the child's drive to grow, and rapid progress is made.

If interpretation is to help the child make meaning and gain knowledge to be used in problem solving, then it must be delivered in a way the child can use. This requires the therapist to do two things. One is to translate the sometimes complex thoughts and emotions behind the child's verbal and nonverbal responses to the Theraplay activities into language the child can actually understand. Language that is developmentally appropriate. The other is to deliver interpretations in a stepwise and systematic way so the child is not overwhelmed. To facilitate this, the author has developed the following model derived from the work of Lowenstein (1951, 1957), Devereaux, (1951), Bibring, (1945), and Lewis (1974).

*Reflections*
This first category of interpretation includes two subcategories, content reflections and motive reflections. Content reflections are those statements therapists make to identify the thoughts or feelings behind what their child clients do or say. When the child looks or acts angry or yells, the therapist simply says, "You seem very angry." When the child tells a story, the therapist makes the underlying fantasy explicit. Content reflections are not restatements. They add new material. The therapist does not say "You seem nervous" when the child has just said "That made me nervous." Motive reflections are explicit statements of the child's reason(s) for saying or doing a particular thing. "I think you just threw your M&Ms on the floor to let me know you don't want me to feed you. You can feed yourself!" Because motive reflections involve a greater level of attribution on the part of the therapist, they are considered somewhat more intense than content reflections and, as such, should be used more carefully.

Reflections serve several purposes. First, they demonstrate for the child the therapist's interest in the thoughts and feelings behind the action. As such, they help educate the child as to how the Theraplay process will unfold. Second, they help expand the child's affective vocabulary. By using reflections, therapists provide children with the words they need to express their innermost thoughts and feelings more accurately and effectively. Third, by replacing some of the child's behavior with words, the therapist helps reduce the child's tendency to act out both in session and in the real world. Lastly, they give therapists the opportunity to validate their perceptions of the child's emotional state. When a therapist reflects incorrectly, children tend not only to negate what the therapist has said but to spontaneously correct it. This provides the therapist with information the child might not have otherwise volunteered.

*Present Pattern*
At this level the therapist is simply identifying overt or covert repetitions in the child's verbal and nonverbal reactions to the Theraplay activities. The therapist should operationalize the repetition as clearly as possible and give examples of how these have been manifested. The patterns may be very concrete: "This is the third time you started to cry when we were playing peek-a-boo." "The last few sessions you have started out by telling me how stupid our sessions are." Alternatively, the patterns may be thematic "Just today, you wanted to quit hide-and-seek, moved away when we were using the lotion, and threw the M&Ms on the floor when we were feeding each other." The primary purpose of such statements is to help children see their behavior as meaningful and psychologically significant, as well as being consistent over time rather than as just a series of random events. Once these consistencies are labeled, then solutions generated to resolve any one of the problems in a cluster can be more easily generalized to the other, similar behaviors. This lays the groundwork for subsequent interpretations. Initially, the therapist would label repetitions of behavior within sessions; later patterns across sessions would be identified.

*Simple Dynamic*
At this level therapists draw connections between (a) the child's thoughts, affects, and motives as previously reflected and (b) previously identified patterns of behavior.  For example, the therapist might suggest that the child who withdrew from each of the activities as previously described did so because being nurtured or taken care of felt scary or dangerous. "I think you get really scared when I am being sort of mushy-nice to you, and so you try to pull away. That way you go back to being the boss. You can show me you don't need me to take care of you." Once the child has become accustomed to the therapist making simple dynamic interpretations for in-session behavior, he or she can proceed to making simple dynamic interpretations of behavior observed across sessions. At this point the therapist is moving toward more traditional types of interpretation by helping the child understand the dynamics of his or her behavior in the recent past. Through simple dynamic interpretation, the child is encouraged to see the continuity of affects and meanings across behaviors. Children are sensitized to the internal feelings, processes, and motivations that guide their behavior. Because simple dynamic interpretations are built off of the two previous levels of interpretation, each of which the child has come to accept independently, acceptance of the interaction of the two is less likely to be resisted (O'Connor, 2000, p. 292).

*Generalized Dynamic*
These interpretations connect children's in-session behavior to their out-of-session behavior. The therapist points out the similarities between the child's patterns of thinking, feeling, and behaving across contexts. For example, the therapist might point out how the child's tendency to withdraw from mushy-nice interactions stems from a fear that dependency will leave him or her vulnerable to neglect or abuse. "It seems like you worry people will only be nice for a little while and then they will stop and hurt your feelings. If you stop first you can't be disappointed, and that makes you feel a lot safer."

*Genetic*
This category includes two types of interpretations. One type is interpretations of the origins of the child's current problems. These are the most traditional form of interpretation, as they are structured and delivered so as to provide children with insight into the root of their problems. The other type is interpretations of the child's significant organizing beliefs. These are core beliefs the child holds that are rooted in early, usually repetitive experience. As examples, consider the abused child who now believes the world is a dangerous place and all adults are potential abusers, or the neglected child who believes he or she is unlovable and worthless. These beliefs derive from the child's genetic experience and are often the primary reason the child cannot or will not change his or her behavior. To change would engender intolerable cognitive dissonance. To the child with a fear of being nurtured, the therapist might suggest that the fear is connected to the belief that he or she is truly, fundamentally unlovable. That fundamental belief might, in turn, be linked to the child having been constantly disappointed by his

or her mother during their early interactions when she was abusing substances. The therapist then goes on to help the child accurately evaluate the reality of his or her cognitions versus the overwhelming negative effect of the mother's behavior.

Interpretations are usually offered in the sequence just listed; however, in formulating them, the therapist usually works backward. That is, the therapist will first develop hypotheses about the etiology of the child's problems and the child's core beliefs (genetic). The therapist will validate these with examples of the child's behavior as reported in the intake (generalized dynamic). Next, the therapist will develop ideas of how these behaviors and feelings may manifest in session (simple dynamic, pattern, and reflection). Having developed these hypotheses, the therapist will watch for those things that either confirm or negate the original hypotheses and interpret accordingly. As previously stated, the hypotheses are continuously re-evaluated and refined as the therapy progresses. The levels of interpretation are also listed in accordance with the frequency with which they will be used in session. Therapists will reflect on a nearly continuous basis while they may make only a few genetic interpretations over the course of the child's entire therapy.

The entire interpretive process is designed to identify the ways in which children's early experience has created cognitive distortions that make it difficult for them to get their needs met in the here and now. Once identified, the therapist helps the child engage in problem solving to reduce this interference. This might mean helping children reframe their worldviews to better fit the reality of their current and hopefully more positive life situation. It might also mean helping children to find ways of getting their needs met despite the limitations still present in their familial relationships. Whatever the target outcome, being able to engage children in functional problem solving is the ultimate goal of the interpretive process.

## Termination

For children with attachment-related difficulties, the end of therapy can be particularly difficult. They come to therapy because they have difficulty forming relationships. In therapy they find the capacity to trust and attach, often forming very close bonds with their therapist. Then, just as they feel truly connected and are, therefore, considered healthy, they discover the therapeutic relationship is going to end. For many, this triggers substantial regression in an effort to preserve this significant connection. The inherent difficulties created by ending therapy with these children can be mediated by implementing four strategies:

1. *The use of a therapy contract from the outset of treatment lets children know to expect therapy to end when certain improvements are attained.* If these improvements are operationalized in a way the child can really grasp them, and if they are periodically assessed with the child as therapy progresses, then children are more likely to both see the end approaching and to appreciate their role in deciding when they are ready to end.

2. *This population requires substantial advance notice of termination.* It would not be unreasonable to give them four to eight sessions' notice and to mark these sessions in some very concrete way, such as indicating the remaining sessions on a calendar given to the child and parent.

3. *The therapist must work to generalize the child's attachment to at least one important adult in their lives outside the playroom.* This is where the Theraplay strategy of involving parents very early on can be helpful, as it ensures termination will not take place until the child has experiences with the parent superceding the therapist in the conduct of the sessions.

4. *Having a final session in which the child's gains are celebrated in a going-away party can help the child focus on the positive aspects of ending therapy as opposed to the difficulties.* This celebration is common in both Theraplay and ecosystemic play therapy, and it can be particularly effective if the final session is planned jointly by the parent and child, with the therapist taking the role of a guest at the party. This turns all control for the session over to the parent and child, minimizes the role of the therapist, and prepares everyone for life after therapy.

## Case Example

The elements of a combined Theraplay and ecosystemic play therapy approach are well illustrated in the following case example.[7] Tony was 5 years old when he was brought to therapy. He and his younger brother had been adopted six months earlier by a couple with no other children. The boys had been freed for adoption by the courts when it became clear their birth mother would not be able to provide them with adequate care. Before being freed for adoption the boys had been in and out of the child welfare system several times subsequent to episodes of severe neglect by their birth mother. At the time of referral, Tony's adoptive parents were very concerned about his apparent failure to develop any connection with them since coming into their home. They described him as incredibly independent, distant, and controlling. He did what he wanted, when he wanted. He was rarely difficult or significantly oppositional, but rather he seemed to go about his business as if the parents weren't there. He took excellent care of his younger brother but seemed to resent how close his brother was becoming to their new parents. Despite his pseudo-mature behavior, Tony showed signs of being in great distress. He often seemed anxious and regularly wet the bed. He also became quite upset if he couldn't direct a particular interaction or if things did not proceed as he expected them to.

A brief intervention specifically designed to facilitate Tony's rapid development of an attachment to his adoptive mother was initiated. The eight sessions combined many Theraplay elements, with an art/story project and considerable

---

[7] This case is a composite drawn from the treatment of several children with attachment-related difficulties by several different therapists.

interpretation. The first three sessions consisted of a great deal of very physical interaction between Tony and the therapist, with the mother present in the room. The mother was told she could join the play or observe it, as she felt comfortable. Initially, Tony seemed enormously pleased with these interactions. The therapist held Tony, tickled him, tossed him playfully in the air, and wrestled with him. These simple physical activities incorporated all of the Theraplay dimensions. They were highly structured and controlled by the therapist. They were challenging in the sense they pushed Tony to engage in behaviors outside of his comfort zone. They were very engaging, as Tony was continuously interacting directly with the therapist. And, finally, they were nurturing through the therapist's use of verbal reinforcement and playfulness.

Although he was having fun during these interactions, Tony struggled to control every moment of the sessions. As the therapist lovingly yet firmly maintained control of the interactions, Tony became more aggressive. Interestingly, he never tried to withdraw from interacting with the therapist. Tony's mother reported that no matter how enraged Tony had been during the sessions, he never complained about them, seemed happy afterward, and looked forward to the next session. Tony's aggression peaked in the third session. The therapist opened the door to let Tony and his mother into the playroom. Tony, who had been playing quietly in the waiting area, launched a full-out physical attack on the therapist. The therapist immediately moved to contain Tony and to provide support and reassurance as Tony raged. Through all of this, Tony's mother sat motionless, stunned by the intensity of Tony's anger.

Before discussing the resolution of this very difficult session, the interpretive material the therapist was delivering along with the activities will be presented. Throughout these first three sessions the therapist tried to help Tony connect the feelings he was experiencing in the therapy to the thoughts and fears related to his very problematic early attachment experiences. The interpretive material was delivered in two formats. The majority was conveyed directly to Tony as the sessions progressed. At the same time, the therapist built a metaphor that integrated the issues Tony was facing into a coherent fantasy tale.

**Reflections** (Sessions 1–8): (1) You know you are very smart. (2) You like feeling powerful. (3) You like to be the boss. (4) Wow, you are so angry. (5) Behind all that anger you seem pretty scared. (6) You sure do seem to worry a lot.

**Pattern Interpretations** (Sessions 1–2): (1) You hardly ever let your Mom do anything on her own without giving her directions. (2) You hardly ever let anyone play with you in a fun way. You only want to play-fight. (3) Every time you come to session, you want to be the boss. This pattern was also conveyed through a *metaphor*: "It is like there is an angry dragon that lives inside you and wants to be the boss all the time so he can protect you and keep you safe."

**Simple Dynamic** (Sessions 1–5): (1) I think you believe Mom won't do a good job if you don't tell her what to do. (2) It seems like it is hard for you to be the boss if you are having fun, so you don't let yourself have fun. (3) Play-fighting is one way of playing and still feeling powerful. (4) But being the boss seems like an even better way of feeling powerful and safe. *Metaphor*: "The problem is the dragon has become too strong, so he doesn't just protect you, he even keeps people from getting close enough to love you. And, *you* really want to be loved."

**Generalized Dynamic** (Sessions 1–2): (1) That is why you hardly ever want your new Mom and Dad to take care of you or be nice to you. It would mean you weren't the boss anymore, and then you wouldn't be safe. (2) It is the same reason you don't like to let your teacher be the boss. (3) It is even the reason you never let any other kids be the boss when you play. *Metaphor*: "That is why the dragon doesn't want your new Mom and Dad to be nice to you. He would lose his power, and he is worried if that happens you won't be safe. But that dragon is part right and part wrong. He is right about losing his power, but he is wrong about you being able to be safe. You will be safe now because you have a new mom and dad to protect you. So if all the grown-ups are really nice to you, then the dragon won't have any more power, and he won't be able to stop people from loving you. So Mom, Dad, and you and I are going to keep being nice no matter how hard the dragon fights. We'll all prove you don't need him to keep you safe anymore."

**Genetic Interpretation** (Session 3): Because your birth mom and dad never took very good care of you and your brother, you decided you needed to be the grownup and do all the taking-care-of. That was good because it helped make sure you got some of the things you needed, but it was also bad because it made you tired and mad—so mad you never wanted grown-ups to come near you ever again. *Metaphor*: "The dragon was made out of all the bad things that happened to you. He was there to protect you and make you strong. But now you have a Mom and Dad who love you, and the dragon is losing his power. He still thinks he needs to fight to keep you safe, but now his fighting just makes it hard for you to enjoy the love Mom and Dad have to give. It is time for you to thank the dragon and let him know you want your new Mom and Dad to love you and protect you now."

After this genetic interpretation was delivered in the third session, Tony completely stopped fighting and began to cry. He sobbed as if he was in agony, and the therapist immediately placed him in his mother's lap. The therapist encouraged Tony's mother to nurture and kiss him and tell him he was safe and loved. Mother and child snuggled together for about 20 minutes as Tony slowly stopped crying and molded against his mother.

Immediately upon entering the playroom for the fourth session, Tony announced that the dragon was gone. The therapist playfully asked him, "Vacation or gone for good?" Tony replied, "Packed his bags and left for good." Tony's mother reported an amazing change in Tony's behavior since the last session. She said he was constantly affectionate and physical with her and his father. He seemed happy and relaxed. He had even begun to join the rest of the family in their activities.

## Conclusion

Theraplay and ecosystemic play therapy share many underlying assumptions and therapeutic techniques. Both focus heavily on the types of developmental issues underlying the difficulties experienced by children with attachment disorders. Theraplay emphasizes right-brain, experiential, emotional and social activities. The goal is to provide the child with corrective experiences that do not depend on language based processing. Ecosystemic play therapy advocates a balance between corrective experience and language-based processing matched to children's developmental level. That is, developmentally younger children are engaged in more experiential therapeutic activities, whereas developmentally older children are engaged in more language-based processes. Furthermore, ecosystemic play therapy advocates the use of language-based processes with all children in order to facilitate generalization of gains made through experiential learning. Both models have a great deal to offer children who have attachment-related problems. Based on the information presented in this chapter, it seems a combination of the two may be even more effective than either one on its own.

## References

American Psychiatric Association. (2000). Diagnostic and statistical manual of mental disorders (4th ed., text revision; DSM-IV-TR). Washington, DC: American Psychiatric Association.

Anderson, H., & Goolishian, M. A. (1992). The client is the expert: A not knowing approach to therapy. In K. J. Gergen & S. McNamee (Eds.), *Therapy as a social construction* (pp. 25–39). Newbury Park, CA: Sage.

Bibring, E. (1945). Psychoanalysis and the dynamic psychotherapies. *Journal of the American Psychiatric Association, II,* 745–770.

Booth, P., Christensen, G., & Lindaman, S. (2005). *Marschak interaction method: A structured observational technique to assess the quality and nature of the parent-child relationship (preschool and school age)* (rev. ed.). Chicago, IL: The Theraplay Institute.

Booth, P., & Jernberg, A. (2010). *Theraplay: Helping parents and children build better relationships through attachment based play,* (3rd ed.). San Francisco, CA: Jossey-Bass.

Bronfenbrenner, U. (1979). *The ecology of human development: Experiments by nature and design.* Cambridge, MA: Harvard University Press.

Bundy-Myrow, S., & Booth, P. (2009). Theraplay: Supporting attachment relationships. In K. O'Connor & L. Braverman (Eds.), *Play therapy theory and practice: Comparing theories and techniques* (pp. 315–366). Hoboken, NJ: Wiley.

Devereaux, G. (1951). Some criteria for the timing of confrontations and interpretations. *International Journal of Psychoanalysis, 32,* 19–24.

Elliott, R. (1984). A discovery-oriented approach to significant change events in psychotherapy: interpersonal process recall and comprehensive process analysis. In L. Rice & L. Greenberg (Eds.), *Patterns of change: Intensive analysis of psychotherapy process.* New York, NY: Guilford Press.

Eron, J. B., & Lund, T. W. (1996). *Narrative solutions in brief therapy.* New York, NY: Guilford Press.

Fonagy, P., Steele, M., Steele, H., Moran, G., & Higgitt, A. (1991). The capacity for understanding mental states: The reflective self in parent and child and its significance for security of attachment. *Infant Mental Health Journal, 12*(3), 201–218.

Gerhardt, S. (2004). *Why love matters: How affection shapes a baby's brain.* New York, NY: Brunner-Routledge.

Giorgi, A. (1983). Concerning the possibility of phenomenological psychological research. *Journal of Phenomenological Psychology, 14* (2), 129–169.

Herrick, J. (2005). *Humanism: An introduction.* Amherst, NY: Prometheus.

Hesse, E. (1999). The Adult Attachment Interview: Historical and current perspectives. In J. Cassidy & P. Shaver (Eds.), *Handbook of attachment: Theory, research & clinical implications.* New York, NY: Guilford Press.

Hughes, D. (1997). *Facilitating developmental attachment: The road to emotional recovery and behavioral change in foster and adopted children.* New York, NY: Jason Aronson.

Hughes, D. (1998). *Building the bonds of attachment: Awakening love in deeply troubled children.* New York, NY: Jason Aronson.

Jernberg, A., & Booth, P. (1999). *Theraplay: Helping parents and children build better relationships through attachment based play* (2nd ed.). San Francisco, CA: Jossey-Bass.

Landreth, G. (2002). Therapeutic limits setting in the play therapy relationship. *Professional Psychology: Research and Practice, 33*(6), 529–535.

Lewis, M. (1974). Interpretation in child analysis: Developmental considerations. *Journal of the American Academy of Child Psychiatry, 13*, 32–53.

Lowenstein, R. (1951). The problem of interpretation. *Psychoanalytic Quarterly, 20*, 1–14.

Lowenstein, R. (1957). Some thoughts on interpretation in the theory and practice of psychoanalysis. *The Psychoanalytic Study of the Child, 12*, 127–150.

Mahler, M. (1967). On human symbiosis and the vicissitudes of individuation. *Journal of the American Psychoanalytic Association, 25*, 740–763.

Mahler, M. (1972). On the first three subphases of the separation-individuation process. *International Journal of Psycho-Analysis, 53*, 333–338.

Marschak, M. (1960). A method for evaluating child-parent interaction under controlled conditions. *The Journal of Genetic Psychology, 97*, 3–22.

Marschak, M., & Call, J. D. (1966). Observing the disturbed child and his parents: Class demonstrations for medical students.

*Journal of the American Academy of Child Psychiatry, 5*, 686–692.

O'Connor, K. J. (1983). The color-your-life technique. In K. O'Connor & C. Schaefer (Eds.), *Handbook of Play Therapy*, Vol. 2. (pp. 251–258). New York, NY: Wiley.

O'Connor, K. J. (1993). Child, protector, confidant: Structured group ecosystemic play therapy. In T. Kottman & C. Schaefer (Eds.), *Play therapy in action: A casebook for practitioners* (pp. 245–280). Northvale, NJ: Jason Aronson.

O'Connor, K. J. (1997). Ecosystemic play therapy. In K. O'Connor & L. Braverman (Eds.), *Play therapy theory and practice: A comparative presentation* (pp. 234–284). New York, NY: Wiley.

O'Connor, K. J. (2000). *The play therapy primer* (2nd ed.). New York, NY: Wiley.

O'Connor, K. (2002). The value and use of interpretation in play therapy. *Professional Psychology: Research and Practice, 33*(6), 523–528.

O'Connor, K. J. (2005). Ecosystemic play therapy. *Japanese Journal of Psychiatry, 19*(3), 273–284.

O'Connor, K. (in press) Ecosystemic play therapy. In C. Schaefer (Ed.), *Foundations of play therapy* (2nd ed.). Hoboken, NJ: Wiley.

O'Connor, K. J., & Ammen, S. (1997). *Play therapy treatment planning and interventions: The ecosystemic model and workbook.* San Diego, CA: Academic Press.

O'Connor, K. J., & New, D. (2002). The color-your-life technique. In C. Schaefer & D. Cangelosi (Eds.), *Play therapy techniques* (2nd ed., pp. 245–256). Northvale, NJ: Jason Aronson.

O'Connor, K., & New, D. (2003). Ecosystemic play therapy. In C. Schaefer (Ed.), *Foundations of play therapy.* New York, NY: Wiley.

Polan, H. J., & Hofer, M. (2008). Psychobiological origins of infant attachment and its role in development. In J. Cassidy & P. Shaver (Eds.), *Handbook of attachment: Theory, research and clinical applications* (pp. 158–172). New York, NY: Guilford Press.

Schaefer, C. E. (2011). *Foundations of Play Therapy* (2ed.). Hoboken, NJ: Wiley.

Schore, A. (2001). Minds in the making: Attachment, the self-organizing brain, and developmentally-oriented psychoanalytic psychotherapy. *British Journal of Psychotherapy, 17*, 299–328.

Schore, A. (2005). Attachment, affect regulation, and the developing right brain: Linking developmental neuroscience to pediatrics. *Pediatrics in Review, 26*, 204–217.

Schore, J., & Schore, A. (2008). Modern attachment theory: The central role of affect regulation in development and treatment. *Clinical Social Work Journal, 36*, 9–20.

Siegel, D. (1999). *The developing mind: How relationships and the brain interact to shape who we are.* New York, NY: Guilford Press.

Siegel, D. J. (2002). An interpersonal neurobiology of the developing mind: Contingent communication and the development of a coherent self. Paper presented at the meeting of the UCLA Extension and Lifespan Learning Institute on Attachment: From Early Childhood through the Lifespan, Los Angeles, CA.

Siegel, D., & Hartzell, M. (2003). *Parenting from the inside out.* New York, NY: Penguin Putnam.

Simpson, J., & Belsky, J. (2008). Attachment theory within a modern evolutionary framework. In J. Cassidy & P. Shaver (Eds.), *Handbook of attachment: Theory, research and clinical applications* (pp. 131–157). New York, NY: Guilford Press.

Slade, A. (1994) Making meaning and making believe: Their role in the clinical process. In A. Slade & D. Wolf. *Children at play: Clinical and developmental approaches to meaning and representation.* New York, NY: Oxford University Press.

Spitz, R. (1946) Anaclitic depression. *Psychoanalytic Study of the Child, 2*, 313–342.

Wood, M., Quirk, C., & Swindle, F. (2007). *Teaching responsible behavior: Developmental therapy-developmental teaching for troubled children and adolescents* (4th ed.). Austin, TX: ProEd.

# Integration of Child-Centered Play Therapy and Theraplay

**17**

Chapter

## *Evangeline Munns*

## Introduction

The current trend in play therapy appears to increasingly be toward an integration of different treatment models. This marriage is a comparatively easy one if many similarities exist between the models. However, this chapter will focus on integrating two models that are diametrically opposite to each other in their techniques. In child-centered play therapy (nondirective), the therapist follows the lead of the child, who initiates interactions (through role-playing), makes decisions, and determines the pace of play. Theraplay® (directive) has the child follow the therapist's lead, who makes the decisions and is in charge of the nature and duration of the activities. Needless to say, integrating these two models can be a challenge!

Regardless of what models are followed, it is important for all play therapists to be guided not only by the developmental level of the child but also by current brain research. This is particularly true when working with young children, in whom there is such rapid brain growth. We now have the technology (PET scans, MRIs, etc.) to be able to study the living brain. Such research reveals that the greatest growth of the human brain occurs in utero beginning during the last trimester of pregnancy and extends to the second year after birth. (The number of neural connections in a young child's brain is 50% greater than in an adult's brain and is two and a half times more active [Doidge, 2007].) There is an extra spurt of growth of neuronal connections during the first year, which is followed by the pruning of connections that are not used, where they fade or die away. (This extra spurt and pruning of connections happens in adolescence as well.) By the end of the fifth year, nine-tenths of the brain is developed. What happens during this crucial time where the brain is rapidly growing and is most plastic will have a lifelong impact. This is of particular concern for children coming from deprived, neglectful, or abusive backgrounds, who most often have insecure attachment patterns with their parents. These children are often referred to play therapists.

Play therapists also need to be aware of the features of the right and left brain (Nicholson and Parker, 2009; Sunderland, 2006), which change as children grow older. During the first three years of life, the right hemisphere is dominant. The right hemisphere processes sensorimotor experiences, emotional and social feelings, and is associated with creativity. The left hemisphere processes language, deals with logical thinking, and becomes dominant after three years.

Different parts of the brain develop sequentially. The lower or reptilian or more primitive part of the brain is the first to mature. It controls our survival systems, such as breathing, heart rate, digestion, sexual urges, and the instincts to "fight, freeze, or flee" when danger is detected. It also forms a base for the organization of the middle (mammalian, limbic, or emotional) brain, which governs our emotions. The middle part of the brain in turn needs to be well organized for the proper maturation of the higher brain (the neocortex and cortex), which governs our abstract, logical thinking, problem solving, reasoning, and judgment.

This suggests that when we are working with young children, we need to reach them through methods that are in line with their developing brains. In other words, nonverbal methods, rather than cognitive, verbal ones, should be emphasized for the very young. Bruce Perry, a neuroscientist, states that verbal therapy alone will never reach or alter the middle brain or brain stem (Perry & Szalavitz, 2006). He has developed a neurosequential program where he meets the child at his or her emotional age (regardless of the client's chronological age). If the child has come from an abusive or deprived background right from infancy, Perry will start by giving that child the experiences that an infant needs at that age, such as rocking, rhythm, touch (through massage), Theraplay activities, and those creating positive, repetitive patterns. Later he introduces therapies to that same child that help to organize his or her emotional or middle brain, such as psychodrama, sand play therapy, play therapy, art therapy, EMDR, and so on. Lastly, he will use the more verbal cognitive therapies that stimulate the higher brain, such as cognitive therapy, narrative therapy, and so on.

Perry's emphasis on touch at the beginning part of his therapy program is also in line with the fact that the tactile system is the most advanced sensory system in the newborn (Gerhardt, 2004) and that a baby explores his or her world largely through touch in the beginning. Children need touch in order to thrive (Brazelton, 1990; Brody, 1993; Field, 2000; Nicholson & Parker, 2009). A baby's self-concept begins with the way he or she is handled and touched (lovingly or harshly?) (Ford, 1993). Oxytocin and opioids are hormones that can be released in the brain through warm physical connections such as cuddling, rocking, caressing, and massage, which help calm the arousal system in the child. Research shows that early parenting experiences of the child are important factors in determining whether stress chemicals (cortisol) are strongly activated on a regular basis in later life. Whether a child is calmed down or left in distress determines his or her later ability for self-regulation (Gerhardt, 2004; Sunderland, 2006). Poor self-regulation has been associated with many social, emotional, and behavioral difficulties in both children and adults (Schore & Schore, 2008).

It is important for children not only to learn how to self-regulate their stress responses, but also they need to learn how to let go and experience "joy juice" (Sunderland, 2006). The brain has a genetic system for joy, but it needs to be activated by intervention with others (Panksepp, 1998). To feel heights of joy, the body's arousal system is activated by high levels of adrenalin, which increases heart and breathing rates (activation of lower brain) and releases optimal levels of hormones like dopamine and opioids (feel-good hormones). Optimal arousal of "joy juice" can lead to a sense of delight and heights of happiness. These peak experiences can make changes in the brain. In later life, these early experiences contribute to spontaneity, feelings of optimism, motivation, and hope (Sunderland, 2006).

In summary, when we choose our models of play therapy, it is important to remember that when we work with young children, particularly from birth to 3 years of age, we are interacting with them when their brain is developing most rapidly and therefore is most plastic, when the right hemisphere is dominant and when attachment to others is at its strongest growth (Schore, 2001, 2005). Children also need warm, affectional, physical contact in order to grow and thrive (Nicholson & Parker, 2009) and to achieve optimal arousal and self-regulation. The importance of paying attention to the development of the right hemisphere is supported by research that indicates that the stress from insecure attachments and/or maltreatment in childhood affects the right brain in particular. Furthermore, right brain deficits are associated with poor empathy capacity, poor ability to perceive the emotional states of others, and poor ability to appraise the internal cues of bodily states, leading to poor self-regulation (Schore & Schore, 2008).

## Rationale for the Integrative Approach

Two models were chosen to focus on in this chapter: Theraplay and child-centered play therapy. Sometimes children need both approaches, which is especially true with young children. For example, a child may have inner conflicts and issues that may be best expressed through child-centered play therapy, but he or she also may have fairly severe attachment and/or relationship problems with troubled parents or siblings that could be best addressed through a model like Theraplay. Furthermore, Theraplay is a treatment method that is in line with the development of the right hemisphere of the brain, because it emphasizes physical contact and strives for optimal arousal and calming of the child, leading to self-regulation. On the other hand, child-centered play therapy fosters the healing of another side of the child. It helps the child to work through inner conflicts and fears, helping the child to master them and to create his or her unique solutions to some of the most troubling aspects of life.

Child-centered play therapy strives to bolster feelings of independence, confidence, strength, and self-knowledge, all traits that are needed for good mental health. Both models focus on the child-therapist relationship as a way of developing trust and a way of learning to connect to another human being in an optimal way. Furthermore, Theraplay actively involves the parents, with goals of helping them to become more attuned and appropriately responsive to their child, as well as enhancing their attachment to each other. Child-centered play therapy has similar goals through the extension of its model through filial therapy (which is described later).

## Child-Centered Play Therapy

Child-centered play therapy is well known to practioners in the play therapy field around the world. It has a history dating back to Virginia Axline's (1947) adaptation of the Rogerian client-centered (nondirective) approach with adults. Gary Landreth (1991) is the best-known proponent of Axline's method. He adopted her eight basic principles within his child-centered play therapy. There is a strong underlying belief that all children have an innate striving for growth. They have a capacity for self-healing, self-direction, and self-actualization. The therapist, through the relationship with the child, provides the environment for this growth to take place. (Note that the core belief of capacity for self-healing is shared by Theraplay.) The eight principles of child-centered play therapy are as follows (Landreth, 1991, p. 77):

1. The therapist is genuinely interested in the child and develops a warm, caring relationship.
2. The therapist experiences unqualified acceptance of the child and does not wish that the child were different in some way.
3. The therapist creates a feeling of safety and permissiveness in the relationship, so the child feels free to explore and express the self completely.
4. The therapist is always sensitive to the child's feelings and gently reflects those feelings in such a manner that the child develops self-understanding.
5. The therapist believes deeply in the child's capacity to act responsibly, unwaveringly respects the child's ability to solve personal problems, and allows the child to do so.
6. The therapist trusts the child's inner direction, allows the child to lead in all areas of the relationship, and resists any urge to direct the child's play or conversation.
7. The therapist appreciates the gradual nature of the therapeutic process and does not attempt to hurry the process.
8. The therapist establishes only those therapeutic limits that help the child accept personal and appropriate relationship responsibility.

In child-centered play therapy, all eight principles are followed, particularly the one relating to following the child's lead. This method has been used with children from 2.5 years of age (at an age when some children can symbolize) to 12 or 13 years of age. It has been applied to a wide range of social, emotional, and behavioral disordered children, from those that are withdrawn, anxious, or depressed to the acting-out, impulsive child.

Typically, the child and therapist enter a playroom. where there is a large variety of toys designed to help the child play out his or her conflicts, fears, and wishes. The therapist creates a supportive, accepting atmosphere, and by tracking what the child does and reflecting on the child's feelings, helps the child to gain insight. Through the therapist's reflections, the child feels "felt" and understood. Limits are set by the therapist that help the child to gain self-control and self-regulation. The relationship between the therapist and child is crucial, because it creates the atmosphere for the child to increase his or her trust and to feel safe enough to explore deep-seated feelings. Weekly sessions usually last about 1 hour for at least six months to one or two years. The parents are not actively involved, but feedback is given to them approximately once every four to six weeks.

There is an extension of child-centered play therapy called filial therapy, where parents are very much involved, which was developed originally by the Guerneys in 1964 (Ryan and Bratton, 2008). Two main approaches to filial therapy are the ones devised by Bratton and Landreth (Bratton, Landreth, Kellam, & Blackard, 2006; Landreth & Bratton, 2005), which includes 10 sessions, and VanFleet's 14-session (or longer) model (VanFleet, 2005). Parents are taught the eight basic principles of child-centered play therapy and are coached in using these principles in play therapy sessions with their children. Parents are taught empathic listening and responding, as well as structuring and limit setting. Parental goals include becoming more attuned to their children, growing in their awareness of their children's needs, and learning how to respond more appropriately. Parents are taught as a single parent, as a couple, or in parental groups. Several checkups during the year are planned for after treatment ends.

Many research studies (including the use of randomized control groups) support the efficacy of this method. For reviews and meta-analysis of research studies for play therapy, including filial therapy, see Bratton et al. (2005) and LeBlanc and Ritchie (2001).

## Theraplay

Theraplay is a short-term, structured form of play therapy, where the therapist leads and the child follows. No toys are used. Theraplay tries to replicate the interactions that normally occur between parents and their young children in a positive, joyful atmosphere. There is an emphasis on healthy physical contact. It is geared toward right hemisphere development (Booth & Jernberg, 2010; Munns, 2009). An agenda is preplanned, based on the child's needs, which are previously determined by an in-depth developmental and family history of both the child and each parent, as well as the use of assessment tools such as the Marschak Interaction Method (MIM), where child and parents interact as they perform a series of semi-standardized tasks (DiPasquale, 2000). The MIM gives a picture of family dynamics, problems, and strengths. Goals are formulated together by the therapist and parents.

Theraplay is based on attachment theory, whose premise rests on the idea that a child's first relationship with his or her chief caregiver forms the template for all other relationships later in life. If this relationship is not secure, then difficulties in social and emotional adjustment are likely to arise throughout life (Bowlby, 1998). Research from around the world supports this theory (Fonagy, 2003; Rutter, 1994). Theraplay tries to go back to the roots of attachment (Munns, 2000, 2009). If a child has experienced an insecure or disrupted attachment from very early on, then the therapist will choose activities that one might do with a very young child: In other words, the therapist meets the child at his or her emotional level, providing nurturing activities that hopefully will provide the child with corrective experiences. This might mean cradling and singing to the child while feeding him or her a lollipop, juice box, or baby bottle, and later, as the child progresses, including more chronologically age-appropriate activities. This is in line with Dr. Perry's neurosequential programming (described previously), which he has successfully used with severely traumatized clients (Perry and Szalavitz, 2006).

Theraplay is applicable to the full age range, from infants to toddlers, preschoolers, latency-aged, adolescents, adults and the elderly, but it fits in especially well with young children. The aims of Theraplay are to enhance the parent-child attachment relationship, to increase trust and self-esteem, and to help parents become more attuned, empathic, reflective, and responsive to their children. (These goals are similar to filial play therapy.) In addition, Theraplay strives for optimal arousal of the child (e.g., to calm and soothe the dysregulated child and for more stimulating, joyful play with the withdrawn, passive, or depressed child). Parents learn to regulate their children's emotions, which later leads to their own self-regulation.

Theraplay has been used with a wide range of emotional, social, and behavioral problems (as child-centered play therapy has), but it is especially suitable for children who have attachment problems, such as those found in children coming from adoptive, step, foster, and institutionalized homes. It has been associated with significant changes in autistic children (Bundy-Myrow, 2000; Goodyear-Brown, 2009; Lindaman and Booth, 2010; Schlanger, 2010).

Theraplay is basically nonverbal, where no interpretations are made and no probing questions are asked, although reflections of how the child might be feeling (similar to child-centered therapy) are sometimes made. Problems are not talked about with the child, and there is an emphasis on noticing his or her positive attributes and strengths. This is very self-esteem building.

Initially, parents observe the therapist with their child from a one-way mirror or corner of the room in the first three or four sessions. (With very young children who may protest being separated from their parents, the parents are directly involved right from the first session.) When possible, an interpreting therapist remains with the parents to answer their questions and to make the parents more aware of their child's feelings and reactions. In the following 8 to 12 sessions (sometimes more with very troubled clients), the parents directly interact with their child under the guidance of the therapist. As the sessions progress, an increasing number of activities are led by the parents. They are also encouraged to practice Theraplay activities of their choosing at home. (It is important to check that this homework is done.) During the last session, there is a party to celebrate the family's progress and strengths. Four checkups are held during the year after therapy ends.

Each Theraplay session lasts about 30 minutes (group Theraplay sessions last about 1 hour). An optional (but recommended) 30-minute session of parental counseling is sometimes added, where a debriefing of the session takes place and progress at home and school is discussed. This can be a very important addition, where parents can become more sensitive, empathic with their child's needs, and more self-reflective as they gain objectivity regarding their own feelings and how their own childhood relationships can impact with their present interactions with their children (intergenerational transmission of attachment patterns [Zeanah, 1994]).

Theraplay activities are based on four underlying dimensions: structure, engagement, nurture, and challenge (Munns, 2008):

*Structure*
In normal situations the parent is in charge of the child's world, especially the young child, so the child's environment becomes safe and predictable. Structure helps the child to feel secure. Following rituals and routines, and setting boundaries and limits creates a rhythm in the child's life and helps promote a regulation of his or her feelings, which eventually leads to self-regulation.

In Theraplay, structure is created by the therapist being in charge, having a definite beginning and end to each session, following an agenda, as well as rules such as "no hurts." This dimension is especially needed by ADHD, impulsive, or dysregulated children, tyrants, parentified children, or those with behavior disorders. Examples of structuring activities are: Follow the Leader, Red Light, Green Light, Simon Says, and so on. (For an extensive list and description of Theraplay activities, see Munns, 2000, 2009, and Booth & Jernberg, 2010.)

*Engagement*
Parents often engage their children in happy ways that bring a shared time of joy and laughter ("joy juice"). Simple games such as peek-a-boo are well-known ways of connecting with young children and, in the process, children learn that surprises can be fun. They also learn that they can be a source of delight to their parents.

In Theraplay, engagement is used as a way to connect to the child. At times this means intruding into the child's space, but this is done in a playful way with a sensitivity to the child's possible reactions of anxiety or fear. Therapists strive to make engaging activities mutually enjoyable. However, if the child's anxiety becomes apparent, his or her feelings are reflected, and another way is found or the activity is modified so it becomes more comfortable to the child. Activities are not forced on the child.

Examples of engagement are This Little Piggy Went to Market, mirroring movements of each other (great for fostering attunement), blowing cottonballs to each other on a pillow, hiding complimentary notes on the child for the parents to find and read out loud, and so on. Engagement is especially needed for withdrawn, shy, fearful, or depressed children, those with strong defenses such as autistic children, or those with an obsessive-compulsive disorder.

*Nurture*
This is the most important dimension of all, and it is needed by all children the world over. In order for a child to survive and thrive, he or she will need nurturing. This is also a dimension that is crucial for a child to feel valued, loved, and cared for. In order for the child to develop an "inner working model" (Bowlby, 1998) that is positive and strong, that child will have had to experience adequate nurturing from his or her chief caregiver. Normally, parents nurture their children in hundreds of ways: feeding, cradling, embracing, caressing, kissing, generally being warm and affectionate and loving, while also providing for adequate care of their child, especially when their child is sick or stressed. When parents respond consistently and responsively to their child's cues for nurturance, they help establish a secure base for their child (Sunderland, 2006).

In Theraplay, nurturing is expressed through a variety of ways, such as feeding the child his or her favorite snack, powdering or lotioning of "hurts," cradling and rocking a child while singing a special song and feeding him or her a lollipop, juice box, or bottle, giving manicures, pedicures, and so on. Nurturing activities are geared toward the child's emotional age.

All children in Theraplay receive nurturing in every session, but this dimension is especially emphasized with children who have come from deprived, neglectful, or abusive backgrounds. Because nurturing often involves touch, the therapist must be extra sensitive to heightened anxiety from children who are afraid of physical contact, such as those who have been abused or are tactile defensive due to sensorimotor difficulties. Steps toward a deconditioning of this fear must be small and gently handled. If the child indicates "no," then the therapist must stop, reflect the child's fear, and find a different way that is more acceptable to the child. No force must be used.

Nurturing is also recommended especially for behavior-disordered and aggressive children who are constantly in trouble, and for those who are pseudo-mature (parentified) who have lost their childhood.

*Challenge*
Challenging activities, when mastered, lead to self-confidence and feelings of competency. The child learns that taking risks can lead to feelings of strength (as long as the tasks are within the child's capabilities). Challenging tasks are often tension releasing, so in Theraplay they are used with aggressive children (e.g., "paper punch").

In Theraplay, challenges are geared to the child's developmental abilities and are often cooperative. Examples of challenging activities are imitating an increasingly difficult sequence of clap patterns, pillow push, hockey game by blowing cotton balls, three-legged walk, watermelon seed spitting contest, and so on. Challenging tasks in Theraplay often create a lot of laughter. Children who are fearful, anxious, timid, withdrawn, or overprotected need appropriate challenging tasks in order to stretch themselves and grow.

Theraplay has an increasing number of research studies to support it, including the use of randomly assigned control groups using standardized pre- and post-test measures. For research reviews, see Coleman (2010), Wardrop and Meyer, (2009), and Munns (2008). Two trends have consistently emerged from this research: Theraplay can significantly improve the adjustment of behavior-disordered children, including lowering their levels of aggression, and Theraplay can heighten children's self-esteem.

## Practical Implementation of the Integrative Approach

Several questions need to be considered when integrating different therapeutic approaches to the same child. What does the child need most at this particular time? If working with parents, one needs to ask, Do the parents need their own therapeutic work as well? Should this come first? Can an integration of different therapeutic approaches be confusing for the child, parents, and also the therapist (especially the inexperienced therapist)? It is obvious that the therapist will need to be thoroughly trained in both models first and know the strengths and limitations of both. If one is using both approaches in the same sessions, how do you decide when you will use one or the other?

A comparatively easy solution to some of these questions is simply to use one approach for a number of sessions and then to use a different method for a second set of sessions, or to use one method for say the first part of the session and a different one for the last part of the session. This last method is briefly described in the first case illustration. It is followed by another case illustration that is more difficult, where two methods were integrated throughout the same session.

## Case Example

### Case A

A very withdrawn, quiet, 5-year-old boy was referred for child-centered play therapy, because he was extremely passive and did not move or make decisions unless he was told what to do by his teachers. He appeared frozen and was hypervigilant. This behavior was evident in the playroom, where he would stand and not engage with any of the toys for many weeks. The therapist was accepting and patiently waited for him to feel safe and secure enough to behave more freely. After several months, with little change in his behavior and a decision by the family to move, it was decided to try 20 minutes of Theraplay first in a different room followed by 40 minutes of child-centered play therapy in the play therapy room with the same therapist who was trained in using both methods. This combination brought some remarkable results. The child was actively engaged, challenged, and nurtured in Theraplay (he did not need any structuring). His overall behavior and emotional expression became more spontaneous.

In the child-centered sessions, he started to more freely explore the room and he played with a variety of toys. One was a baby doll that he undressed and then, taking a pretend needle from the medical kit, he pricked the baby's bottom fairly viciously, over and over again. (This child had had many medical procedures in the past.) More information from the family revealed that this child had witnessed domestic violence, where his father had pushed his mother down the stairs. From brain research (Perry and Szalavitz, 2006), we know that children who experience trauma can have an instinctive response of "fight, flight, or freeze" under severe stress. This little boy could not fight or flee, so he became frozen. Through both Theraplay and child-centered play therapy, he gradually became more normalized in his behavior. The emphasis in this case was on child-centered play therapy, because the child had a lot of underlying issues to work through, and he needed to learn to make his own decisions.

The more difficult way of integrating different therapeutic models is when the therapist uses both models at the same time in the same session. The following case will illustrate this where Theraplay was emphasized, but child-centered play therapy also played an important part.

## Case B

A 4-year-old child who had been assessed and diagnosed as autistic and developmentally delayed was referred to our play therapy services, because she was extremely withdrawn, passive, and avoided interacting with either adults or peers. Many people had approached her, but she rarely responded. Mary played alone, lining up toys in rows, showing little imagination or creativity in her play. She became an isolated figure in the classroom. Her eye contact was brief, and her facial expression was flat. Mary was basically mute except for occasional single words and echolalia, where she repeated phrases of people speaking to her. She used a flat, monotone voice. Occasionally she would hum to herself. Loud noises frightened her (sound of a lawn mower). Her perseveration was evident in her play and also in her tendency to jump for hours (if allowed to do so) on a miniature trampoline. When adults gave her clear directions, she was obedient and cooperative. Her parents reported that at home she often did nothing.

The Marschak Interaction Method was administered, which included both parents and Mary in a series of tasks designed to assess parent-child relationships (DiPasquale, 2000). This assessment revealed that although the parents were warm, supportive, and caring toward Mary, they also put tremendous pressure constantly on her to speak (she had received speech therapy in the past) and for achievement in the majority of the tasks. Her father in particular was overdirecting and overcontrolling to the point that Mary tuned him out. There was little relaxation and a lot of tension. Added to this, it was learned that both paternal and maternal grandparents were also trying to constantly elicit speech from her.

The therapist felt that Mary needed child-centered play therapy where, with a supportive therapist who put no pressure on her, she could make her own decisions and hopefully engage in more imaginative play and work out her issues in her own way. However, in the therapist's past experience, doing nondirective play therapy with autistic children brought very little change after months of such therapy with this population. This was a worry. With the parents' constant pressure for her to talk, it was evident that the parents needed to be included in therapy with her. Their relationship had to change. Both models of filial and Theraplay included work with parents. However, the father was strongly obsessive compulsive and highly anxious, so it was felt that Theraplay might be more suitable for him. Mary needed the direct engagement that Theraplay could give her to stimulate her in a playful way.

Goals for Theraplay were for the parents to simply enjoy their child, to accept her unconditionally, with no expectations for her to speak or achieve. Other goals were to enhance the attachment between Mary and her parents, to increase their sensitivity and attunement to her needs, to engage her in playful, joyful ways that would help to free her emotionally and motorically, as well as increasing her self-confidence. Additional goals for Mary were to increase her assertiveness, to be less passive, to overcome some of her fears, and to be more open to interacting with people. Engagement, nurture, and challenge were the dimensions to be emphasized. At the beginning of treatment, the therapist asked the parents to completely stop trying to teach her any language, and this request was to be extended to all relatives as well, for the duration of her treatment.

Before Theraplay started, the therapist spent many weeks sitting beside Mary in her classroom, giving her full attention and accepting whatever she did using a modified form of nondirective play therapy where little tracking or reflections were given. Because this child seemed so easily overwhelmed by adults, the therapist simply wanted to establish a quiet, comfortable rapport with her in surroundings that she was familiar with. One day as she was molding some play-dough, Mary turned to the therapist and said "cookie" and offered it to the therapist. This was a breakthrough and turning point, where Mary started giving the therapist more eye contact and a few smiles. It was decided that Mary was now ready for Theraplay and would not be afraid to leave her classroom and go with the therapist to her office (the Theraplay room). She walked cheerfully, hand in hand down a long hallway to the therapist's office.

The first Theraplay session went well. She seemed fairly relaxed, cooperated fully, and even seemed to enjoy some of the activities (e.g., being picked up and swung around in a circle, which elicited a big smile). Each session started with a welcome song, followed by a checkup where the therapist noticed her positive features ("What have you brought today? I see you have your shiny hair, blue sparkling eyes, and when you smile—guess what?—there's a big dimple right there!"). This was followed by checking for hurts or boo-boos on her hands and gently powdering or lotioning them. These three activities always occurred in every session, as did the feeding of snacks and a goodbye song at the end of the session. A typical agenda looked like this:

Welcome song

Checkup

Lotioning of hurts

Play-dough trophies (play-dough prints of body parts such as hands, ears, etc.

Imitating clap patterns (including touching each other's hands)

"Ring Around the Rosie" holding hands as we circled

Blowing and catching soap bubbles

Push me over and pull me up (to help her be more assertive)

Feeding of a snack

Goodbye song

The therapist tried to maintain a balance of quiet, calming activities with more vigorous, exciting activities. A balance of activities where there was close physical contact and those where there was distance, when both therapist and Mary moved about the room, was also planned.

By the fourth session, Mary's parents and an interpreting therapist started to observe the sessions behind a one-way mirror. (Ordinarily, parents start observing three or four sessions right from the beginning. However, this was the first time the therapist had used Theraplay with an autistic child, and she did not want anyone to observe her at the beginning.) By the sixth session, more challenging activities were introduced, such as balancing a bean bag on her head while walking, pushing each other with a pillow, playing peek-a-boo with a pillow, and so on. In the seventh session, two more challenging activities were introduced: jumping from various heights into the therapist's arms (Mary was afraid of heights) and cradling her in the therapist's arms while singing a special song about her. Her mother cried while observing this and stated that Mary had never allowed her to do this in the past.

In the eighth session, the parents and therapist entered a Theraplay session for the first time. Previous to their coming in, the therapist and Mary hid under a blanket and called out "come find us." Mary echoed "find us." (She had already started to be more expressive verbally beforehand; i.e., she had said "ready set" at the beginning of the swinging activity.) Much to everyone's surprise, Mary invented a hide-and-seek game by walking into a closet, closing the door, and then peeking out. She repeated this again and again. Everyone was delighted at her showing some iniative. From this moment on, following her lead whenever she initiated anything became a priority (child-centered play therapy). The following sessions still focused primarily on doing Theraplay activities, but everyone was sensitive to letting her lead if she chose to do so.

In the ninth session, more active activities that included everyone continued to be played out, such as wheelbarrow walk, hopping across the room, stacking hands, cotton ball fight, and cotton ball sooth. Nurturing activities such as playing beauty parlor were also included.

The 10th session was another turning point. When hiding under the blanket, Mary spontaneously called out "Mummy, daddy, find us." In the activity Circle Magnets (where everyone sits in a circle and, while singing, keeps getting closer until there is a group hug at the end), Mary spontaneously sang the second and third verse of "Jack and Jill" by herself. Everyone looked at her in amazement. No one had known that she knew this song. (During this time, the therapist, who was also a psychologist, administered an intelligence test used for assessing deaf children, called the Leiter Performance Scale, and Mary scored in the average range.) With this information and Mary's amazing performance in the Theraplay sessions (she spontaneously sang the second and third verses of "Ba, Ba, Black Sheep" and other songs in other sessions), the therapist encouraged a young, motivated teacher to spend more one-on-one time with Mary in the classroom, knowing that there was so much more potential to this little girl than previous assessments in the past had given her credit for. Her parents were also encouraged to do Theraplay activities at home at least once a week for 30 minutes. They were guided to be sensitive to Mary's cues, particularly to be perceptive of what she enjoyed and what made her anxious or afraid, and never to force her in any way. Unconditional acceptance and just taking delight in what she did were key approaches.

The 16th and final session was celebrated with a party where the family's favorite activities were included and often led by the parents. Special food and drink were brought in by the parents (Mary spontaneously shared some of her food with her father). Small remembrance gifts were exchanged. The dates for four Theraplay checkups during the year were planned for. By this time, Mary was much more involved in the classroom, was more open to responding to social contact by others, and was more receptive and alert toward learning in general. She also seemed happier, showing many more smiles and even occasional laughter. She moved more freely and with more confidence.

In each of the checkups during the year, Mary related to the therapist as if she had just seen her yesterday and was open and eager to see the therapist. She continued with her positive gains throughout the years. When Mary was 9 years old, the mother requested another checkup, because Mary kept asking to see the therapist. This request was granted, and during this checkup Mary continued to be eager and happy in her interactions with the therapist. Another contact with Mary was made when she was 12 years old. The therapist had been invited to Mary's home to discuss, with the executive of a parent group for autistic children, the possibility of teaching Theraplay to other parents. Mary greeted the therapist at the door with a big smile and was able to converse very appropriately. She talked about a friend at school: "Well, I have a friend in school, who tried out for the school choir. But she didn't make it. I felt so sorry for her." The therapist was so happy for her—she had a friend and she could show empathy for her!

At 21 years old, Mary had graduated from high school, had taken extra training at a technical school, and had started her own business (with her parents' help). The therapist was invited to the opening of her business and was greeted at the door by Mary, who said "I remember you—you used to sing "Hello Mary, hello Mary" (the opening welcome song of the Theraplay sessions when she was 4 years old). To this day Mary runs her own business, has direct physical contact with her clients, has a few friends, and has traveled extensively with her parents, as well as traveling alone and also with friends. She has spoken about being autistic at conferences and other groups. In a local newspaper, an article was written by a reporter who had interviewed Mary's mother, who stated; "Dr. Munns performed miracles with an approach called Theraplay. By the age of 6 years, Mary was transformed from a frail girl with a lost, preoccupied air to a smiling, laughing, talking child—still occasionally withdrawn, hand flapping and obsessively jumping—but a world away from how she had been. Today she runs her own business, and has 300 clients. She regularly speaks to symposiums and workshops and offers her insights to parent support groups throughout the city" (Zarzour, 2010, p. 3).

## Conclusion

Integrating Theraplay and child-centered play therapy is an ideal combination when working with young children, especially if they are very young. In the infant to 3-year-old population, children cannot easily express their needs or fears, so nonverbal therapies are most appropriate. Because the right brain is dominant at that age, which also coincides with the greatest growth of the brain and strongest attachment growth, it seems logical to incorporate play therapy models that are attachment based, such as Theraplay and filial therapy (which represents child-centered play therapy).

Young children need both a directive and a nondirective approach. They love to be engaged by direct, playful interactions with an adult (like Theraplay), and their brains are hard-wired for those kind of interactions, but they also need space and time where they can do what they want to do and in this process discover who they are and their relationship to the world around them. Having periods of following the child's lead is very important, especially with a 2-year-old who is at a stage of exploration and striving for independence (e.g., "me do"). Adults should let that happen, even in a structured approach. However, young children also need direction from adults to keep their world safe, secure, and predictable and to help them learn to self-regulate. This duplicates normal interactions between parents and their small children, which appears to be a dance where parents follow the child's lead and at other times will initiate interactions and be the leaders (Stern, 1995).

Whatever method is followed, directive or nondirective, the therapist has to be sensitively attuned to the child's nonverbal as well as verbal cues, needs to be empathic, must give the child unconditional acceptance, and somehow transmit a feeling to the child that he or she has strengths and potentialities for positive growth. It is strongly recommended that before a therapist tries to integrate different models that he or she receive training and have experience in both methods so that the strengths and limitations of each method is known and what aspects of each model are best suited for specific populations.

# References

Axline, V. (1947). *Play therapy*. Cambridge, MA: Houghton Mifflin.

Booth, P. B., & Jernberg, A. M. (2010). *Theraplay: Helping parents and children build better relationships through attachment-based play* (3rd ed.). San Francisco, CA: Jossey-Bass.

Bowlby, J. (1998). *A secure base*. New York, NY: Basic Books.

Bratton, S. C., Landreth, G. L., Kellam, T., & Blackard, S. (2006). *Child-parent relationship therapy (CPRT) treatment manual. A 10-session filial therapy model for training parents*. New York, NY: Routledge.

Bratton, S. C., Ray, D., Rhine, T., & Jones, L. (2005). The efficacy of play therapy with children. A meta-analytic review of the outcome research. *Professional Psychology Research and Practice, 36*(4), 376–390.

Brazelton, T. B. (1990). Touch as a touchstone: Summary of the round table. In K. E. Barnard & B. Brazelton (Eds.), *Touch: The foundations of experience*. Madison, CT: International Universities Press.

Brody, V. A. (1993). *The dialogue of touch: Developmental play therapy*. Treasure Island, FL: Developmental Play Therapy Associates.

Bundy-Myrow, S. (2000). Group theraplay for children with autism and pervasive developmental disorder. In E. Munns (Ed.), *Theraplay: Innovations in attachment-enhancing play therapy*. Northvale, NJ: Jason Aronson.

Coleman, R. (2010). Research findings that support the effectiveness of theraplay. In P. B. Booth & A. M. Jernberg (Eds.), *Theraplay: Helping parents and children build better relationships through attachment-based play* (3rd ed., pp. 85–97). San Francisco, CA: Jossey-Bass.

DiPasquale, L. (2000). The Marschak Interaction Method. In E. F. Munns (Ed.), *Theraplay: Innovations in attachment-enhancing play therapy* (pp. 27–51). Northvale, NJ: Jason Aronson.

Doidge, N. (2007). *The brain that changes itself*. New York, NY: Penguin Books.

Field, T. (2000). *Touch therapy*. New York, NY: Churchill Livingstone.

Fonagy, P. (2003). The development of psychopathology from infancy to adulthood: The mysterious unfolding of disturbance in time. *Infant Mental Health Journal, 24*(3), 212–239.

Ford, C. W. (1993). *Compassionate touch: The role of human touch in healing and recovery*. New York, NY: Simon & Schuster.

Gerhardt, S. (2004). *Why love matters: How affection shapes a baby's brain*. New York, NY: Brunner-Routledge.

Goodyear-Brown, P. (2009). Theraplay approaches for children with autism spectrum disorders. In E. F. Munns (Ed.), *Applications of family and group theraplay* (pp. 69–80). New York, NY: Jason Aronson.

Guerney, B. (1964). Filial therapy: Description and rationale. *Journal of Consulting Psychology, 28*(4), 303–310.

Landreth, G. L. (1991). *Play therapy: The art of the relationship*. Muncie, IN: Accelerated Development.

Landreth, G. L., & Bratton, S. C. (2005). *Child-parent relationship therapy (CPRT): A 10-session filial therapy model*. New York, NY: Routledge.

LeBlanc, M., & Ritchie, M. (2001). A meta-analysis of play therapy outcomes. *Counseling Psychology Quarterly, 14*, 149–163.

Lindaman, S., & Booth, P. B. (2010). Theraplay for children with autism spectrum disorders. In P. B. Booth & A. M. Jernberg (Eds.), *Theraplay: Helping parents and children build better relationships through attachment-based play* (3rd ed.). San Francisco, CA: Jossey-Bass.

Munns, E. F. (2009). *Applications of family and group theraplay*. New York, NY: Jason Aronson.

Munns, E. F. (2008). Theraplay with zero to three-year-olds. In C. E. Schaefer, S. Kelly-Zion, J. McCormick, & A. Ohnogi, *Play therapy for very young children* (pp. 157–170). Northvale, NJ: Jason Aronson.

Munns, E. F. (2000). *Theraplay: Innovations in attachment-enhancing play therapy.* Northvale, NJ: Jason Aronson.

Nicholson, B., & Parker, L. (2009). *Attached at the heart: Eight proven parenting principles for raising connected and compassionate children.* New York, NY: iUniverse.

Panksepp. J. (1998). *Affective neuroscience.* New York, NY: Oxford University Press.

Perry, B. D., & Szalavitz, M. (2006). *The boy that was raised as a dog.* New York, NY: Basic Books.

Rutter, M. (1994, October). Clinical implications of attachment concepts: retrospect and prospect. Paper presented at the International Conference on Attachment and Psychopathology, Toronto, Ontario, Canada.

Ryan, V., & Bratton, S. C. (2008). Child-centered play therapy for very young children. In C. E. Schaefer, S. Kelly-Zion, J. McCormick, & A. Ohnogi, *Play therapy for very young children* (pp. 25–66). Northvale, NJ: Jason Aronson.

Schlanger, R. (2010). *For the love of Melissa.* Bloomington, IN: AuthorHouse.

Schore, A. N. (2001). The effects of early relational trauma on right brain development and affect regulation and infant mental health. *Infant Mental Health Journal, 22*(1-2), 201–269.

Schore, A. N. (2005). Attachment, affect regulation, and the developing right brain: Linking developmental neuroscience to pediatrics. *Pediatrics in Review, 26,* 204–217.

Schore, J. R., & Schore, A. N. (2008). Modern attachment theory: The central role of affect regulation in development and treatment. *Clinical Social Work Journal, 36,* 9–20.

Stern, D. N. (1995). *The motherhood constellation: A unified view of parent-infant psychotherapy.* New York, NY: Basic Books.

Sunderland, M. (2006). *The science of parenting.* New York, NY: Dorling Kindersley.

VanFleet, R. (2005). *Filial therapy: Strengthening parent-child relationships through play* (2nd ed.). Sarasota, FL: Professional Resource Press.

Wardrop, J., & Meyer, L. (2009). Research on theraplay effectiveness. In E. F. Munns (Ed.), *Applications of family and group theraplay* (pp. 17–24). Northvale, NJ: Jason Aronson.

Zarzour, K. (2010). Mom shares story of autism. *The Thornhill Liberal,* May 15, p. 3.

Zeanah, C. (1994, September). Intergenerational transmission of relationship psychopathology: A mother-infant case study. Paper presented at the International Conference on Attachment and Psychopathology. Toronto, Ontario, Canada.

# An Integrative Humanistic Play Therapy Approach to Treating Adopted Children With a History of Attachment Disruptions

| 18 |
| :---: |
| Chapter |

## *Sue C. Bratton, Kara Carnes-Holt, and Peggy L. Ceballos*

## Introduction

Attachment theory is a well-established framework for understanding social-emotional development and for conceptualizing the nature of a child's primary relationships. Since Bowlby's (1969) pioneering observations on human attachment behavior, researchers and clinicians have been interested in understanding and applying attachment principles in child therapy (Cassidy & Shaver, 2008; Heard & Lake, 1997). A secure attachment during early childhood is associated with mental health and satisfying relationships, whereas insecure attachments have been linked to a host of psychosocial disorders across the life span (Belsky & Fearon, 2002; Fearon, Bakermans-Kranenburg, Ijzendoorn, Lapsley, & Roisman, 2010; van der Kolk, 2005). Attachment problems arise from a variety of often complex factors that result in inconsistency or loss of the attachment relationship with the primary caregiver. Fostered and late-adopted children are particularly at risk for attachment-related problems that can range from subtle to severe. Children who experience attachment disruptions in their caregiving relationships during the first year of life are at greater risk for adverse effects throughout their development (Perry & Szalavitz, 2006), hence the need for relationship-based, early intervention that optimally includes intense parental involvement as part of the overall treatment plan (Hughes, 2006; Forbes & Post, 2006; Purvis, Cross, & Sunshine, 2007; Siegel & Hartzell, 2003).

This chapter begins with a rationale for an integrative approach to treating attachment difficulties. The application of humanistic and attachment theory in an integrative play therapy intervention is illustrated through a complex case involving a late adopted child who had experienced multiple attachment disruptions. Central to this approach is the significant involvement of parents/caregivers in the therapeutic process. We propose that, whereas a humanistic approach provides the primary framework for conceptualization and practice, an understanding of attachment theory and an awareness of attachment dynamics in the therapist-child and parent-child relationships informs and enhances treatment.

## Rationale for Integrative Approach

Essential to the humanistic approach to play therapy is the belief in the healing nature of the therapist-child relationship and the conditions and attitudes necessary for an effective therapeutic alliance (Rogers, 1961). Attachment theory places a similar value on the significance of the quality of the parent-child relationship. The importance of a secure, predictable relationship in helping children develop the capacity for self-regulation is emphasized in both. Wilson and Ryan (2005) discussed the similarities of nondirective play therapy and optimal infant socialization that occurs in a healthy parent-child relationship. We propose that a humanistic play therapy approach following the child-centered play therapy (CCPT) principles and procedures outlined by Landreth (2002) provides a child with the experience of an attuned relationship that provides a secure base from which the child can feel safe to explore, create, and make sense of past and current experiences.

### Humanistic Play Therapy Principles and Practice

Bratton and Ray (2002) defined humanistic play therapy as belief in (a) the phenomenal world of the child; (b) the child's natural striving toward growth and maturity; (c) the child's capacity for self-evaluation, self-regulation, self-direction, self-responsibility, and socialization; and (d) the importance of the therapist-child relationship in facilitating the child's dynamic growth and healing. Although Axline was the first to apply these principles in play therapy, Clark Moustakas (1953) and, more recently, Louise Guerney (1983) and Garry Landreth (1991, 2002), have made significant contributions to the understanding and practice of humanistic play therapy approaches in the United States. CCPT is the most well-known humanistic play therapy approach in North America. The humanistic principles and procedures outlined in this chapter are aligned with those detailed in Landreth's (2002) text on CCPT.

In practice, CCPT offers a clear method of treatment, in which the relationship between child and therapist is the catalyst for all healing change. The child's experience within the therapeutic relationship is the factor that is most meaningful and vital. The therapist conveys attitudes of genuineness, unconditional positive regard, and empathy that if experienced by the child facilitates the child feeling accepted and safe to fully express self and move toward more positive functioning. This process allows the therapist to "experience in a very personal and interactive way the inner dimensions of the child's world" (Landreth & Bratton, 2000, p. 5). Axline (1947) described this process as one in which the play therapist grants the child the freedom to be, without evaluation or pressure to change. Following CCPT principles described by Axline (1947) and revised by Landreth (2002), the therapist develops a warm relationship with the child, accepts the child unconditionally, allows permissiveness within the relationship, acknowledges the child's feelings, respects the child's capacity to solve problems, trusts the child's inner direction, recognizes the gradual nature of the child's process, and establishes minimal limits.

Filial therapy, developed by Bernard and Louise Guerney in the early 1960s (Guerney, 1969), expanded the practice of CCPT to include parents in the treatment process. Landreth (1991, 2002) developed a more structured, time-limited filial therapy model, which was recently formalized into a text, *Child Parent Relationship Therapy* (CPRT; Landreth & Bratton, 2006) and a manualized treatment protocol (Bratton, Landreth, Kellam, & Blackard, 2006). In this model, parents receive training and direct supervision in the basic methodology of child-centered play therapy within a small support-group format. Parents conduct weekly, supervised play therapy–type sessions with their child, learning to convey acceptance, empathy, and encouragement, as well as master the skills of effective limit setting. CPRT empowers parents to be therapeutic caregivers to their children and helps facilitate the attachment bond, which is critical for adoptive families. CCPT and CPRT both have a substantial research base to support their utility with a broad array of target issues (Bratton, Ray, Rhine, & Jones, 2005; Bratton, Landreth, & Lin, 2010; Baggerly, Ray, & Bratton, 2010; Ray & Bratton, 2010), but research specific to this population is needed. Carnes-Holt (2010) investigated the effects of CPRT with 61 caregivers of adopted children in the only controlled outcome study to date to examine humanistic play therapy procedures with this population. She found that training caregivers in CCPT skills had a statistically significant beneficial treatment effect on reducing child behavior problems and stress in the parent-child relationship, as well as increasing parental empathy.

## Attachment Theory

Infants born into this world depend on their primary caregiver for survival. When the caregiver consistently meets the infant's needs for sustenance, nurturance, and safety, the infant grows to trust that her caregiver can be counted on to meet her needs (Heard & Lake, 1997). According to Bowlby (1980), children who have experienced this type of responsive relationship develop a secure attachment to their primary caregiver, who serves as a secure base from which the child can explore the world. This attachment process is intrinsically connected to the holistic development of the child. Through interactions in the primary attachment relationship, the infant develops the capacity for emotional self regulation (Schore, 2003). A secure foundation of a safe, predictable, and attuned relationship provides the needed socio-emotional framework for individuation and independence (Schore, 1994). This type of relationship develops the framework for the child's perception of self, relationships, and the world—or what Bowlby (1969) referred to as the internal working model. A secure attachment provides the resources for the child to develop meaningful interpersonal relationships in the future (Bowlby, 1980; Schore, 1994; Siegel & Hartzell, 2003).

> *Intimate attachments to other human beings are the hub around which a person's life revolves, not only when he is an infant or a toddler or a schoolchild but throughout his [sic] adolescence and his [sic] years of maturity as well, and on to old age. From these intimate attachments a person draws his [sic] strength and enjoyment of life and, through what he [sic] contributes, he [sic] gives strength and enjoyment to others. (Bowlby, 1980, p. 442)*

Siegel and Hartzell (2003) discussed the essential role of attunement in secure attachment. Attunement is often communicated through nonverbal expressions between caregiver and child, in which the caregiver's internal state is aligned with the child's internal experience. The attuned caregiver is seen as emotionally responsive, and consistent. Attunement is the foundation for the child's ability to seek a sense of holistic balance of body, emotion, and mind (Siegel, 2007). Thus, a sense of integration begins to develop in children by the means of the child-caregiver relationship. The child can begin to feel a sense of internal congruence as well as satisfaction in developing interpersonal connections with others.

Fundamental to attachment theory is the notion that variation in the quality of caregiving by a parent, such as emotional availability, acceptance, sensitivity, and responsiveness, particularly during times of distress, will predictably lead to varying degrees of secure or insecure attachment behaviors in the child (Cassidy, 1999). As described above, secure attachment develops in the midst of an attuned relationship that facilitates repeated experiences of love, safety, and trust. Unfortunately, all children do not experience this type of relationship. Although attachment disruptions can result from a variety of factors, ranging from difficult pregnancies and medical complications to emotional neglect and physical abuse, foster care and other non-relative placements account for a growing number of children whose primary attachment bond has been broken (Hinshaw-Fuselier, 2004). "Loss of a primary attachment figure represents a loss of everything to a child: loss of love, safety, protection, even life itself" (James, 1994, p. 7). Children who experience multiple caregiver losses in their early development are at significant risk for the development of insecure attachment.

Insecure attachments are typically categorized as avoidant, ambivalent, or disorganized (Bowlby, 1980; Goldberg, 1995; Schore, 1994). Avoidant attachment is commonly manifested when the child experiences repeated rejection and emotional unresponsiveness from the caregiver. As a result, the child adapts to these repeated experiences by avoiding an emotional connection and a sense of closeness with the primary caregiver. The anxious-ambivalent or resistant pattern of attachment is characterized by a relationship between parent and child in which the parent is inconsistently attuned to the child's emotional needs. Due to unreliable and unpredictable caregiving, the child cannot be confident that her needs will be met; hence, the child experiences a sense of anxiety and exhibits approach/avoidance behavior with caregivers. A third category, disorganized attachment style, is often characterized by caregiver interaction styles that are repeatedly experienced by the child as chaotic and frightening. Feelings of intense terror can overwhelm the child, with the result that the child often functions from an alarm state.

Disruption in the early caregiving relationship has been widely acknowledged as traumatic to the developing child, often resulting in significant neuro-developmental consequences (Perry, 2006). "At the core of traumatic stress is a breakdown in the capacity to regulate internal states" (van der Kolk, 2005, p. 403). A child who lacked attentive and protective parenting is continually searching for a way to achieve a felt sense of safety, commonly manifested in hypervigilance (Perry, 1994). Increased fear, sensory processing issues, difficulty self-regulating, disorder of memory, and short-term memory loss are some of the consequences present in the lives of children who have experienced attachment breaks and interpersonal trauma (Forbes & Post, 2006; Hughes, 1999; Purvis et al., 2007). When traumatized children experience their environment as unpredictable and chaotic, their anxiety and distress increases (Perry, 1994) and results in what is commonly referred to as the fight, flight, or freeze response.

The fight, flight, or freeze response originates in the amygdala which signals the rest of the brain as a guide of how to respond to stressful situations. Repeated early interpersonal traumas significantly compromise the regulatory ability of the amygdala, resulting in a myriad of outward behaviors and emotions that can range from a child quietly rocking in a corner to a child exhibiting intense aggressive behaviors (Perry, 1994; Siegel & Hartzell, 2003). Children who have previously experienced inconsistent care, neglect, and abuse perceive that, in order to be safe, they must control their environment (Hughes, 1999). This control may manifest through behaviors such as extreme tantrums, aggression, indiscriminate affection, and isolation from others. These are the survival skills the child has developed as a way to maintain personal safety and control.

Attachment disruptions impede the holistic development of the child and often result in developmental lags, particularly in the social emotional realm. Informed treatment planning must take into account the often varied development needs of the child. Perry (2006) communicated this difficulty when talking with the adoptive parents of a young child:

> *The challenge is that, in one moment, you will need to have expectations and provide experiences that are appropriate for a five-year-old, for example, when teaching him a specific cognitive concept. Ten minutes later, however, the expectations and challenges will have to match those for a younger child, for example, when you*

*are trying to teach him to interact socially. He is, developmentally, a moving target. That is why parenting these children is such a frustrating experience. One moment you are doing the correct thing and the next you are out of sync. (p. 223)*

In summary, the attachment process is intrinsically connected to the holistic well-being of the child. Attachment theory provides a lens for understanding the child's social emotional development and experience of primary relationships. Additionally, an understanding of attachment dynamics in the therapist-child and parent-child relationships provides the clinician with greater sensitivity to the child's needs (Ryan, 2004).

## Application of Integrated Approach

### Case Example

The following case provides a glimpse into the process of an integrative humanistic play therapy approach with a young child who presented with a complex history of multiple attachment disruptions. This case illustrates how an understanding of attachment theory informs the humanistic clinician's conceptualization and understanding of the child and the therapeutic process, which in turn guides clinical decision making. Furthermore, relationship dynamics between therapist and child are explained from both a humanistic and attachment perspective. The child participated in play therapy and Child Parent Relationship Therapy (CPRT) with the first author for a total of 55 sessions over a 20-month period, including 16 supervised play sessions with his parents. The playroom space and materials used in this case were consistent with Landreth's (2002) recommendations to facilitate a wide range of expression and included play materials representative of the child's bicultural experiences.

Although individual play therapy is the focus of this chapter, regular parent consultation, CPRT/filial therapy training with the parents, and collaboration with school professionals were essential components of treatment. Regrettably, the scope of this chapter prevents a full description of these systemic interventions. Specifically, this case illustrates the child's movement toward (a) trusting that primary adults (therapist and parents) in his life could be counted on to consistently respond to his needs, (b) integration of his early experiences into his self-concept, (c) increased levels of self-acceptance and self-regulation, and (d) enhanced developmental functioning in all areas, particularly in the social and emotional realms. Identifying information has been changed to protect the child and his family.

*Identifying Features of the Client*
Andy presented as a much smaller than average 6-year-old male (by American norms) who was of Chinese descent. He was referred to play therapy by his adoptive parents, both of whom are of Anglo descent. Before being adopted

at 4 years old, he lived at an orphanage in China, where he was given the name of Dom. He had been abandoned at the orphanage when he was approximately 1 year old by a temporary caregiver. He was currently living with his adoptive parents, Carol and Tom (both 45 years of age), a 13-year-old stepsister, Ann (biological child of parents), and a 7-year-old stepbrother, Chris, who was adopted from China when Andy was 5½ years old. At the time of intake, Dom had just completed kindergarten, and he had recently decided he wanted to be called Andy, the American name he was given at the adoption proceedings.

*Developmental History*
Very little is known about Andy's developmental history before adoption. Orphanage records revealed that when Dom was a small baby, his birth mother abruptly abandoned him to a neighbor under the pretense of running an errand, and that the neighbor kept him for an unspecified length of time before leaving him at the orphanage at what officials guessed to be around the age of 1 year old. Records stated that Dom never talked, but that he was an affectionate and cute baby and child. His developmental milestones were not recorded, but he was mostly toilet trained at the time of adoption. His gross motor skills and coordination were reported by his adoptive parents to be above average. When Carol and Tom first met Andy in the orphanage, they noticed that he appeared cross-eyed, but that he seemed able to focus when they came close to him. Andy had just turned 4 years of age when Carol and Tom brought him from China to join their family. A checkup by the family pediatrician determined that Andy's eye condition was so severe that he could see very little. After being in the United States a little over one week, he underwent major eye surgery. Carol recalled the week after surgery as very stressful for Andy and for her. As part of his eye treatment, Andy wore eyeglasses with a very strong correction.

Within a month of his arrival, 4-year-old Andy was enrolled in the prekindergarten program at the school where Carol was an administrator. He was described as "extremely affectionate, clingy, and shy" and as "not wanting to be away from Carol—ever!" At age 5, Andy was enrolled in kindergarten at the same school, at which time he began exhibiting anger outbursts and uncontrollable crying, but not to the extent that his parents reported at intake.

*Presenting Complaints*
During an initial phone consultation with Andy's mother, she reported concerns about his mood swings, violent outbursts, intense separation anxiety, running away, and stealing. Secondary concerns included speech and learning delays, eating and sleeping difficulties. Carol's overwhelming stress was evident in her voice. I scheduled her and Tom for an intake and allotted 2 hours to gather a thorough psychosocial history as well as to provide them with emotional support. My initial contact with Andy's parents focused on forming a strong therapeutic alliance and empowering them to see themselves as vital partners in the therapeutic process. Both parents attended the intake,

but Carol, who was clearly more stressed, provided the majority of information. She briefly relayed what little she knew of Andy's early developmental history (described in the preceding section) and explained her major concerns about her son's current behavior.

Socially, Andy was described as "acting younger than his age." At home, his preference was to stay with his mother or play with his newly adopted brother. Carol and Tom expressed concern about Andy's language development. They reported that he did not speak his first word until several months after he came to live with them. Carol also thought it was strange that Andy never talked about his experiences in China. Recently, when she decided she needed to broach the subject, he refused to discuss that he was adopted or that he had lived anywhere other than with them. Carol asked if it was possible that he had blocked out his early memories from the orphanage. I provided Andy's parents with a brief explanation about implicit and explicit memory (Badenoch, 2008), which they found helpful. I explained that in future meetings we would discuss related issues that would help them better understand their son, but for now, regardless of what Andy remembered or did not remember, it was important that they simply listen and accept his story.

The majority of the intake focused on Andy's mood swings, his excessive reaction to being separated from his mother, and what Carol called her son's out-of-control rages. Carol reported that Andy purposely damaged things during his rages and cited several extreme examples. She described physically restraining him until he calmed down, adding that Andy generally wanted her to continue to hold him and cuddle after an episode. Carol and Tom were confused by Andy's behavior toward Carol—excessively clinging much of the time and moments later pushing her away or trying to hurt her, followed by his need for Carol to hold him.

A formal assessment by the school district five months before his referral for play therapy confirmed significant language and cognitive delays, for which he currently received special education services. In addition, Andy had been diagnosed by the school psychologist with Reactive Attachment Disorder (RAD; American Psychiatric Association, 2000). Based on information on RAD obtained from an Internet search, Carol was alarmed that Andy was fated to have life-long difficulties.

While Carol and Tom's description of Andy's current behavior and early history were consistent with diagnostic criteria for this disorder, including Andy's ambivalent—and what seemed to them as contradictory—response to them, I explained that it made sense that Andy's early history had prevented him from developing a sense of how to get his needs met from caregivers in an appropriate manner. Rather than view Andy as having a severe disorder, I encouraged them to view his current difficulties as a response to his inconsistent and disrupted early caregiver experiences—difficulties that together we would work to help Andy overcome. I was encouraged that Carol and Tom seemed to recognize that Andy's behavior stemmed from his early experiences and genuinely wanted to understand how to help him. I explained that helping them learn how to better understand and respond to Andy's often contradictory and developmentally regressed social-emotional needs would be an important part of our work together. I emphasized that the entire family needed help, not just Andy, and coached them on how to explain about their family coming to counseling. I let them know that I would use similar language in explaining the times I met with them for consultations. Carol agreed that she would benefit from meeting with a counselor while Andy was in play therapy to help her cope with her high level of life stress.

**Discussion.** During this initial consultation, I believed that I had forged a strong connection with Andy's parents and that they would be active partners in the therapeutic process. Our discussions confirmed that frequent parent consultations to provide Carol and Tom with education and support were much needed. As our relationship strengthened, and they knew that I was on their side (not just Andy's), exploring Carol and Tom's own attachment history and how that naturally impacted their parenting of Andy would be an important element of our work together. I believed it would be helpful for them to view Andy's behavior and their response through a framework of attachment. Furthermore, based on their interest, I provided Tom and Carol with additional information on the impact of early traumatic experiences on brain development and how that might be affecting Andy's current functioning. Providing Tom and Carol with this type of information proved useful in their accepting Andy's behavior as normal given his history. Adopting this view strengthened their appreciation of the crucial role that they played in helping him heal from his early experiences. The scope of this chapter prevents more than a cursory mention of the neurobiological effects of early trauma. Bonnie Badenoch (2008), Bruce Perry (2006), and Daniel Siegel (1999, 2010) provide useful resources for understanding the impact of early trauma on the developing brain, as well as examples that mental health professionals can easily adapt to educate caregivers.

Andy's diagnosis of RAD seemed to be a source of Carol's view of Andy as damaged. Late-adopted children often present with a wide range of disruptive behaviors, making it difficult to assess and implement the most appropriate therapeutic interventions. The diagnosis of RAD has become common to explain the disruptive behaviors exhibited by foster and adopted children. According to Perry (2006, p. 205), an accurate diagnosis of RAD is rare and supports the notion that RAD may be overdiagnosed in this population of children. The authors of this chapter prefer, initially, to take a more conservative approach to conceptualizing children who present with symptoms similar to Andy's. If a diagnosis must be rendered, it is often more fitting to explore a diagnosis such as post-traumatic stress disorder (PTSD) to communicate the traumatic effect that attachment disruptions can have on the child, as opposed to RAD, which indicates that the child has an inability to attach to another individual. We find it more helpful for parents to view their child as attachment challenged (or similar wording) due to their early, insecure attachment history. Andy's behavior suggested the possibility of early abuse or neglect, in addition to known attachment disruptions. His contradictory approach-avoidance behavior described by Carol and Tom is often seen in children who experienced maltreatment in their first years of life. Lieberman and Van Horn (2005), experts in treating the effects of early trauma, explained its effect on attachment: "The child's normative tendency to seek protection from the parent is violated by the stark realization that the parent is the source of danger. The child is torn between approach and avoidance, between seeking comfort and fighting off danger" (p. 23).

*Case Conceptualization and Treatment Plan*

The following conceptualization was based on a thorough intake assessment that included parent interview, developmental history, measurement of stress in the parent-child relationship, and formal and informal parent- and teacher-reported assessments of Andy's socioemotional development and behavioral functioning. A play observation between Carol and Andy was conducted approximately six weeks after treatment began to assess attachment, patterns of interaction, and how Carol responded to behavior management issues. A discussion of assessments and findings specific to each is omitted because of space limitations.

Andy was displaying many of the symptoms one would expect from a child with his history: indiscriminate affection with relative strangers, incessant fear of his adoptive mother leaving him, difficulty going to sleep and staying asleep, hoarding (he refused to eat much but wanted to save his food for later), and hypervigilance and extreme sensitivity to noise (likely exacerbated by his inability to see much during the first four years of his life). Perry (1994) explained that hypervigilance is typically seen in children like Andy who, because they lacked attentive and protective parenting in the first years of life, are continually scanning their environment for a way to achieve a felt sense of safety. Andy's early experiences were characterized by a series of abandonment and loss of primary caregivers, first his mother, next the neighbor who cared for him for several months, and then various caregivers that came and left the orphanage. Finally, Andy lost his cultural identity and the only home he could remember in his young life. It was impossible to assess the quality or consistency of Andy's attachment experience with his early caregivers, but his multiple losses are a major concern. These experiences occurred during the time in Andy's development when separation from caregivers typically creates anxiety and confirmed for Andy that his fears were real—his significant caregivers (mother/neighbor) left and did not come back. These early traumatic events likely compounded the impact of his hospitalization and brief separation from his new mother shortly after he arrived in the United States.

Based on Andy's behaviors described by his parents, and consistent with my experiences as Andy and I began our relationship, I guessed that his early attachment experiences had been inconsistent—sometimes his needs had been responded to, his cries had been soothed, and other times they had not. He seemed to view the world as sometimes safe and other times unpredictable and scary. These inconsistent early experiences with primary caregivers seemed to have resulted in two internalized and contradictory messages regarding his worth and what he needed from his caregivers: (1) "Sometimes you meet my needs. I cannot let you out of my sight, you might not come back when I need you. I have to make you like me so you will not want to leave me. I need you," and (2) "I don't trust you. I cannot depend on you. I must not be worthy of being loved and cared for. I have to take care of myself. I don't need you." These messages represented what Bowlby (1969) referred to as the internal working model of a child presenting with a predominate ambivalent insecure-anxious pattern of attachment (Ainsworth, Blehar, Waters, & Wall, 1978). Thus, Andy approached relationships with ambiguity, which was very puzzling to Tom, and even more so to Carol, who felt rejected and confused when Andy pushed her away. This response is common among adoptive parents who are faced with the challenge of developing a relationship and helping the child experience that relationships can be safe and trusting. Confusion, frustration, rejection, and heartache often become part of the adoptive parents' daily life when it appears that their child continues to reject them, sabotaging the relationship (Purvis et al., 2007; Ryan, 2004).

Helping Carol and Tom realize that Andy's current behavior, especially his response to them, stemmed from his early attachment experiences would be critical to Andy's successful treatment. I believed that they would be able to be more accepting of Andy and more responsive to his underlying needs if they could begin to view Andy's behavior as expected given his experience, rather than as a failure on their part. Adoptive parents often resort to blaming either themselves or the child, and familial relationships can quickly deteriorate. Hughes (2006) discussed the potentially adverse effect that an insecurely attached child can have on the adoptive parents:

> *Her anger, rejection, withdrawal, defiance, and indifference may activate within the parent doubts about their parenting abilities. Sensing that they are failing as parents, these parents are not likely to feel safe while with their child. Their worth, value and abilities are being questioned continuously. They are at-risk for becoming angry, tense, withdrawn, discouraged, and indifferent to their child. (p. 4)*

Carol and Tom's understanding and acceptance of Andy's underlying needs would only be the beginning of what Andy needed from them in order to heal. Children with an early complex trauma history involving attachment breaks need comprehensive treatment that directly involves caregivers. Research suggests that early relationship experiences are a powerful influence on brain development—both positive and detrimental. For children who have had negative and/or inconsistent caregiving, new research suggests that once-per-week therapy is insufficient to change and reinforce the new neuropathways in the brain (Siegel, 2010; Perry, 2008). Therefore, I believed it would be essential to educate Andy's parents about his need for consistent and repetitive positive relationship-based experiences with them, and to help them be cognizant of the time, repetition, and patience involved for lasting change in how he viewed himself and his primary relationships.

*Play Therapy Treatment Objectives*

Because of Andy's history of extreme difficulty separating from Carol, before my first meeting with Andy, Carol and I talked by phone to discuss alternative plans for her to come to the playroom with Andy if he was too anxious or frightened to go on his own. I further emphasized that it was very important that each week she be sitting exactly where Andy had left her when we returned to the reception area after our sessions. I used every opportunity to emphasize how important structure, consistency, and predictability were to Andy developing a felt sense of safety and security. As a result of our discussions, we decided that Carol would bring Andy for a brief visit to meet me and introduce him to the playroom in Carol's presence. The goal was to be sensitive to his needs for predictability and what I guessed would be a need to have his mother close by in a new situation. I reminded her to read Andy the book I had given her and to offer the explanation about the family getting help so everyone would get along better.

My initial objective was to establish a responsive and predictable therapeutic relationship in which Andy would feel secure and safe enough to explore his experiences, including those that in the past had been too threatening to admit to awareness. Axline (1947), considered the first to utilize humanistic principles in play therapy, described this optimal play climate as "good growing ground," a safe and protected space where the child can fully experience and integrate all aspects of self and potential for growth.

I guessed that it would not be easy to provide the kind of authentic relationship that this little boy needed in order to feel safe. His experiences had told him otherwise. It was my job to provide Andy with a reparative experience—one in which he would come to perceive me as a caregiver figure who was trustworthy, consistent, and predictable, and who would not leave him prematurely. I knew that along with consistency in our relationship, establishing a predictable structure in the playroom would create the sense of security that Andy would need in order to perceive me as someone he could trust. From trust he would grow to count on me to be a reliable and predictable caregiver figure in his life. Only then would Andy feel safe enough to explore and express all of his experiences. I would need to be patient in developing this kind of relationship with Andy, whose experience had taught him that relationships were not consistent, safe, or secure. A child with a previous history of attachment breaks and traumas is often confused and frightened at the opportunity to have a consistent interactive relationship. An overactive and highly sensitive amygdala is common in children with early experience such as Andy; therefore, I reminded myself that Andy would likely be approaching this new relationship from a place of fear rooted in the primary part of his brain.

An additional objective was for Andy to experience in our relationship what Rogers (1961) described as the conditions necessary for facilitating change: genuineness, empathy, and warmth or unconditional regard—a relationship in which he did not have to earn my approval or acceptance by impressing me or being overtly affectionate (his mode of connecting when we first began our relationship). My hope was that as Andy experienced congruence and unconditional acceptance in our relationship, he would begin to alter his self-perception of damaged, not worthy of love, or "no-good," to one of lovable and worthy of positive regard. In this way, he would begin to revise his perception of how he viewed himself, others, and relationships. I believed that by providing Andy with this kind of experience, he would be ready for the most critical therapeutic task of all, to experience this kind of relationship with his adoptive parents. As Andy grew to allow himself to fully experience and trust his parents' unconditional love for him, he would no longer feel the need to push them away for fear that they would eventually leave him.

### Treatment Objectives for Involving Caregivers

Equally important to my objectives for my work with Andy in the playroom were my goals for providing system support. Andy's current family situation was a significant strength, one that I would build on during Andy's therapy. Carol and Tom seemed amenable to participating in additional parent or family therapy services that I knew would be essential, and when timed appropriately, would ultimately be the most healing component of Andy's treatment. Initially, I planned to incorporate regular parent consultations with Carol every two to three weeks to provide support and education, as well as to help her develop a better understanding of Andy by describing themes I observed in his play, the connection between his play and his early experiences, and how these themes were relevant to his behavior at home and school.

My first priority in our parent consults was to address safety issues related to Andy's violent outbursts. Based on their positive response to information on the impact of early trauma on brain development, I planned to explain that Andy's heightened amygdala was likely causing Andy to react from a state of fear and insecurity. Other ideas included helping Carol and Tom become more attuned to what precipitated the events, as well as developing strategies that they could implement to prevent or deescalate the situation. One strategy that I expected would be useful was to help Carol identify times throughout the day when Andy seemed receptive to being touched or held in a loving and playful manner, rather than waiting for Andy to get his holding needs met during the aftermath of his rages.

Helping Andy's parents learn how to establish a healthy attachment with their son would be critical to his healing, therefore Child Parent Relationship Therapy (CPRT; Landreth & Bratton, 2006) would be a key element in our overall treatment plan. Additional goals that would be addressed through CPRT included: (1) normalize Carol and Tom's behavioral and emotional response to Andy's behavior problems and help them feel supported and empowered; (2) foster a greater understanding of Andy's needs, including the impact his attachment experiences had on his development and current functioning; (3) enhance parent-child attunement through creating mutually enjoyable and developmentally responsive interactions; (4) help Carol and Tom learn to be consistent in responding to Andy's needs, including his regressive and aggressive behaviors in ways that communicated safety and acceptance; and

354 Integrative Play Therapy

(5) strengthen Carol and Tom's parenting skills and confidence in responding to Andy's unique and often challenging needs.

Finally, I knew that involving Andy's teacher as part of the treatment team would provide additional opportunities for Andy to experience repetitive positive experiences from an important caregiver. At my next meeting with Andy's parents, I planned to discuss my concerns about Andy's school placement and explain how I would work with Andy's teacher and other school staff as needed. In light of Andy's behavior, learning, and speech difficulties in the past school year, and what appeared as significant delays in his social and emotional development, I proposed the idea that Andy repeat kindergarten with the same teacher, who seemed sensitive to his regressed developmental needs. I hoped that this school placement would provide Andy with more opportunities to experience a sense of safety, security, and predictability in his life, and in this way, optimize his social, emotional, and cognitive development.

*Course of Treatment and Assessment of Progress*
Selected vignettes from the play therapy process are described to illustrate an integration of humanistic and attachment principles in practice. The scope of this chapter, again, prevented inclusion of other, equally significant happenings in the therapeutic process that contributed to Andy's successful treatment.

I first met Andy at a brief visit, during which I introduced him to the playroom with his mother present. While I had given Carol a children's book to read to him that explained play therapy, I believed that Andy would feel more secure if he had firsthand experience with me and the playroom before our first session. This turned out to be a helpful strategy. Andy was excited about all the toys, picking out ones he planned to play with "next week." I ended our meeting by showing him that there were two ways he could get from the waiting room to the playroom and that he could choose which way he wanted to go.

**Sessions 1–10.**   Andy was sitting in his mother's lap when I greeted him in the waiting room to take him to the playroom for our first session. I was not surprised that he seemed anxious. I leaned down and made eye contact and said, "Hi, Andy. Hi, Carol. Andy, remember I showed you and your mom the playroom last week. It's time for us to go back to the playroom and play." (He smiled and shook his head up and down.) As if right on cue, and following the instructions I had given her, Carol stated, "Andy, I'll be right here waiting for you when you get through playing!" He looked at me, and then looked at his mother. I quickly added, "You can choose for us to run to the playroom or walk." His face lit up, and he jumped up and said "Run!" as he took off down the hall with me running behind him trying to catch up. That started a weekly ritual of Andy running to beat me to the playroom. Although I gave Andy the choice of running or walking to the playroom to take his focus off of separating from his mother, I was surprised he went so easily, given Carol's report of Andy's difficulty separating from her.

Andy's first four sessions were characterized by his need to gain my approval and affection by impressing me and by overt demonstrations of affection, which included touching me, patting my head, and putting his face right up next to mine. Based on his early history, it was not a surprise that he acted overly familiar with me. Andy would have to experience my genuine and unconditional acceptance firsthand before he could come to see himself as inherently worthy, without needing to prove himself.

As might be expected from a traumatized child, Andy was initially hyper-vigilant to every noise he heard in and outside of the playroom. These disruptions made it difficult for him to focus. It was no wonder that learning was so difficult for Andy! The fifth session marked a shift in Andy's play. He was now feeling safe enough to leave my side and explore the playroom. Andy noticed two items that would prove to be favored objects throughout most of our sessions: the flashlight and the baby bottle. He first experimented with the flashlight, delighting in turning the lights out and shining the light so we could see each other. Next, he took the baby bottle and filled it with water from the sink, sucking contentedly on it for approximately the last third of our session. When I reminded Andy that we had 5 minutes left to play, he went to the sandbox and climbed in. He laid back against the edge and sucked on the bottle with a glazed look on his face.

When I announced that our time was up, Andy shook his head with the bottle still in his mouth, letting me know that he wasn't ready to leave. I was patient and restated the limit as I leaned down to his level and made eye contact and gently, yet firmly, reflected his desire to stay longer. "Andy, I know that you'd like to stay longer, but our time is up for today. You can drink some more from the bottle next week." I repeated similar statements three more times, letting him know I understood he was having a hard time leaving today. Still, Andy shook his head and remained in the sandbox. Often, this is a time when you need to be firmer in your tone of voice, but I sensed that there was something different about this experience. I realized in that moment that I wished Andy didn't have to leave either, but I knew that it was important that he experience the consistency and predictability of our time together. I bent down even closer to him and said, with all the empathy I was feeling, "Andy, I wish we didn't have to leave either, but we do. It's time for us to go back to the waiting room where Mom is." Focusing my responses on our relationship, rather than on Andy's behavior, seemed to be what he needed—a lesson that I shared with Carol in our next parent consultation. This brief but powerful interaction with Andy reminded me how important it is for me to trust my experience with children—that when I do, they let me know what they need from me.

During session six, Andy began to use the flashlight as a way of connecting with me in a more genuine and playful way. He turned out the lights, came very close, and shone the flashlight between our faces, saying, "I see you." I responded, "You see me, and I see you." He repeated what I said, and giggled, to which I repeated my response again. He repeated this interaction multiple times, seeming to enjoy the rhythm of our interaction. Andy had found a way to connect with me in our own unique and spontaneous way, not determined by what he thought he needed to do to win my approval. This became one of many what seemed like infant-mother games that Andy would initiate over time.

During session seven, Andy began to paint for the first time, painting all the colors on top of each other to make a blob of brownish-black. The following brief interaction seemed to reveal Andy's inner conflict between his wants, wishes, and needs and trying to please others, especially the most significant person in his life, "Mommy."

> **A:** *"Mommy be mad."* (*As he began to use his hands to smear the paint*)
>
> **S:** *"You're worried that Mommy will be mad."*
>
> **A:** *"Messy"* (*As he went to the sink and washed the paint off hurriedly*)
>
> **S:** *"You're worried that mom wouldn't like it if you got messy."* But before I could get the words out, he began to take his shoes off and looked over at me as if to ask my approval.
>
> **S:** *"Looks like you're not sure if that's okay. In here you can decide if you want to take off your shoes."* Andy quickly took off his shoes, picked up the paintbrush, and then proceeded to paint the bottom of his feet and his hands, enjoying the feel of the brush (much like the sensorimotor play of a younger child).
>
> **A:** *"Tickles"* (*a big smile on his face*)
>
> **S:** *"You like how that feels."*
>
> **S:** *"Andy, we have one minute left to play. It's time to wash up to go home."* (I was careful to make sure that we washed all the paint off his feet and hands before we went back to the waiting room to prevent potential guilt feelings that Andy might experience if Carol reacted adversely to a "messy Andy").

During our parent consult in week eight, Carol announced that Andy's "stealing" was now happening at school as well as at home. Andy's concern last week about being messy and his mother being mad now made more sense in light of Carol's obvious upset about Andy's behavior. My first priority was to help Carol (and others) to reframe how they viewed Andy's behavior. It seemed obvious that Andy's stealing, as described by Carol, was not malicious. I asked Carol to consider describing his behavior as, "taking things that belong to others" instead of "stealing" when talking to Andy (and others). I explained that her description of the events and Andy's response when confronted were consistent with what one would expect from much younger children, who simply see something they want or need and take it. I reminded her of a toddler's worldview, "If I want it, it's mine!" She agreed that if Andy were 2 years old that she would not see his behavior as stealing. Carol and I devised a plan for how to respond to Andy at home and at school if and when he initiated this behavior again. To ensure consistency, Carol and I met with Andy's teacher at school to discuss the plan, and Carol also elicited school administrators' help. We all approached this as if Andy's behavior was a function of development and that our job as adults was to help further his development by helping him learn the concept of ownership and people's related feelings about their property. Andy's parents and the school were instrumental in helping Andy move through this phase over the next several weeks.

*Discussion.* My sense of Andy's socioemotional level of functioning was confirmed by the infant/toddler way in which he tried to connect with me in our early sessions. However, of concern, his behavior also indicated that he had learned to use this strategy indiscriminately to initiate relationships with others, including strangers like me. I made a note to discuss my concern with Carol at a later time. Andy's enjoyment of the rhythmic interaction with the flashlight was another indication of his need to regress to meet what I guessed were his early unmet needs. Even my strategy for helping Andy go to the playroom was one I would use with a toddler. I quickly gave a simple choice between two physical activities that we could do together.

Andy's emotional and physiological response to sucking the bottle seemed to indicate an early unmet need that was greater than merely the satisfaction he seemed to get from sucking. It is common that children with early trauma and attachment disruptions experience gaps in their development in which they did not successfully master a stage before being expected to move to the next stage, which often exacerbates emotionally based disruptive behaviors. Developmental stages are built on one another. It is imperative in treatment that children are given the freedom and opportunity to regress to early developmental stages and meet those needs in healthier and more adaptive ways so they can progress through the next developmental stages. This is an essential component to the attachment and developmentally informed treatment of young children. Because Andy's sucking seemed to be meeting a core need that included nurturance, I decided to provide a small pitcher of juice in the play kitchen area, so that he could use juice instead of water to fill the bottle if he chose. From that time forward, he always chose juice, often referring to it as "my special juice." Sucking the bottle was a prominent feature of Andy's play throughout most of our sessions, peaking around session 35 and lessening in intensity and frequency in later sessions.

Andy's worry about getting messy and "mommy be mad" were likely related to sensing that his mother was upset about the stealing at school and further exacerbated by his early experiences. The fears of children with attachment disruptions are often amplified and may be perceived as irrational and unwarranted by caregivers and therapists. Remembering that the child's internal working model of self and relationships is rooted in feeling rejected and undeserving of being in relationship can help his parents empathize with the child's perceptions of various experiences. For Andy, this desire to please his mommy is much deeper than the fear of getting in trouble if he gets paint on his clothes. This need to please is rooted in his core survival skills connected to the belief that "I must make this caregiver happy so that I will not be abandoned again and left alone in this unpredictable and often scary world." For children with insecure attachment, their fundamental need for safety and acceptance often underlies more obvious play behaviors. An understanding of attachment dynamics permits the therapist to consider alternative views of the child's needs expressed through play; and with greater awareness of the child's fundamental need comes the potential that the therapist can respond to the heart of the issue with intentionality, understanding, and above all genuine empathy of the child's experience.

Helping Carol reframe how she viewed Andy's stealing helped her normalize his behavior. Carol's role as an administrator at Andy's school understandably complicated her response. It seemed particularly helpful that I met with school staff to explain my conceptualization of Andy's behavior and his socioemotional functioning. In addition, I explained that stealing is a common behavioral symptom of many children with attachment disruptions and challenges (Hughes, 2006) and is one form of an external behavior that is used to soothe an internal state of stress and dysregulation (Forbes & Post, 2006, p. 50). Children with trauma histories often have difficulty self-regulating because of the lack of a secure early attachment relationship that is directly involved in regulatory development. This explanation seemed to strengthen Andy's teacher's resolve to help provide him with a consistent and positive nurturing experience.

**Sessions 11–24.**   This phase was intense, moving from chaos and struggle to the beginnings of self-acceptance and mastery. During sessions 11 to 13, Andy's level of agitation was at an all-time high. One of his favorite items in the playroom was a cowboy hat that had a whistle attached by a string. He loved wearing the hat as he marched around the room, and rhythmically blew the whistle. At the beginning of session 11, Andy immediately took the hat/whistle behind the theater where he thought he was out of sight, cut the whistle off, and stuffed it in his pocket. His play was highly disorganized, and he was clearly distressed. I was having difficulty being with him in this experience and found myself wanting to rescue him. I had to work very hard to not let my need to protect Andy from these difficult feelings interfere with his need to work through this in his own way. When I let Andy know we had one minute left, he went straight to the door with obvious relief. At this point the whistle was still in his pocket. I gently responded, "Andy, I think maybe you put the whistle in your pocket when you were playing with it earlier. Remember the toys stay in the playroom." First, he shook his head "no" to indicate he did not have the whistle. I responded, "Maybe you should check to make sure." He reached into his pocket and said, "I forgot," and handed it to me. I put it over by the hat and let him know, "It will be right here for you next week."

Andy's play in session 12 was very similar, but with an even higher level of agitation as he waited for the session to be over, so he could once again attempt to leave the playroom with the whistle. During session 13, with the whistle already pocketed, Andy spent 15 minutes throwing toys, repeating, "no good, no good." I reflected, "Nothing seems to be going right today." He seemed to calm down for a moment, and with less intensity than before, he hit himself in the head (with his hand) and said, "stupid." While I knew this moment was significant, I was unsure of what Andy needed from me. I went over to him and reflected, "Andy, I know you're upset about something, but you're not for hitting." I paused, and feeling the need to respond in a more authentic and congruent manner, I added, "It is my job to take care of you and keep you safe in the playroom."

Afterward, I struggled with whether my response was coming from my own need or from a sensitivity to Andy's experience and what he needed from me in that moment. He paused and looked up to me and quietly said, "I want to go." I was torn between putting an end to his struggle (and mine) and the need to maintain the structure and consistency of our time together. In that moment I realized that I trusted Andy to figure out what he needed to do, so I held firm and replied with all the empathy I was feeling for this little boy, "Andy, I know that you're having a hard time in the playroom today, but we have 20 minutes left, and then it will be time to go." He insisted, "I don't want to play anymore." I replied softly, "That's up to you. You can decide whether you want to play or not." Andy did not try to leave, but every few minutes he looked at the clock and asked me how much time we had left. When I told him we had 1 minute left, he went straight to the door. Just as I was about to state the limit about the whistle staying in the playroom, Andy reached in his pocket and pulled it out and handed it to me, looking directly in my eyes. I held out my hand and smiled gently, but no words came to me. I hoped that I communicated nonverbally what was in my heart.

In session 14, Andy's play changed dramatically. He no longer had a need to try and sneak the whistle out of the playroom. The doubt and shame prevalent in the last three sessions had been replaced by greater autonomy, spontaneity, and freedom. He wore the hat and whistle during the entire session and spent much of the time marching and smiling broadly as he blew the whistle as loud as he could. Carol reported that Andy was no longer taking things at school and that he had mostly stopped this behavior at home.

Andy's play over the next 10 sessions was characterized by greater spontaneity in self-expression and increased positive affect. For a child who had begun therapy so hypersensitive to what he needed to be in order to win others' approval, this movement was just what I had hoped for. During this time, he found the "baby" dolphin and chose it to become a central figure in his play. He often carried "baby" around while he played or gave it to me to hold. He determined that the dolphin was a "he" and was especially gentle with it.

It was also during this time period that he introduced his favorite game, "hide and find." With the exceptions of a few breaks, this was a game that Andy delighted in up until our termination, sometimes spending more than half of our session in this activity. From the first time he introduced this activity with, "Close eyes, I hide," I sensed that this game was very important to our relationship. I wanted to play my part just the way he needed me to, so I inquired, "How will I know when you're ready?" Andy said, as if obvious, "Count to 10," and after I did, "Find me!" he yelled. I slowly began to look for him. I was wondering to myself, does he need me to find him easily or take a long time? Because of his abandonment issues, I was thinking that how I responded to my task of finding him was vital. In a soft voice, I asked, "are you going to be easy to find or hard to find?" Andy paused a minute and said,

"Hard!" So, I began a long search around the room, amplifying my movements and efforts to find him, often exclaiming variations of, "I bet you're over here. Hmm, not here. You hid really good. I wonder where you are?" When he would giggle, I would reflect, "I hear something, you must be over there." Each time we played this out, no matter whether he chose to be easy to find or hard to find, he always gave me clues to let me know when he was ready to be found.

Again, Andy had chosen a playful and increasingly intimate way to deepen our relationship and work through his early experiences of what I had guessed to be an inconsistent response to his nurturing needs. He was learning that I could be trusted to consistently respond to what he needed. Through this experience and his experience of being with a loving family, I hoped that Andy would begin to see the world as secure and predictable—a place where he could depend on adults to keep him safe and respond appropriately to his needs. Andy was clearly working on attachment and trust issues that I believed could be more effectively addressed by involving Carol and Tom in Andy's play therapy. We discussed starting CPRT/filial therapy training in the near future so that Andy could play out his attachment needs with his parents. Carol reported that Andy was making good progress, including a reduction in his violent outbursts, a marked decrease in stealing, and fewer sleep problems.

*Discussion.* The tumultuous phase in Andy's therapy was once again an example of the amplified and deeply rooted internal working model that is present in Andy's play and verbal messages. His view of himself as "no good" represents his struggle to accept himself, and is likely connected with the belief from his implicit memory system (rooted in experience) that he is not acceptable and lovable by others. His early attachment and developmental experiences created neuropathways in his brain that hindered his ability to accept himself and feel valued and accepted by others. Andy's approach to the therapeutic relationship is parallel to how he approached his relationships with others in everyday life. Andy's predominate anxious-ambivalent attachment style served as his current blueprint for relationship dynamics. This is representative in Andy's patterns of relating to me, fluctuating from seeking to please me and establish a connection in our first 10 sessions to these weeks of agitation, distress, and emotional distance.

He had also learned that he could not count on caregivers to protect him, keep him safe, and regulate his difficult emotions. His difficulty with self-regulation is evident in his internal struggle between realizing that although he wanted the whistle, it was not his (just as outside of the session, he was struggling with understanding this concept on a larger scale). The combined impact of Andy being able to play out his struggles in the safety of the playroom with me as a supportive witness and his parents' and teachers' changed attitude and response to his behavior at home resulted in an almost complete halt in the stealing behavior. The playroom experience between child and therapist is often viewed as a microcosm of how the child operates in day-to-day life. And from a child-centered perspective, what is lived in the playroom can be generalized to real life (Landreth, 2002). Andy clearly demonstrates this principle. As he learns he can choose to play with the whistle and give it back, he learns to regulate his emotions and bring himself under control.

A child-centered approach to play therapy creates an environment for Andy to be in the lead and control the pace of the play experience. As he demonstrates in his choice of "hide and find," this approach allows Andy the freedom to explore when and how to be in relationship with others. I trust his inner wisdom and do not push or rush this process, so that Andy will continue to feel safe to explore relationship dynamics. The authors of this chapter have informal data from our experiences that various forms of hide-and-seek play are very common in children with trauma and attachment histories. It appears that this play activity is often the child's attempt to integrate early experiences and perhaps to modify an insecure attachment style. Andy is beginning to shift his perception and consider the possibility: "What if I am worth finding?" "Does a caring adult want to find me and be in relationship?" "Do I want to risk being found?"

**Sessions 25–35.** Sessions 25 through 28 marked the introduction of another significant play theme in which he began to use the dress-up clothes trunk as a central part of his play. Andy's play was highly organized and purposeful. He clearly had a plan in mind. He began by first taking everything out and trying on most of the clothes to see how he looked, often dressing us both like "girls." He ended this play sequence each week with a ritual of putting the burning flashlight in the trunk, along with the baby dolphin, and closing the lid. Before he left the playroom, he would open the lid to make sure the light was still on. He seemed to gain a great deal of satisfaction from his play during these weeks, and I conveyed that I understood its importance. It was during this time that Carol reported that Andy was showing more interest in what he was like as a baby. He wanted to watch television shows with babies in them and look at pictures of babies, and he would ask, "Was that me?" "Did I look like that?"

As our play sessions continued, Andy's play was primarily focused on issues related to attachment and mastery. His play showed increased levels of reciprocity and sharing. He delighted in inventing several variations of baby-like games in which he directed me to touch and count his fingers and toes while I spun him around in a chair. He combined his need for sucking with having me sit close to him and spin or rock the chair while he sucked. The intimacy, genuineness, and congruence in our relationship reached an all-time high, which I knew meant that he was ready to allow a deeper level of intimacy with his parents.

During this time, he also began to express negative feelings toward me directly. One day I was 15 minutes late for a session, and he wouldn't look at me as we walked to the playroom (no running today!). When we entered the playroom, he looked at me and then kicked the inflatable bop bag. I reflected, "Seems like you might be mad that I was late. It's okay to tell me that you're mad." Andy shook his head slightly as if to say he was not mad. I wanted him to know that it was okay for him to be angry at me and that our relationship could recover. I bent down to Andy and gently said, "You were expecting me to be here today when I was supposed to, and I wasn't. I'm sorry." (something I should have said earlier!). Although I believed that we had forged a strong therapeutic alliance in which Andy had grown to trust me, it seemed that Andy's anxiety and fear of abandonment and rejection was triggered by my being late. Again, I knew that it would only be through living these moments out that he could begin to trust that relationships could recover from momentary breaks.

In keeping with our plan, Carol and Tom began intensive CPRT training following the treatment protocol outlined by Bratton, et al. (2006). Coinciding with play therapy sessions 30 to 35, I met with Carol and Tom for twice-weekly CPRT sessions for six weeks, scheduled to end just before their two-week family vacation. During the initial training period, Tom chose to conduct play sessions with Andy, while Carol worked with their other adopted son, Chris. Carol and Tom and I decided that this was a good opportunity to focus on helping Andy develop a closer bond with Tom, in hopes of relieving Carol of her full-time parenting role with Andy. Before beginning home play sessions, Carol and Tom completed five play sessions at the clinic under my direct supervision. Andy played out some of the same themes with his Dad that he played with me, particularly doctoring the baby and sucking from the baby bottle. I had prepared Tom for the possibility that Andy might want to suck from the bottle, but Tom struggled to accept that behavior from his son who had just turned 7 years old. He understood that it was important to Andy and that he should be accepting, but he remained skeptical. We role-played how Tom could respond that would convey his acceptance and encourage Andy to involve him in his play. However, in their first home play session when Andy initiated sucking from the bottle, it became obvious that Tom was struggling to accept his son's need to suck. What ultimately seemed to help most was asking Tom to remember when Anne, his now 14-year-old biological daughter, was a baby and how he had enjoyed holding her close and giving her a bottle. Andy had not had the opportunity to have that experience with him or Carol (and maybe not with anyone). Both Tom and Carol were motivated students and became fairly proficient in demonstrating the CCPT play skills taught in CPRT. They agreed to continue their play sessions during their two-week vacation at the beach.

*Discussion.*    Because attachment disruptions indicate the presence of a relationship-based problem, CPRT's focus on the parent-child relationship seems to make it an appropriate therapeutic treatment modality for helping adoptive families respond to the challenge of establishing and maintaining a secure attachment relationship. The philosophy of CPRT emphasizes the unique experience of each child and the child's innate capacity for healing. Parents are taught the fundamental skills of child-centered play therapy, thus Andy's parents would be learning to respond to him in ways that were consistent to his experience with me in play therapy. Understandably, caregivers often have difficulty accepting regressed behavior that children may exhibit during special playtimes. The discrepancy between the child's emotional age and chronological age can be difficult for a caregiver to witness during special playtimes. Supporting and educating caregivers on how to respond to the child based on his or her emotional age rather than chronological age fosters a systemic developmentally responsive treatment for the child. When a caregiver understands that during special playtimes the child is playing out his or her needs, the caregiver can learn to respond with attunement and acceptance, the road of healing.

**Sessions 36–46.** Themes of attachment, trust, and mothers/babies (often looking for each other) continued over the next 11 weeks. Andy's play became more complex and imaginative. During this time, Andy often had difficulty leaving the playroom. Another significant happening was the arrival of an exchange student from Andy's birth country, who would be living with them over the next year. Andy referred to him as "my new big brother," and his arrival seemed to be an impetus for Andy to more directly address issues around his adoption and his cultural identity.

Session 36 marked Andy's first attempts to play out what seemed to be experiences that were directly related to his abandonment by his birth mother and his orphanage experience. Andy took the baby dolphin and for the first time buried it deep in the sand. He abruptly left it there and began to hammer nails in the log for the first time in several weeks. I saw this behavior as a play disruption, a sudden shift from play that seems to hold specific meaning for the child in response to anxiety or discomfort (Findling, Bratton, & Henson, 2006). When children deal with traumatic material, it can be retraumatizing, thus it was important for Andy to approach this at his own pace. Later he went back to the sandbox and looked at me and said, shaking his head, "Don't know where he is." I simply reflected, "Not sure where he is," not knowing who it was that didn't know where the baby was. I waited patiently to see if a story would unfold. Andy took the large dolphin (which I interpreted as a mother/caregiver figure) and a few other caregiver-figure animals (a seal, walrus, and polar bear) off the shelf and placed them carefully in the sandbox. He again abruptly went back to hammering (an activity that he had long ago mastered). After I announced that we had 5 minutes left, Andy went to the sandbox and hurriedly moved the mother animals all around on top of the sand as if they were all looking for the baby, then had the large dolphin dig down and find the baby and exclaim, "There he is!" I reflected, "Looks like he's happy that they found him." (Inside, I was struggling with staying with Andy's expression of wanting his mother to find him and knowing that will not happen. My need to try and protect him from being hurt had surfaced again.) I wondered if Andy's play represented wishful thinking that maybe he could go back and find his mom (or remembered "mother figure").

On two occasions Andy initiated play with two mother dolls with different skin colors, but both times abandoned his play after a brief period of time. Using animals rather than people figures to make sense of his adoption experience seemed to provide Andy with the safety and distance he needed.

Over the next several weeks, Andy was preoccupied with babies and mothers. The playroom had several sets of animal families grouped together by family. He readily identified the babies and separated them from the mother-figures, devising various scenarios of what happened next. Often he would place the babies across the room from the mothers, sometimes out of sight behind the puppet theater. At times the babies could not find the mothers, and other times the mothers could not find the babies. In Andy's play there were always more babies than mothers, which seemed to reflect his orphanage experience. Another theme that emerged was that the baby dolphin began to receive better care than the other babies, who often were thrown down from the shelf, but the baby dolphin was always gently handed to me to hold. Andy returned to burying the baby dolphin deeply in the sand, but with a different story line this time. For the first time he identified the large dolphin as a mother and then handed it to me as if I knew what I should do. It seemed very important that I get my part right!

> **S:** *"Show me what you want me to do." (I said this in a soft voice that clearly conveyed he was the director of this play.)*
> **A:** *"Look for baby."*
> **S:** *"Is he going to be hard to find or easy to find?"*
> **A:** *"Hard." (I started to look in the sandbox.)*
> **A:** *"No—everywhere, not here." (Now, I understood, I was supposed to search for the baby dolphin like I searched for Andy when we played hide and find.)*
> **S:** *"I may need some help if you want me to find him." (After I had spent a long time looking for the baby and not getting a sense of what Andy needed from me.) I was not sure who I represented (birth mother, orphanage caregiver, or maybe even Carol), neither did I understand if he wanted me to find the baby or not, so I was careful to let him fully direct this play sequence. Andy never did direct me to find the baby, but he seemed to enjoy that I was methodically looking all over the playroom.*
> **S:** *"I'm looking everywhere I can think to look, but I can't find him. I wonder where he is?" (Andy looked at me and shrugged his shoulders.)*
> **S:** *"I don't know where he is either, but I'm going to keep looking. I'm not giving up."*

Andy seemed content that I (mother dolphin) looked everywhere and never gave up. He also seemed satisfied with or resigned to the fact that in this session the mother never found the baby. Andy seemed to be integrating his previous experiences into a positive memory of being wanted and special, even if his mother had left him. Just before we left the playroom each week, Andy was always careful to return the dolphin to its place on the shelf. It seemed important to him that the baby was left in its safe and predictable spot.

Sessions 43 to 45 marked a brief but tumultuous shift in Andy's play, with a marked increase in expression of negative affect. During session 45 in particular, he was clearly feeling conflicted about something. His anger was expressed more directly toward me, although I suspected it was transference of his feelings toward his mother. During our last 5 minutes of a play session, Andy initiated the spinning game with a new twist: he filled the bottle with juice, took his glasses off, and scooted the chair so it was touching my legs and then showed me how he wanted me to just barely move the chair back and forth (felt like rocking). He laid across the chair and contentedly sucked while he gazed into my eyes with a glazed look. It was a very intimate moment—the kind he needed to be having with Carol and Tom. I made a mental note to talk with Carol about taking a break from play therapy and beginning filial therapy in the next couple of weeks.

When Andy and I returned to the reception area, Carol was insistent that she needed to talk to me before they left. I bent down to let Andy know that his mom and I would be back in 15 minutes and that he would stay with the receptionist while we were gone. Andy grabbed his mom around the legs and stated adamantly that he didn't want her to go and was not going to let her go. Although on the surface his words and actions conveyed one message, I had the strongest sense that the real issue was that he did not want me to hear what he thought his mother was planning to say to me. I knelt down beside Andy and whispered where only he could hear, "Andy, there's nothing your mom could say to me that would ever change how I feel about you." Although, in general, I believe that my actions with children speak much louder than my words, I sensed that Andy needed to hear what was in my heart. I knew that he experienced my acceptance of him as unconditional, at least within the protected space of the playroom, but his past experiences told him that things can (and will) change. He looked at me for a few moments as if he was deciding if I was telling the truth, then smiled at me as if to say "Okay" and went over to watch the cartoon playing in the waiting room. Our relationship had passed a test.

Andy's academic performance and behavior at school were bothering Carol, and her frustration was carrying over to home, where she was already feeling overwhelmed by her parenting responsibilities as a result of Tom traveling more than usual for work. Her escalating level of stress was an indication that I needed to shift my focus to strengthening the relationship between Carol and Andy and at the same time provide Carol with some much-needed parental support. Carol was initially unsure about taking a break from play therapy to focus on filial therapy, but I emphasized to her that right now Andy needed her more than he needed me. Coincidentally, I sensed at this moment that Carol needed me as much or more than Andy did. We decided that she would begin filial play sessions with Andy in two weeks during our regularly scheduled appointment time.

*Discussion.*    Andy's play disruption after burying the dolphin is an example of Andy's ability to self-regulate his intense feelings and emotions. He regulated and self-soothed by taking a break from this intense and meaningful play before returning to play that seemed highly significant in making sense of his early attachment and trauma experiences. This scenario is a prime example of the humanistic philosophy of trusting the child's therapeutic pace and inner wisdom and resources for healing. Andy's use of animal figures to represent what seems like his early caregivers seemed to create the distance and safety he needed. Because trauma is often stored fragmented in the brain, it is important that children develop a coherent narrative, accessing the explicit memory system of experiences so that this can be integrated into a sense of self. It appears that Andy's use of the animals to make sense of his adoption experience was the beginning of integrating this story into his life's narrative. Providing toys and materials for his narrative allowed Andy to approach frightening, confusing, and emotionally charged memories at his own pace (Busch & Lieberman, 2007, p. 162). Andy's curiosity in understanding his early experience of loss of caregivers indicated to me that he was ready to make his life story book with his parents' help—something Carol and I had discussed numerous times.

I was puzzled by the shift in Andy's mood, from expression of anger one minute to intensely intimate the next, yet, I trusted that he knew what he needed. I worked hard to be fully present and trust my experience to guide my response. I trusted the strength of our relationship, but I also knew that Andy's early experiences might cause him to question whether it was possible for this relationship to be different from others. Often children with disrupted attachment histories will unconsciously create stress and chaos as a sense of safety rooted in the prior insecure attachment framework, because in the past, rejection is what felt most predictable. Because therapy was progressing in a positive direction, I wondered if Andy may have been experiencing a need to briefly regress and test whether this relationship was truly unconditional and accepting.

**Sessions 47–50.** For the next four weeks, I coached and supervised Carol's play sessions with Andy during what was typically our play therapy hour. I spent time supporting her worries about Andy and about being a good enough mother for him. We actively worked on increasing her enjoyment and acceptance of Andy for who he was, school difficulties and all. Carol reported feeling much less stressed, and we both agreed that Andy's behavior had improved markedly by the end of the four weeks. A return to filial play sessions proved to be just what Carol and Andy needed. In sessions 49 and 50, the three of us met together before Andy and Carol's play session, and they shared what they had added to Andy's adoption story book. Andy was excited about his "new big brother" and added pictures from their shared country of origin. Working on this together also seemed to help Andy address his concerns about his "big brother" going back to China in a little over a month. With the end of the school year five weeks away, Carol and I decided that the end of the school year would be a good time to end treatment, at least for now.

**Sessions 51–55.** Planning for the ending of therapy is important for all children, but even more so for children who have had multiple experiences of abandonment and loss. I knew that how I approached the ending of our relationship would be critical in order that Andy not perceive me as yet another important adult (and female) who was leaving him. I explained to Carol that I would meet with her and Andy briefly before Andy's play session in the following week to talk with both of them about termination. Because Andy and I had such a long-standing relationship, I decided that five weeks seemed like an appropriate termination phase.

Andy's play during our final sessions together was primarily constructive and showed his mastery over the playroom. He did not introduce any new play and seemed to be replaying our time together, almost like fast-forwarding a favorite home movie. When I went to meet Andy in the waiting room for our last time together, he showed me the cupcake he had brought for us to share. He clearly had a plan as he raced to the playroom ahead of me. He directed me to light the candle on the cupcake and sing Happy Birthday, after which he blew the candle out and said, "Do it again!" Andy's birthday was two months away, but he seemed to have found a perfect way to celebrate our ending and, at the same time, his beginning. After the 12th round of Happy Birthday, he said that we could now eat the cupcake, and he carefully cut it in half with a play knife from the kitchen.

After I gave the notice that there were 5 minutes left in the session, he came back and sat down by me. Then Andy looked up at me and said, "I won't see you." I assured him that although we would not see each other for awhile, he could always call me. I wrote down the clinic phone number and gave it to him. Then, he looked up at me for a few moments and said quietly, "You might need to call me." I leaned over and quietly replied, "Sounds like you are worried about us not seeing each other. Anytime you need me or want to come back here, you can call or tell your mom." Then Andy responded with a big smile, "I know! I give you my phone number," as he wrote the number and gave it to me. I smiled in response and exclaimed, "Now we both know how to call each other if we need to." Andy seemed very satisfied that he had figured this out—it was important for him to know that although I would not physically be with him that I was not abandoning him—that I would be available if he needed me.

Andy then jumped up and ran behind the puppet theater and yelled, "Guess where I am?" (without turning out the lights). I stood up to begin our usual ritual of "hide and find," prepared to search all around the room for him, when after just a few moments (not waiting for me to find him as he had always done in the past), he jumped from behind the puppet theater, threw his arms wide in the air, and with a huge smile on his beautiful face, exclaimed, "HERE I AM!" I could not have summed it up any better! I responded by throwing my arms in the air and exclaimed, "Yes, THERE YOU ARE!" Andy was free; he no longer needed me, at least for this stage of his development. His relationship with his parents had been strengthened, and he seemed to feel mostly secure in being able to count on them to meet his needs and to love him no matter what. I believed that Andy was well on his way to fully becoming all that he was meant to be.

*Discussion.*   Andy's reliving our time in the playroom together during our final sessions in some ways felt like he was making a coherent narrative of his play therapy experience. In our final session, Andy showed me that he had figured out appropriate ways to express emotions, self-regulate, and even maintain a relationship. The way that Andy navigated ending our relationship seemed to create a sense of security for him that if we needed each other, we both knew how to find each other again. His ability to understand the concept that even though he will not see me every week he knows I will still be accessible when he needs me demonstrates his emotional and developmental progress throughout therapy. And finally, his exclamation, "Here I am!" illustrates poignantly that Andy discovered through experience that he is a child worth finding and connecting with in a caring relationship.

## Conclusion

This case has illustrated an integrative humanistic approach to play therapy with a late adopted child to demonstrate the complexity of treating children who have experienced multiple attachment disruptions in their early development. Whereas attachment theory facilitated a greater understanding of Andy's relationship dynamics and informed treatment, humanistic philosophy provided the foundation for conceptualizing and guiding the process of play therapy. Andy's movement toward healing and more positive functioning is believed to be a function of his experience within the therapeutic relationship, first with the therapist and ultimately with his parents. For children with a complex attachment history, their ability to benefit fully from treatment is dependent on the therapist's success in engaging their caregivers in the therapeutic process. Andy's parents represented a significant strength and a vital element in the success of this case. Andy's case is a poignant example of the child's inherent tendency to form secure and intimate relationships and to move toward mastery, growth, and healing, when they are provided what Axline (1947) referred to as "good growing ground." (p. 10)

## References

Ainsworth, M. D. S., Blehar, M. C., Waters, E., & Wall, S. (1978). *Patterns of attachment: A Psychological study of the Strange Situation.* Hillsdale, NJ: Erlbaum.

American Psychiatric Association. (2000). *Diagnostic and statistical manual of mental disorders* (4th ed., text revision; DSM-IV-TR). Washington, DC: American Psychiatric Association.

Axline, V. (1947). *Play therapy: The inner dynamics of childhood.* Boston, MA: Houghton Mifflin.

Badenoch, B. (2008). *Being a brain-wise therapist: A practical guide to interpersonal neurobiology.* New York, NY: W.W. Norton.

Baggerly, J., Ray, D., & Bratton, S. (Eds.). (2010). *Child-centered play therapy research: The evidence-base for effective practice* (pp. 267–294). Hoboken, NJ: John Wiley.

Belsky, J., & Fearon, R. (2002). Infant-mother attachment security, contextual risk, and early development: A moderational analysis. *Development and Psychopathology, 1,* 293–310.

Bowlby, J. (1980). Attachment and loss: Loss, sadness and depression. London, England: Pimlico.

Bowlby, J. (1969) Attachment and loss. Vol. I: Attachment. London, England: Pimlico.

Bratton, S., Landreth, G., Kellam, T., & Blackard, S. (2006). *Child Parent Relationship Therapy (CPRT) treatment manual: A 10-session filial therapy model for training parents.* New York, NY: Routledge.

Bratton, S., Landreth, G., & Lin, Y.D. (2010). Child Parent Relationship Therapy (CPRT): A review of controlled-outcome research. In J. Baggerly, D. Ray, & S. Bratton (Eds.), *Child-centered play therapy research: The evidence-base for effective practice* (pp. 267–294). Hoboken, NJ: Wiley.

Bratton, S., & Ray, D. (2002). Humanistic play therapy. In D. Cain & J. Seeman (Eds.), *Humanistic psychotherapies: Handbook of research and practice* (pp. 369–402). Washington, DC: American Psychological Association.

Bratton, S., Ray, D., Rhine, T., & Jones, L. (2005). The efficacy of play therapy with children: A meta-analytic review of treatment outcomes. *Professional Psychology: Research and Practice, 36*(4), 376–390.

Busch, A. L., & Lieberman, A. F. (2007). Attachment and trauma: An integrated approach to treating young children exposed to family violence. In D. Oppenheim & D. F. Goldsmith (Eds.), *Attachment theory in clinical work with children: Bridging the gap between research and practice* (pp. 139–171). New York, NY: Guilford Press.

Carnes-Holt, K. (2010). *Child-parent relationship therapy (CPRT) with adoptive families: Effects on child behavior, parent-child relationship stress, and parental empathy.* Published doctoral dissertation, University of North Texas, Denton, TX.

Cassidy, J. (1999). The nature of the child's ties. In J. Cassidy, & P. Shaver (Eds.), *Handbook of attachment: Theory, research, and clinical applications.* New York, NY: Guilford Press. (pp. 3–20).

Cassidy, J., & Shaver, P. (Eds.). (2008). *Handbook of attachment: Theory, research, & clinical applications* (2nd ed.). New York, NY: Guilford Press.

Fearon, R., Bakermans-Kranenburg, M., Ijzendoorn, M., Lapsley, A., & Roisman, G. (2010). The significance of insecure attachment and disorganization in the development of children's externalizing behavior: A meta-analytic study. *Child Development, 81*(2), 435–456.

Findling, J., Bratton, S., & Henson, R. (2006). Development of the trauma play scale: An observation-based assessment of the impact of trauma on the play therapy behaviors of young children. *International Journal of Play Therapy, 15*(1), 7–36.

Forbes, H., & Post, B. (2006). *Beyond consequences, logic, and control: A love-based approach to helping attachment-challenged children with severe behaviors.* Orlando, FL: Beyond Consequences Institute.

Goldberg, S. (1995). Introduction. In S. Goldberg, R. Muir, & J. Kerr (Eds.), *Attachment theory: Social, developmental and clinical perspectives.* NY: Routledge.

Guerney, B. (1969). Filial therapy: Description and rationale. *Journal of Consulting Psychology, 28*(4), 304–310.

Guerney, L. (1983). Client-centered (nondirective) play therapy. In C.E. Schaefer & K. O'Connor (Eds.), *Handbook of play therapy.* New York, NY: Wiley.

Heard, D., & Lake, B. (1997). *The challenge of attachment for caregiving.* London, England: Routledge.

Hinshaw-Fuselier, S. S. (2004). Pathways to Disorganized Attachment in Infancy: Are Maternal Depressed Mood and Disruptive Life Events Meaningful Contributors? (Doctoral Dissertation, The University of Texas at Austin. Retrieved from http://repositories.lib.utexas.edu/bitstream/handle/2152/2015/hinshawfuseliers042.pdf;jsessionid=89FE306A9863F2F756E49732B0820CA6?sequence=2

Hughes, D. A. (1999). Adopted children with attachment problems. *Child Welfare, 78*(5), 541–561.

Hughes, D. (2006). *Building the bonds of attachment* (2nd ed.). Lanham, MD: Jason Aronson.

James, B. (1994). *Handbook for treatment of attachment-trauma problems in children.* Lexington, MA: Lexington Books.

Landreth, G. L. (2002). *Play therapy: The art of the relationship* (2nd ed.). New York, NY: Routledge.

Landreth, G. (1991). *Play Therapy: The art of the relationship.* New York, NY: Routledge.

Landreth, G. L., & Bratton, S. C. (2006). *Child parent relationship therapy (CPRT): A 10-session filial therapy model.* New York, NY: Routledge.

Landreth, G., & Bratton, S. (2000). Play therapy. *Counseling and Human Development, 31*(1), 1–12.

Lieberman, A., & Van Horn, P. (2005). *Don't hit my mommy: A manual for child-parent psychotherapy with young witnesses of family violence.* Washington, DC: Zero to Three Press.

Moustakas, C. (1953). *Children in play therapy.* New York: McGraw-Hill

Perry, B. D. (1994). Neurobiological sequelae of childhood trauma. Post-traumatic disorders in children. In M. Murburg (Ed.), *Catecholamine function in posttraumatic stress disorder: Emerging concepts* (pp. 253–276). Washington, DC: American Psychiatric Press.

Perry, B. D. (2006). Applying principles of neurodevelopment to clinical work with maltreated and traumatized children: The neurosequential model of therapeutics. In N. B. Webb (Ed.), *Working with traumatized youth in child welfare* (pp. 27–52). New York, NY: The Guilford Press.

Perry, B. D. (2008). The neurosequential model of therapeutics. Retrieved from www.childtrauma.org

Perry, B. D., & Szalavitz, M. (2006). *The boy who was raised as a dog and other stories from a child psychiatrist's notebook.* New York, NY: Basic Books.

Purvis, K., Cross, D., & Sunshine, L. (2007). *The connected child: Bring hope and healing to your adoptive family.* New York, NY: McGraw-Hill.

Ray, D., & Bratton, S. (2010). What the research shows about play therapy: 21st century update. In J. Baggerly, D. Ray, & S. Bratton (Eds.), *Child-centered play therapy research: The evidence-base for effective practice.* Hoboken, NJ: Wiley.

Ryan, V. (2004). Adapting non-directive play therapy for children with attachment disorders. *Clinical Child Psychology and Psychiatry, 9*(1), 75–87.

Rogers, C. (1961). *On becoming a person.* Boston, Houghton, Mifflin.

Schore, A. (1994). *Affect regulation and the origin of the self.* Hillsdale, NJ: Erlbaum.

Schore, A. (2003). *Affect regulation and the repair of the self.* New York, NY: Norton.

Siegel, D. J. (1999). *The developing mind: Toward a neurobiology of interpersonal experience.* New York, NY: Guilford Press.

Siegel, D. J. (2007). *The mindful brain: Reflection and attunement in the cultivation of well-being.* New York, NY: Norton.

Siegel, D. J. (2010). *Mindsight: The new science of personal transformation.* New York, NY: Bantam Books.

Siegel, D., & Hartzell, M. (2003). *Parenting from the inside-out: How a deeper self-understanding can help you raise children who thrive.* New York, NY: Jeremy P. Tarcher/Putnam.

van der Kolk, B. (2005). Developmental trauma disorder. *Psychiatric Annals, 35,* 401–408.

Wilson, K., & Ryan, V. (2005). *Play therapy: A non-directive approach for children and adolescents* (2nd ed.). Oxford, England: Balliere Tindall.

# Author Index

## A

Abidin, R. R., 45, 49, *57*
Accordino, D. B., 226, *238*
Accordino, M. P., 226, *238*
Achenbach, T. M., 272, *293*
Ackerson, J., 208, 212, *221*
Ainsworth, M. D. S., 246, 247, 249, *261*, 267, 281, *293*, 351, *368*
Ainsworth, M. S., 157, *173*
Alexander, F., 6, *15*
Alexander, J., 250, *261*
Algina, J., 39, 44, 47, *57*, *58*
Allen, V. B., 212, *223*
American Psychiatric Association, 178, *192*, 244, 247, 255, *261*, 271, *293*, 297, *322*, 348, *368*
Ammen, S., 304, 308, *323*
Anchin, J. C., 14, 15, *15*
Anderson, H., 301, *322*
Andrews, J. D. W., 13, *15*
Antshel, K. M., 100, *103*
Arkowitz, H., 6, 7, 9, 10, *15*
Arnkoff, D. B, 33, *35*
Ashby, J. S., 225, 226, 235, 238, *238*, *239*
Asher, S. R., 95, 101, *104*
Atkinson, D. R., 4, *16*
Avenevoli, S., 183, *192*
Axline, V., 25, *34*, 42, *57*, 266, *293*, 328, *339*, 343, 352, *368*
Axline, V. M., 98, *103*, 108, 115, *126*, 210, *221*
Azar, S. T., 156, 157, *173*

## B

Badenoch, B., 348, 349, *368*
Baggerly, J., 115, *126*, 343, *368*
Bahl, A., 41, *58*
Bahl, A. B., 41, *57*
Bainum, C., 62, *72*
Baker, S., 27, *34*
Baker, W. L., *263*

Bakermans-Kranenburg, M., 341, *369*
Balachova, T., *57*, *261*
Baldwin, L. M., 254, *262*
Bandura, A., 227, *238*
Barber, B. K., 157, *173*
Barcley, K. H., 212, *221*
Barker, C., *295*
Barker, C. H., 40, *57*
Barkley, R. A., 251, 252, *261*
Barlow, D. H., 40, *57*
Barnes, K. T., 157, *173*
Barnes, M., 212, *223*
Barnett, D., *261*
Barrett, P. M., 208, 209, *222*
Barry, T. D., 100, *103*
Barth, R. P., 250, 252, 253, *261*
Bauermeister, J. J., 39, *58*
Baumrind, D., 41, *57*, 157, *173*
Beck, A., 227, *238*
Beck, A. T., 109, *126*, 130, *150*
Beck, J. S., *150*
Becker-Weidman, A., 255, *261*
Beelmann, A., 101, *104*
Beidel, D. C., 100, *103*
Beitman, B. D., 13, *15*
Belsky, J., 157, *173*, 298, *324*, 341, *368*
Benedict, H., 28, 29, *34*
Berg, I. K., 62, 65, 66, *72*
Bergin, A. E., 9, *15*, 23, *34*
Bergman, A., *263*
Berk, M. J., 107, 110, *127*
Berk, M. S., 137, *151*, 180, *193*
Bernal, G., 39, *58*
Bernstein, J. E., 212, *222*
Bettner, B. L., 231, *239*
Beutler, L. E., 8, 11, 12, 14, *15*, *17*
Bibring, E., 315, *322*
Bickman, L., 4, *16*
Bifulco, A., 273, *293*
Birk, L., 8, *15*
Bishop, D. S., 254, *262*
Blackard, S., 329, *339*, 343, *369*

# SUBJECT INDEX

## A

AAI (Adult Attachment Interview), 273–274
AAPT (animal-assisted play therapy), 165
ABFT (attachment-based family therapy), 252
Abreaction, 63
Abused children, *see* Maltreated and neglected children
Academic achievement, 226
Acceptance, 158–159, 166
Accountability, 7–9
Acting out behaviors, 202
Actualization, of self, 99
Adaptive coping strategies, 137–140
Adaptive perfectionism, 226
Adler, A., 5, 6, 154
Adlerian play therapy (APT), 225–227, 229–238
  and bibliotherapy, 210, 221
  case example of CBTPT integration with, 233–238
  cognitive-behavioral play therapy integration with, 232–233
  theoretical concepts and principles of, 229–232
Adlerian theory, 226–227
Adolescents:
  filial therapy for, 164
  mood disorders in, 178–179
  noncompliance in, 61
  play therapy for, 71
Adopted children, 341–368
  attachment disorders in, 297
  attachment therapies for, 250
  case example of humanistic play therapy for, 346–368
  coercive therapies with, 249–250
  filial therapy for, 167
  humanistic play therapy for treatment of, 341–346
  transitions in lives of, 167–169
Adoptive parents, 245, 257, 352

Adult Attachment Interview (AAI), 273–274
Affect:
  and cognition, 122
  co-regulation of, 140
  regulation of, 188–190
Age:
  in ecosystemic model, 304
  for filial therapy, 164
  for sandtray therapy, 61
  in Theraplay model, 304, 330
  of traumatized children, 200
Aggressive play, 170
Ainsworth, M. D. S., 246, 247, 249, 267
Alexander, F., 6–7
Algina, J., 47
Alternative Families CBT, 108
Altruism, 97
Ambivalent attachment, 352
American Professional Society on the Abuse of Children (APSAC), 251
Ammen, S., 308
Amygdala, 345
Anchin, J. C., 14
Anger, 118
Animal-assisted play therapy (AAPT), 165
Animal therapy, 76, 85, 87
Anomalies, 3–4
*Anthroposophy* (R. Steiner), 76
Antisocial behaviors, 100
Anxieties and fears, 207–221
  and attachment disruptions, 357
  bibliotherapy for treatment of, 210–214
  book selection for children with, 217–220
  in childhood, 208–209
  desensitization to, 131
  interventions for, 214–217
  and resistance in therapy session, 312
  social, 100
  in Worry Wars protocol, 136

Subject Index  **387**

Dreikurs, R., 231
Drisko, J. W., 247
Dry sand, 67
DSM-IV, *see* Diagnostic Statistical Manual-IV-TR
DTORF (Developmental Therapy Objective Rating Form), 309
Dualistic themes, 196
Duncan, B. L., 11, 15
Dunkel, S., 251
Dyadic development psychotherapy (DDP), 254–255
Dyadic Parent-Child Interaction Coding System, Third Edition (DPICS-III), 41, 46
Dyadic sessions, 115
Dynamics of attachment and interest sharing, 267–269

**E**

Early recollection approach, 154
EBCI (Eyberg Child Behavior Inventory), 46
Echo reading, 218
Eclecticism, 8–10, 21
Ecological model, 299
Ecosystemic play therapy (EPT), 297–322
 and attachment problems, 297–299
 model of, 253
 pretreatment process in, 308–311
 as theoretical integration approach, 25–26
 theory and model of, 299–300
 in Theraplay integration case example, 319–321
 Theraplay integration with, 301–308
 and Theraplay model, 300–301
 treatment phases in integrative approach to, 311–319
EFT (emotionally focused therapy), 246
Egalitarian therapeutic relationship, 230
Ego boost, 99
Ego-strengthening activities, 80
Eisenstadt, T. H., 40, 48
Ellis, A., 109, 130
Emotions. *See also* Feelings
 articulation of, 210

denial and suppression of, 158–159
 expression of, 157–158, 314
 identification of, 313–314
 during play, 133
 in traumatized child case example, 110
Emotional blocks, 79, 80
Emotional healing, 77, 80–82
Emotionally focused therapy (EFT), 246
Emotional safety, 166
Emotional womb, 78–80
Emotion regulation:
 with filial therapy, 166
 in mood disorder case example, 190
 for mood disorders, 188–189
 in play therapy, 98
EMP (experiential mastery plan), 26
Empathic listening skill, 163–164
Empathy, 102
Empirically supported treatments (ESTs), 248–249
Enactments, 159–160
Encouragement, 230
Engagement, 331–332
Engaging activities, 301, 313
Environment, 181–182
Epistemology, 13
EPT, *see* Ecosystemic play therapy
Erikson, E., 266
ESTs (empirically supported treatments), 248–249
Evidence-based practices:
 and funding, 22
 play therapy comparisons to, 125
 and psychotherapy integration, 12, 14
Existential factors, 98
Experiential family therapy, 158–159
Experiential interventions, 300–302, 312–313, 315
Experiential mastery plan (EMP), 26
Experiential model, 199–201
Experiential play therapy, 196
Exploration phase, 311
Exploratory interest-sharing system, 268, 275
Exploratory models, 5
Expository books, 218
Exposure-based treatments:
 gradual, 131–132
 in traumatized child case example, 113–114, 123–124

Printed and bound by CPI Group (UK) Ltd, Croydon, CR0 4YY

16/04/2025

14658526-0001